The Joint Commission (TJC) Prohibited
Abbreviations and Notations

Abbreviation	Write
U or u	unit
IU	international unit
qd qod	daily every other day
Trailing zero (X.0 mg) Lack of leading zero (.X mg)	Delete the trailing zero (X) Insert a leading zero (0.X)
MS or MSO$_4$ MgSO$_4$	morphine sulfate magnesium sulfate

Institute for Safe Medication Practices (ISMP)
Dangerous Abbreviations and Notations

Abbreviation	Write	Abbreviation	Write
AD, AS, or AU	right ear, left ear, or both ears	× 3d	for 3 days
OD, OS, or OU	right eye, left eye, or both eyes	SC, SQ, or sub q	subcut or subcutaneous(ly)
BT	bedtime	ss	one half
cc	mL for milliliters	SSI	sliding scale (insulin)
HS	bedtime	µg	mcg
qhs	nightly	> <	greater than less than
qid	4 times a day	+	plus or and
qn	nightly	@	at

Please note: This is a partial list. For a more complete list, refer to www.ISMP.org.

Drug Calculations
Process and Problems for Clinical Practice

ELSEVIER

evolve

:• *To access your Student Resources, visit:*

http://evolve.elsevier.com/BrownMulholland

Evolve® Student Resources for **Brown: Drug Calculations** offer the following features:

- **WebLinks**
  An exciting resource that lets you link to hundreds of websites carefully chosen to supplement the content of your textbook. The WebLinks are regulary updated, with new ones added as they develop.

Drug Calculations

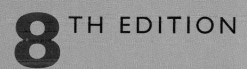

Process and Problems for Clinical Practice

8 TH EDITION

META BROWN, RN, MED

Retired Colonel
U.S. Army Field Hospital
Former Director, Division of Nursing
Gateway Community College
Phoenix, Arizona

JOYCE M. MULHOLLAND, APRN, BC

Nursing Education Consultant, Tucson, Arizona
M.S. California State University,
Long Beach, California
M.A. Arizona State University,
Tempe, Arizona
B.S. Fairleigh Dickinson College,
Rutherford, New Jersey

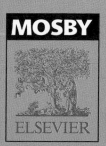

MOSBY

ELSEVIER

MOSBY
ELSEVIER

11830 Westline Industrial Drive
St. Louis, Missouri 63146

DRUG CALCULATIONS: PROCESS AND PROBLEMS
FOR CLINICAL PRACTICE, 8TH EDITION

ISBN: 978-0-323-04576-6

Notice

Knowledge and best practice in this field are constantly changing. As new research and experience broaden our knowledge, changes in practice, treatment, and drug therapy may become necessary or appropriate. Readers are advised to check the most current information provided (i) on procedures featured or (ii) by the manufacturer of each product to be administered, to verify the recommended dose or formula, the method and duration of administration, and contraindications. It is the responsibility of the practitioner, relying on their own experience and knowledge of the patient, to make diagnoses, to determine dosages and the best treatment for each individual patient, and to take all appropriate safety precautions. To the fullest extent of the law, neither the Publisher nor the Authors assumes any liability for any injury and/or damage to persons or property arising out or related to any use of the material contained in this book.

The Publisher

Previous editions copyrighted 2000, 1996, 1992, 1988, 1984, and 1979

Library of Congress Control Number: 2007927351 $52.95

Senior Editor: Yvonne Alexopoulos
Senior Developmental Editor: Danielle M. Frazier
Publishing Services Manager: Jeff Patterson
Senior Project Manager: Clay S. Broeker
Design Direction: Ellen Zanolle

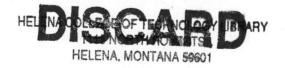

Working together to grow
libraries in developing countries

www.elsevier.com | www.bookaid.org | www.sabre.org

ELSEVIER   BOOK AID
International   Sabre Foundation

Printed in Canada

Last digit is the print number: 9 8 7 6 5 4 3 2 1

Reviewers

Carla H. Appling, MSN, RN
Instructor of Nursing
Covenant School of Nursing
Lubbock, Texas

Deborah L. Freyman, RN, MA, MSN
Nursing Faculty
National Park Community College
Hot Springs, Arkansas

Margaret M. Gingrich, RN, MSN
Associate Professor
Harrisburg Area Community College
Harrisburg, Pennsylvania

Kathleen K. Gudgel, RN, MSN
Instructor of Nursing
School of Health Sciences
Pennsylvania College of Technology
Williamsport, Pennsylvania

Jo A. Voss, PhD, RN, CNS
Assistant Professor
College of Nursing
South Dakota State University
Rapid City, South Dakota

Angela S. Wilson, PhD, RN, BC
Associate Professor, Department Chair
The University of Virginia's College at Wise
Department of Nursing
Wise, Virginia

Preface to Instructors

Drug Calculations was originally designed in the late 1970s as a basic practical resource for nursing students and faculty in classrooms and clinical areas. Since then, the content has been thoroughly reviewed and updated to be useful for refresher courses, practicing nurses in specialty areas, distance-learning students, nurses pursuing independent learning, associate and baccalaureate nursing students, and as practical nurse students.

This book primarily presents the ratio and proportion method, the easiest provable method of dose calculation for the majority of nursing students to master in a short time, and delivers all the necessary material in a simple-to-complex sequence with brief rules, succinct examples, and logical steps to understanding and mastery of the underlying concepts.

A comprehensive, systematic arithmetic self-assessment quiz allows the student to focus on any basic mathematics areas that may need review in preparation for dose calculations.

The first chapter offers a sufficient review of the basic arithmetic needed to solve all the calculations in the text. Students are referred to a general mathematics text if more practice is desired.

The text presents pharmacology principles and selected illustrations to enhance learning relevant to specific calculation areas. The reader is referred to current pharmacology texts, drug handbooks, and clinical skills manuals for complete coverage of those broad subjects.

As in prior editions, answers are completely worked out in the back of the book for all worksheets so that the learner can pinpoint areas of need. Concepts of the nursing process, logical thinking, and critical thinking are employed throughout the text, with highlighted clinical alerts to call the reader's attention to dose-related safety situations in actual practice that have resulted in medications errors. Also, as in prior editions, little emphasis on memorized concepts is encouraged.

Priorities are placed upon patient safety, and proofs and labels are requested for answers to all the basic problems to avoid errors and establish good habits. It is up to the faculty to make a decision about the use of calculators. Our recommendation is that the problems in the basic chapters be worked out in order to reinforce the students' understanding of the process and to enhance their ability to prove their answers. The goal is to be able to function independently without a calculator if that becomes necessary.

New Features for the 8th Edition

- Each chapter has been reviewed and updated for currency and accuracy. More labels and new illustrations for realistic practice have been included.

- Chapter Introductions begin each chapter, providing general discussion of content and helping students focus and prepare for learning.

- More problems, labels, and tables have been added to the revised chapters to give the students additional practice. The Joint Commission requirements for abbreviations have been included in this edition.

- Chapter 3, Safe Medication Administration, has been revised to include a section with critical abbreviation quizzes, a comprehensive summary of safe medication practices, and additional final problems and answers. Chapter 9, Insulin, contains four new worksheets on insulin dosage based on carbohydrate intake and weight, as well as discussion of the new insulin currently on the market.

- A multiple-choice worksheet to reinforce knowledge is included in most chapters. These worksheets give the student the opportunity to use different critical thinking skills to analyze possible answers, discard incorrect responses, and select the correct answer.

- Additional problems have been added to the Multiple-Choice Final and the Comprehensive Final, with answers to help the student evaluate their progress.

- For reader convenience, abbreviations and formulas are located on the inside covers and are consistent with the new standards from The Joint Commission to make medication administration safer and help to eliminate errors.

Ancillaries

Instructor's Electronic Resource for Brown/Mulholland: Drug Calculations: Process and Problems for Clinical Practice, 8th edition: Written to correspond directly with the text, the Instructor's Electronic Resource includes suggestions for classroom and laboratory practice, teaching guidelines, and a test bank organized by chapter with over 150 questions to be used by instructors to develop quizzes, tests, and comprehensive final exams. All components of the CD-ROM are also available and online through Evolve at *http://evolve.elsevier. com/BrownMulholland.*

Dosages and Solutions Computerized Test Bank (Version II): This is a generic test-bank that contains over 700 questions on general mathematics, converting within the same system of measurements, converting between different systems of measurement, oral dosages, parenteral dosages, flow rates, pediatric dosages, intravenous calculations, and more. This Computerized Test Bank is available online through Evolve at *http://evolve.elsevier.com/BrownMulholland.*

Drug Calculations Student CD-ROM (Version III): Completely updated, this user-friendly, interactive student tutorial has a brand new organization and design for easier navigation. It includes an extensive menu of various topic areas within drug calculations such as oral, parenteral, pediatric, and intravenous calculations. It includes exercises in which students can fill in syringes to answer problems. Covering the ratio and proportion, formula, and dimensional analysis methods, this CD contains 565 practice problems, including a comprehensive post-test. It is packaged with every copy of the text.

Acknowledgments

We hope that the users will find that this edition meets their needs. We extend our thanks to all the reviewers and users for their thoughts, time, and excellent suggestions. We followed them whenever practical, timely, and consistent with the style of this text and the needs of a majority of practitioners.

Meta Brown Seltzer thanks Lee Wiysel, RN, CDE, the clinical diabetic education clinician at the John C. Lincoln North Mountain Campus, who provided me with current practices in diabetic education.

Meta Brown Seltzer

Joyce M. Mulholland

Preface to Students

Drug Calculations: Process and Problems for Clinical Practice provides all the information, explanation, and practice needed to competently and confidently calculate drug dosages. A review of basic arithmetic is provided to refresh math skills. The text also provides exclusive coverage of the ratio and proportion method of drug calculation in a full-color workbook format. Take a look at the following features so that you may familiarize yourself with this text and maximize its value:

Worksheets with a series of practice problems follow each section, providing the practice you need to master math calculations.

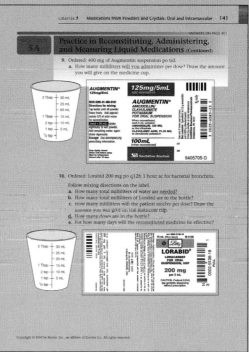

The step-by-step format of problems includes a "proof" step to ensure that you understand the calculation and provide a way to double-check answers.

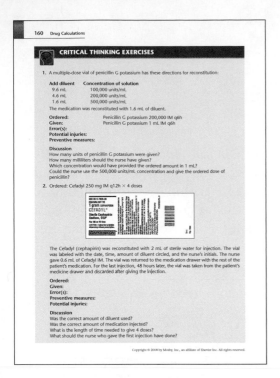

Critical Thinking Exercises at the end of most chapters include various patient scenarios, providing you the opportunity to apply the knowledge you have learned.

Drug Calculations Student CD-ROM (Version III): Completely updated, this user-friendly, interactive student tutorial has a brand new organization and design for easier navigation. It includes an extensive menu of various topic areas within drug calculations such as oral, parenteral, pediatric, and intravenous calculations. It includes exercises in which students can fill in syringes to answer problems. Covering the ratio and proportion, formula, and dimensional analysis methods, this CD contains 565 practice problems, including a comprehensive post-test. It is packaged with every copy of the text. See the sample screen shots below.

Here is an outline of the table of contents for the **Drug Calculations Student CD-ROM, (Version III).**

Look for this icon at the end of the chapters. It will refer you to the **Drug Calculations Student CD-ROM (Version III)** for additional practice problems and content information.

Contents

Detailed Contents

11 Children's Dosages, 293

12 Dimensional Analysis, 327

Drug Calculations
Process and Problems for Clinical Practice

General Mathematics Self-Assessment

Accurate medication dose calculations build on fundamental mathematics knowledge. Solve these basic problems and check your answers on page 361. Chapter 1, General Mathematics, provides a refresher for each type of problem.

Change to whole or mixed numbers.

1. $\frac{9}{2}$

2. $\frac{26}{5}$

Change to improper fractions.

3. $8\frac{1}{3}$

4. $5\frac{2}{5}$

Find the lowest common denominator in the following fractions.

5. $\frac{4}{11}$ and $\frac{1}{8}$

6. $\frac{2}{5}$ and $\frac{5}{9}$

Add the following.

7. $\frac{1}{5}, \frac{1}{6},$ and $\frac{2}{3}$

8. $1\frac{1}{2} + 3\frac{1}{8} + 2\frac{1}{6}$

Subtract the following.

9. $\frac{5}{7} - \frac{1}{3}$

10. $8\frac{1}{4} - 3\frac{3}{8}$

Multiply the following and reduce to lowest terms.

11. $\frac{1}{6} \times \frac{1}{3}$

12. $\frac{2}{8} \times 1\frac{1}{3}$

Divide the following and reduce to lowest terms.

13. $\frac{1}{3} \div \frac{2}{5}$

14. $1\frac{1}{8} \div 2\frac{1}{2}$

Express the following fractions reduced to lowest terms (numbers).

15. $\frac{4}{120}$

16. $\frac{3}{7}$

Write the following as decimals.

17. Twelve hundredths

18. Three and sixteen thousandths

Add the following.

19. 3.04 + 1.864

20. 25.7 + 3.008

Subtract the following.

21. 3 − 0.04

22. 0.96 − 0.1359

Multiply the following.

23. 0.003×1.2

24. 3×0.4

Divide the following and carry to the third decimal place.

25. $201.1 \div 20$

26. $20.6 \div 0.21$

Change the following to decimals and carry to the third decimal place.

27. $\frac{24}{44}$

28. $9\frac{1}{8}$

Find the following percentages.

29. 15% of 63

30. 2% of 4210

Change the following decimals to fractions and reduce to lowest terms.

31. 0.005

32. 0.05

Change the following fractions to a decimal and a percentage.

33. $\frac{17}{100}$

34. $\frac{1}{8}$

Round the following decimals.

	Decimal	Nearest Whole Number	Nearest Hundredth	Nearest Tenth
35.	0.8734			
36.	0.842			
37.	0.553			
38.	0.689			
39.	2.75			

Answer the following questions.

40. What is 25% of 2?   Ans: fraction _____   Ans: decimal _____

41. What is $\frac{1}{4}$ of 2?   Ans: fraction _____   Ans: decimal _____

42. What is 75% of 2?   Ans: fraction _____   Ans: decimal _____

43. Divide 0.5 by 0.25:

44. Divide 0.2 by 0.1:

45. Divide $\frac{1}{100}$ by $\frac{1}{200}$:

General Mathematics

Objectives

- Add, subtract, multiply, and divide fractions and mixed numbers.
- Convert improper fractions and mixed numbers.
- Reduce fractions to lowest terms.
- Create equivalent fractions and compare values.
- Add, subtract, multiply, and divide decimals.
- Compare decimal values.
- Round decimals.
- Convert decimals, fractions, and percentages.

2   3   4   5 mL   6   7   8   9   10 mL

1/2 tsp   1 tsp   1 1/2 tsp   2 tsp

INTRODUCTION

This chapter provides a thorough and easy-to-follow review of the arithmetic needed for accurate medication dose calculations. Many examples, practice problems, and answers related to fractions, decimals, and percentages are offered. Your ability to avoid medication errors and solve medication dose-related problems starts with competence in basic arithmetic. If you need further review, refer to a general basic mathematics text. Mastery of these concepts is essential before you proceed to the following chapters and medication-related calculations.

Fractions

A fraction is part of a whole number. The fraction $\frac{6}{8}$ means that there are 8 parts to the whole number (bottom number, or denominator), but you want to measure only 6 of those parts (top number, or numerator).

The fraction $\frac{6}{8}$ can be reduced by dividing both the numbers by 2.

$$\frac{6 \div 2}{8 \div 2} = \frac{3}{4} \quad \begin{array}{l} \text{numerator} \\ \text{denominator} \end{array}$$

Changing Improper Fractions to Whole or Mixed Numbers

An improper fraction has a numerator that is larger than the denominator, as in $\frac{8}{4}$.

STEPS When the top number (numerator) is larger than the bottom number (denominator), divide the bottom number (denominator) into the top number (numerator).

Write the remainder as a fraction and reduce to lowest terms.

Examples
$\frac{8}{4} = 8 \div 4 = 2$ *This is a whole number.*

$\frac{16}{6} = 16 \div 6 = 2\frac{4}{6} = 2\frac{2}{3}$ This is a *mixed number* because it has a whole number plus a fraction.

4

ANSWERS ON PAGE 362

WORKSHEET 1A — Changing Improper Fractions to Whole or Mixed Numbers

Change the following to whole numbers or mixed fractions and reduce to lowest terms.

1. $\frac{6}{6} =$ 2. $\frac{10}{2} =$ 3. $\frac{13}{4} =$

4. $\frac{14}{9} =$ 5. $\frac{34}{6} =$ 6. $\frac{100}{20} =$

7. $\frac{9}{4} =$ 8. $\frac{120}{64} =$ 9. $\frac{18}{3} =$

10. $\frac{41}{6} =$

Changing Mixed Numbers to Improper Fractions

STEPS Multiply the whole number by the denominator of the fraction.

Add this to the numerator of the fraction.

Write the sum as the numerator of the fraction; the denominator of the fraction remains the same.

Examples $2\frac{3}{8} = \frac{8 \times 2 + 3}{8} = \frac{19}{8}$ numerator / denominator

$4\frac{2}{5} = \frac{5 \times 4 + 2}{5} = \frac{22}{5}$ numerator / denominator

ANSWERS ON PAGE 362

WORKSHEET 1B — Changing Mixed Numbers to Improper Fractions

Change the following to improper fractions.

1. $3\frac{1}{2} =$ 2. $1\frac{1}{6} =$ 3. $4\frac{1}{8} =$

4. $3\frac{7}{12} =$ 5. $13\frac{3}{5} =$ 6. $16\frac{1}{3} =$

7. $3\frac{5}{6} =$ 8. $2\frac{5}{8} =$ 9. $10\frac{3}{6} =$

10. $125\frac{2}{3} =$

Finding a Common Denominator for Two or More Fractions

To add and subtract fractions, the denominators must be the *same*.

Example   Fractions with same denominators

$$\frac{5}{16} - \frac{2}{16} \quad \text{or} \quad \frac{3}{8} + \frac{1}{8} \quad \text{or} \quad \frac{3}{4} + \frac{1}{4}$$

These fractions can be added and subtracted. Each set's value is also easier to compare because of the common denominators.

Example   Different denominators in fractions with the same value as the fractions in example A:

$$\frac{5}{16} - \frac{1}{8} \quad \text{or} \quad \frac{3}{8} + \frac{2}{16} \quad \text{or} \quad \frac{3}{4} + \frac{2}{8}$$

These fractions cannot be added or subtracted until they are converted in *equivalent* fractions with a *common* denominator. The relative value of each set is harder to compare. A *common* denominator is a number that can be divided evenly by *all* the denominators in the problem. It is easier to add or subtract fractions if the lowest common denominator is used.

> **STEP**   Examine the largest denominator in the group to determine whether the other denominators will divide *evenly* into it.

Example $\frac{5}{16}$ and $\frac{1}{8}$: the largest denominator, 16, can be divided by 8 without a remainder. 16 is the common denominator.

Example $\frac{2}{8}$ and $\frac{3}{4}$ and $\frac{1}{2}$: the largest denominator, 8, can be divided by 4 and by 2 without a remainder. 8 is the common denominator.

> **STEP**   If any of the denominators will not divide evenly into the largest denominator, examine multiples (greater than one) of the *largest* denominator to find the lowest number that the other denominators will divide into evenly.

Example $\frac{3}{8}$ and $\frac{2}{3}$ and $\frac{1}{4}$: 3 will *not* divide evenly into 8.

The largest denominator in the group is **8**.

$8 \times 2 = 16$ 3 will *not* divide evenly into 16.

$8 \times 3 = 24$ Both 3 and 4 will divide evenly into **24**.

$8 \times 4 = 32$ 3 will *not* divide evenly into 32.

$8 \times 5 = 40$ 3 will *not* divide evenly into 40.

$8 \times 6 = 48$ Both 3 and 4 will divide evenly into **48**.

Therefore 24 and 48 are common denominators for $\frac{3}{8}$ and $\frac{2}{3}$ and $\frac{1}{4}$, but 24 is the *lowest* common denominator for the three numbers.

Example $\frac{1}{7}, \frac{1}{6}$, and $\frac{1}{3}$

3 and 6 will *not* divide evenly into 7.

Multiples of 7: 14, 21, 28, 35, and 42.
42 is the lowest number that can be divided evenly by 6 and 3. Therefore **42** is a common denominator, the lowest common denominator.

Changing Fractions to Equivalent Fractions

RULES   Whatever you do to the denominator (multiply or divide by a number), you must do the *same* to the numerator so that the value does not change.

To maintain equivalence, the numerator and the denominator must be divided (or multiplied) by the *same* number.

Example $\frac{3}{8}, \frac{2}{3}$, and $\frac{1}{4}$

STEPS   Find the common denominator—in this case 24.

Multiply each *numerator* by the *same* number used to obtain the common denominator for that fraction. Refer to page XXX.

$\frac{3}{8}\underset{(\times 3)}{=}\frac{?}{24}$ $3 \times 3 = 9$ Therefore $\frac{3}{8} = \frac{9}{24}$

$\frac{2}{3}\underset{(\times 8)}{=}\frac{?}{24}$ $2 \times 8 = 16$ $\frac{2}{3} = \frac{16}{24}$

$\frac{1}{4}\underset{(\times 6)}{=}\frac{?}{24}$ $1 \times 6 = 6$ $\frac{1}{4} = \frac{6}{24}$

Reducing Fractions to Lowest Terms

A fraction is in lowest terms when the numerator and denominator cannot be divided by any other number except one.

RULE   To reduce a fraction to *lowest* terms, **divide** the numerator and denominator by the *largest* same whole number that will divide evenly into both. When there are no whole numbers that can be used except one, the fraction is in lowest terms.

The fraction $\frac{6}{8}$ is not in lowest terms because it can be reduced by dividing both the numerator and the denominator by 2, a common denominator. $\frac{3}{4}$ is expressed in lowest terms.

Example $\frac{6 \div 2 = 3}{8 \div 2 = 4}$ Note that both 6 and 8 are divided by 2.

Example $\frac{10 \div 5 = 2}{15 \div 5 = 3}$ Note that both 10 and 15 are divided by 5.

Example $\dfrac{4 \div 4 = 1}{24 \div 4 = 6}$ Note that both 4 and 24 are divided by 4.

$\frac{3}{4}$ and $\frac{2}{3}$ and $\frac{1}{6}$ cannot be further reduced. No other number than one will divide evenly into both the numerator and denominator. They are now in their simplest or *lowest* terms.

CHANGING TO EQUIVALENT FRACTIONS
USING HIGHER TERMS

RULE   To change a fraction to *higher* terms and maintain equivalence, ***multiply*** both the numerator and the denominator by the *same* number.

....

Example $\dfrac{6 \times 2 = 12}{8 \times 2 = 16}$ $\dfrac{6}{8} = \dfrac{12}{16}$

The value has not changed because the multiplier 2 is used for both the numerator and the denominator, and $\frac{2}{2} = 1$.

Multiplying or dividing numbers by one does *not* change the value. Equivalence is maintained.

Addition of Fractions and Mixed Numbers

RULE   If fractions have the same denominator, add the numerators, write over the denominator, and reduce.

....

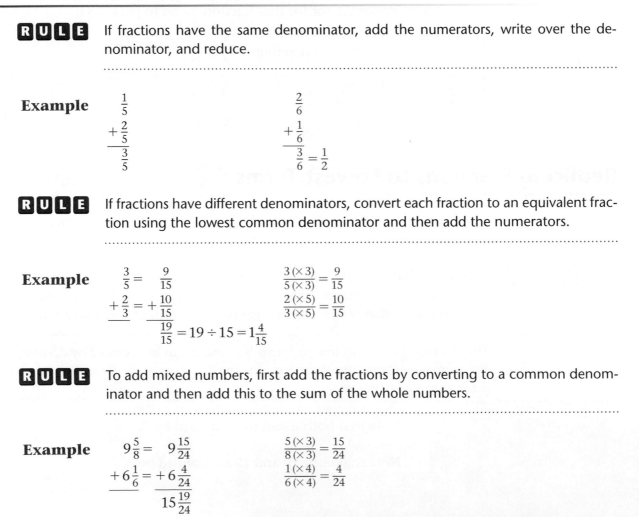

Example
$$\begin{array}{r} \frac{1}{5} \\ +\frac{2}{5} \\ \hline \frac{3}{5} \end{array}$$

$$\begin{array}{r} \frac{2}{6} \\ +\frac{1}{6} \\ \hline \frac{3}{6} = \frac{1}{2} \end{array}$$

RULE   If fractions have different denominators, convert each fraction to an equivalent fraction using the lowest common denominator and then add the numerators.

....

Example
$$\begin{array}{r} \frac{3}{5} = \quad \frac{9}{15} \\ +\frac{2}{3} = +\frac{10}{15} \\ \hline \frac{19}{15} = 19 \div 15 = 1\frac{4}{15} \end{array}$$

$$\dfrac{3\,(\times 3)}{5\,(\times 3)} = \dfrac{9}{15}$$
$$\dfrac{2\,(\times 5)}{3\,(\times 5)} = \dfrac{10}{15}$$

RULE   To add mixed numbers, first add the fractions by converting to a common denominator and then add this to the sum of the whole numbers.

....

Example
$$\begin{array}{r} 9\frac{5}{8} = \quad 9\frac{15}{24} \\ +6\frac{1}{6} = +6\frac{4}{24} \\ \hline 15\frac{19}{24} \end{array}$$

$$\dfrac{5\,(\times 3)}{8\,(\times 3)} = \dfrac{15}{24}$$
$$\dfrac{1\,(\times 4)}{6\,(\times 4)} = \dfrac{4}{24}$$

ANSWERS ON PAGE 362

WORKSHEET 1C

Addition of Fractions and Mixed Numbers

Add the following fractions and mixed numbers, using the common denominator, and reduce to lowest terms.

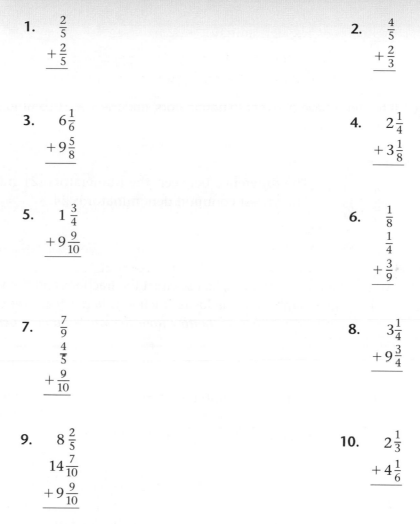

1. $\dfrac{2}{5}$
   $+\dfrac{2}{5}$

2. $\dfrac{4}{5}$
   $+\dfrac{2}{3}$

3. $6\dfrac{1}{6}$
   $+9\dfrac{5}{8}$

4. $2\dfrac{1}{4}$
   $+3\dfrac{1}{8}$

5. $1\dfrac{3}{4}$
   $+9\dfrac{9}{10}$

6. $\dfrac{1}{8}$
   $\dfrac{1}{4}$
   $+\dfrac{3}{9}$

7. $\dfrac{7}{9}$
   $\dfrac{4}{5}$
   $+\dfrac{9}{10}$

8. $3\dfrac{1}{4}$
   $+9\dfrac{3}{4}$

9. $8\dfrac{2}{5}$
   $14\dfrac{7}{10}$
   $+9\dfrac{9}{10}$

10. $2\dfrac{1}{3}$
    $+4\dfrac{1}{6}$

Subtraction of Fractions and Mixed Numbers

RULE   If fractions have the same denominator, find the difference between the numerators and write it over the common denominator. Reduce the fraction if necessary.

Example

$$\begin{array}{r} \frac{27}{32} \\ -\frac{18}{32} \\ \hline \frac{9}{32} \end{array}$$

The difference between the numerators (27 minus 18) equals 9. The denominator is 32.

RULE   If fractions have different denominators, find the lowest common denominator and proceed as above.

Example

$$\begin{array}{r} \frac{7}{8} = \frac{21}{24} \\ -\frac{2}{3} = \frac{16}{24} \\ \hline \frac{5}{24} \end{array}$$

The difference between the numerators (21 minus 16) equals 5. The lowest common denominator is 24.

RULE   To subtract mixed numbers, first subtract the fractions and then find the difference in the whole numbers. If the lower fraction is larger than the upper fraction, you cannot subtract it. *You must borrow from the whole number before subtracting the fraction.*

Example

$$\begin{array}{r} 21\frac{7}{16} \\ -7\frac{12}{16} \\ \hline \end{array}$$

You cannot subtract 12 from 7 because 12 is larger than 7. Therefore you must borrow a whole number (1) from the 21, make a fraction out of 1 $\left(\frac{16}{16}\right)$, and add the 7.

$$\frac{16}{16} + \frac{7}{16} = \frac{23}{16}$$

Because you added a whole number to the fraction, you must take a whole number away from 21 and make it 20. The problem is now set up as follows:

$$21\frac{7}{16} = 20\frac{16}{16} + \frac{7}{16} = 20\frac{23}{16}$$
$$-7\frac{12}{16}$$
$$\overline{13\frac{11}{16}}$$

RULE   Reduce your answer to lowest terms.

ANSWERS ON PAGE 362

WORKSHEET 1D

Subtraction of Fractions and Mixed Numbers

Subtract fractions and mixed numbers, and reduce the answers to lowest terms.

1. $\frac{2}{3}$
    $-\frac{1}{2}$

2. $\frac{27}{32}$
    $-\frac{18}{32}$

3. $10\frac{2}{5}$
    $-6\frac{1}{4}$

4. $7\frac{16}{24}$
    $-3\frac{1}{8}$

5. $6\frac{3}{10}$
    $-2\frac{1}{5}$

6. $\frac{7}{8}$
    $-\frac{1}{3}$

7. $3\frac{5}{8}$
    $-1\frac{3}{8}$

8. $5\frac{3}{7}$
    $-1\frac{6}{7}$

9. 7
    $-1\frac{3}{4}$

10. $2\frac{7}{8}$
    $-\frac{3}{4}$

Multiplication of Fractions and Mixed Numbers

STEPS	Change the mixed number to an improper fraction if necessary.
	Cancel, if possible, by dividing the numerators and denominators by the largest common divisor contained in each.
	Multiply the remaining numerators to find a result, or product.
	Multiply the denominators to find a result, or product.
	Reduce the answer to lowest terms.

Example

$$\frac{4}{5} \times \frac{15}{16} = \frac{\cancel{4}^{\,1}}{\cancel{5}_{\,1}} \times \frac{\cancel{15}^{\,3}}{\cancel{16}_{\,4}} = \frac{3}{4}$$

$$4\frac{1}{2} \times 2\frac{1}{4} = \frac{9}{2} \times \frac{9}{4} = \frac{81}{8} = 10\frac{1}{8}$$

$$6 \times \frac{3}{8} = \frac{6}{1} \times \frac{3}{8} = \frac{\cancel{6}^{\,3}}{1} \times \frac{3}{\cancel{8}_{\,4}} = \frac{9}{4} = 2\frac{1}{4}$$

ANSWERS ON PAGE 363

WORKSHEET
1E

Multiplication of Fractions and Mixed Numbers

Multiply the following fractions and mixed numbers, and reduce the answers to lowest terms.

1. $\frac{1}{5} \times \frac{2}{4} =$

2. $\frac{1}{5} \times \frac{1}{6} =$

3. $1\frac{3}{4} \times 3\frac{1}{7} =$

4. $4 \times 3\frac{1}{3} =$

5. $\frac{2}{4} \times 2\frac{1}{6} =$

6. $5\frac{1}{2} \times 3\frac{1}{8} =$

7. $\frac{3}{5} \times \frac{5}{8} =$

8. $\frac{5}{6} \times 1\frac{9}{16} =$

9. $\frac{5}{100} \times 900 =$

10. $2\frac{1}{10} \times 4\frac{1}{3} =$

Division of Fractions and Mixed Numbers

STEPS   Change mixed numbers to improper fractions if necessary.

Invert the number after the ÷ (division) sign.

Follow the steps for multiplication, and reduce any fractions.

Examples $\frac{1}{2} \div \frac{1}{3} = \frac{1}{2} \times \frac{3}{1} = \frac{3}{2} = 1\frac{1}{2}$

$8\frac{3}{4} \div 15 = \frac{\overset{7}{\cancel{35}}}{4} \times \frac{1}{\underset{3}{\cancel{15}}} = \frac{7}{12}$ *

———————————

*Reducing fractions $\left(\frac{7}{4} \times \frac{1}{3}\right)$ makes the math easier and reduces errors.

ANSWERS ON PAGE 363

**WORKSHEET
1F**

Division of Fractions
and Mixed Numbers

Divide the following fractions and mixed numbers, and reduce the answers to lowest terms.

1. $\frac{1}{5} \div \frac{1}{8} =$

2. $\frac{1}{3} \div \frac{1}{2} =$

3. $\frac{3}{4} \div \frac{1}{8} =$

4. $\frac{1}{16} \div \frac{1}{4} =$

5. $8\frac{3}{4} \div 15 =$

6. $\frac{3}{4} \div 6 =$

7. $2 \div \frac{1}{5} =$

8. $3\frac{3}{8} \div 4\frac{1}{2} =$

9. $\frac{3}{5} \div \frac{3}{8} =$

10. $4 \div 2\frac{1}{8} =$

Value of Fractions

RULE   The smaller the denominator of a fraction, the greater the fraction's value if the numerators are the same.

....

Example   Which would you rather have, $\frac{1}{6}$ or $\frac{1}{9}$ of your favorite candy bar? $\frac{1}{6}$ is greater than $\frac{1}{9}$. It represents a larger part of the whole unit.

$\frac{1}{6}$	$\frac{1}{6}$	$\frac{1}{6}$	$\frac{1}{6}$	$\frac{1}{6}$	$\frac{1}{6}$

= 6 parts   Each $\frac{1}{6}$ part is **larger** than the $\frac{1}{9}$ part.

$\frac{1}{9}$	$\frac{1}{9}$	$\frac{1}{9}$	$\frac{1}{9}$	$\frac{1}{9}$	$\frac{1}{9}$	$\frac{1}{9}$	$\frac{1}{9}$	$\frac{1}{9}$

= 9 parts   Each $\frac{1}{9}$ part is **smaller** than the $\frac{1}{6}$ part.

ANSWERS ON PAGE 363

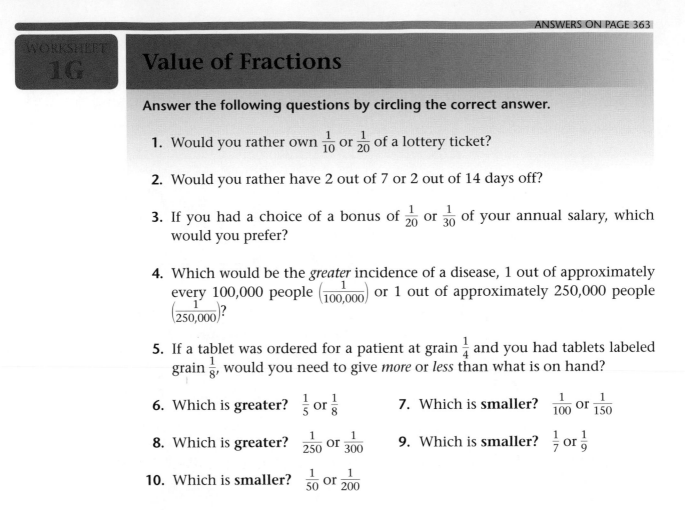

WORKSHEET
1G

Value of Fractions

Answer the following questions by circling the correct answer.

1. Would you rather own $\frac{1}{10}$ or $\frac{1}{20}$ of a lottery ticket?

2. Would you rather have 2 out of 7 or 2 out of 14 days off?

3. If you had a choice of a bonus of $\frac{1}{20}$ or $\frac{1}{30}$ of your annual salary, which would you prefer?

4. Which would be the *greater* incidence of a disease, 1 out of approximately every 100,000 people $\left(\frac{1}{100,000}\right)$ or 1 out of approximately 250,000 people $\left(\frac{1}{250,000}\right)$?

5. If a tablet was ordered for a patient at grain $\frac{1}{4}$ and you had tablets labeled grain $\frac{1}{8}$, would you need to give *more* or *less* than what is on hand?

6. Which is **greater?** $\frac{1}{5}$ or $\frac{1}{8}$ 7. Which is **smaller?** $\frac{1}{100}$ or $\frac{1}{150}$

8. Which is **greater?** $\frac{1}{250}$ or $\frac{1}{300}$ 9. Which is **smaller?** $\frac{1}{7}$ or $\frac{1}{9}$

10. Which is **smaller?** $\frac{1}{50}$ or $\frac{1}{200}$

Value of Decimals

A decimal fraction is a fraction whose denominator (bottom number) is 10, 100, 1000, 10,000, and so on. It differs from a common fraction in that the denominator is *not* written but is expressed by the proper placement of the decimal point.

Observe the scale below. All whole numbers are to the left of the decimal point; all decimal fractions are to the right.

RULES All whole numbers are to the left of the decimal; all decimal fractions are to the right of the decimal point.

To read a decimal fraction, read the number to the right of the decimal and use the name that applies to "place value" of the *last* figure other than zero. Decimal fractions read with a *ths* on the end.

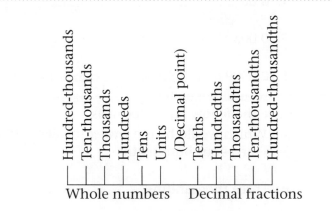

Examples 0.257   = Two hundred fifty-seven thousand*ths*

0.2057   = Two thousand fifty-seven ten-thousand*ths*

0.20057 = Twenty thousand fifty-seven hundred thousand*ths*

RULE For a whole number and a fraction, read the decimal point as an **and.**

Example 327.006 = Three hundred twenty-seven *and* six thousand*ths*

Comparison of Decimals

To determine which decimal is larger or smaller, compare the decimals from left to right, starting with the tenths place value, then the hundredths if needed, and so on.

Examples	0.4 and 0.5	5 is larger than 4. 0.5 is greater than 0.4.
	0.123 and 0.234	2 is larger than 1 in the tenths place so 0.234 is greater than 0.123.
	0.189 and 0.194	Both have 1 in the tenths column, but comparing the hundredths column reveals that the 9 is greater than 8. Therefore 0.194 is greater than 0.189.
	0.34 and 0.269	Avoid distraction because of the difference in lengths. Compare the tenths place value first. 3 is greater than 2. Therefore 0.34 is greater than 0.269.

ANSWERS ON PAGE 364

WORKSHEET
1H

Value of Decimals

Read the following decimals and write out in words.

1. 0.06

2. 0.092

3. 0.005

4. 100.01

5. 0.0009

6. 3287.467

Write the following as decimals.

7. Thirty-four hundredths   _____

8. Three thousandths   _____

9. Eight ten-thousandths   _____

10. Two and seventeen thousandths   _____

11. Five hundredths   _____

12. Four and one tenth   _____

13. Twenty-four and two tenths   _____

14. Fifteen and one hundredth   _____

15. Nine and two ten-thousandths   _____

16. Three and eight thousandths   _____

17. One hundred and eighteen thousandths   _____

18. Eighteen and fifteen hundredths   _____

19. Fifty-five thousandths   _____

20. Thirty-four and one tenth   _____

CLINICAL ALERT

Make it your habit to always insert a zero (0) in front of decimal fractions when a whole number is absent. This draws attention to the decimal and avoids two potentially critical errors: missing the decimal or mistaking it for a number "1."

ANSWERS ON PAGE 364

WORKSHEET
11

Comparison of Decimals

One of the keys to avoiding decimal errors when calculating medication doses is to know at a glance whether the amount you will give is *more* or *less* than the amount provided. Refer to page 15 for a review.

Which is *smaller?* Circle the correct answer.

1. 0.4 or 0.3

2. 0.5 or 0.25

3. 0.125 or 0.25

4. 2.309 or 2.07

5. 1.465 or 1.29

6. 0.5 or 0.37

7. 5.12 or 0.512

8. 0.394 or 0.094

9. 0.005 or 0.015

10. 1.224 or 1.088

Which is *larger?* Circle the correct answer.

11. 0.9 or 0.1

12. 0.07 or 0.7

13. 0.58 or 0.09

14. 0.25 or 0.05

15. 0.001 or 0.1

16. 2.74 or 2.0067

17. 0.147 or 0.31

18. 25.04 or 25.14

19. 0.125 or 0.25

20. 0.75 or 0.075

Addition of Decimals

STEPS	
	Write decimals in a column, keeping the decimal points under each other (A).
	Add as in whole numbers, from right to left.
	Place the decimal point in the answer directly under the decimal points in the numbers to be added.
	Insert zeros as placeholders if desired within the problem after the last number (B).

	A	B	C
Examples	0.8 + 0.5 1.3	1.64 + 2.10 3.74	2.42 + 1.08 3.5∅

REMEMBER   Line up the decimal points.
Remove trailing zeros from the answer (C).

ANSWERS ON PAGE 365

WORKSHEET
1J

Addition of Decimals

Add the following decimals.

1. $0.4 + 0.7 =$

2. $5.03 + 2.999 =$

3. $1.27 + 0.06 + 4 =$

4. $15.6 + 0.19 + 500 =$

5. $210.79 + 2 + 68.41 =$

6. $88.6 + 576.46 + 79 =$

7. $6.77 + 102 + 88.3 =$

8. $79.4 + 68.44 + 3 =$

9. $10.56 + 356.4 =$

10. $99.7 + 293.23 =$

Subtraction of Decimals

STEPS	Write decimals in a column, keeping the decimal points under each other.
	Subtract as in whole numbers, from right to left.
	Place the decimal point in the answer directly under the decimal points in the numbers to be subtracted (zeros can be added *after* the decimal point without changing the value).

Examples

$$\begin{array}{r} 0.604 \\ -\,0.524 \\ \hline 0.08\cancel{0} \end{array} \qquad\qquad \begin{array}{r} 0.500 \\ -\,0.123 \\ \hline 0.377 \end{array}$$

(REMEMBER) Line up the decimal points.

ANSWERS ON PAGE 365

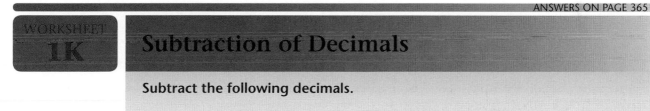

WORKSHEET
1K

Subtraction of Decimals

Subtract the following decimals.

1. $21.78 - 19.88 =$ **2.** $98.4 - 66.5 =$

3. $0.45 - 0.367 =$ **4.** $108.56 - 5.4 =$

5. $34.678 - 0.502 =$ **6.** $7.066 - 0.2 =$

7. $266.44 - 0.56 =$ **8.** $78.567 - 6.77 =$

9. $1.723 - 0.683 =$ **10.** $0.81 - 0.6701 =$

Multiplication of Decimals

STEPS	Multiply as with whole numbers.
	Count the total number of decimal places in the multiplier and in the number to be multiplied.
	Start from the right and count off the same number of places in the answer.
	If the answer does not have enough places, supply as many zeros as needed, counting from right to left as illustrated below. Eliminate trailing zeros in the answer.

Example $2.6 \times 0.0002 =$

$$
\begin{array}{rl}
2.5 & \text{(1 decimal place)} \\
\times\,0.0002 & \text{(4 decimal places)} \\
\hline
0.00050\!\!\!/ & \text{(5 decimal places from right to left in the answer} \\
& \text{before the trailing zero is deleted)}
\end{array}
$$

ANSWERS ON PAGE 365

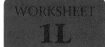

Multiplication of Decimals

Multiply the following decimals.

1. $100 \times 0.5 =$

2. $0.25 \times 2 =$

3. $3.14 \times 0.002 =$

4. $2.14 \times 0.03 =$

5. $36.8 \times 70.1 =$

6. $200 \times 0.2 =$

7. $88 \times 90.1 =$

8. $2.76 \times 0.003 =$

9. $54.5 \times 21 =$

10. $203.7 \times 28 =$

Division of Decimals

Examine the divisor—the number you are dividing by. Is it a *whole* number or a *decimal*?

RULE   If the divisor is a *whole* number, the dividend decimal place is unchanged. Immediately place the decimal point prominently on the answer line directly *above* the decimal point in the dividend. Use zeros in the answer to hold places until you can divide. Prove your answer.

Examples   ■   1.20 ÷ 15

$$
\begin{array}{r}
0.08 \leftarrow \text{Answer} \\
\text{Divisor} \rightarrow 15\overline{)1.20} \leftarrow \text{Dividend} \\
1\,20
\end{array}
$$

■   3.15 ÷ 7

$$
\begin{array}{r}
0.45 \\
7\overline{)3.15} \\
2\,8 \\
\hline
35 \\
35
\end{array}
$$

PROOF (Divisor × answer = dividend)

$$
\begin{array}{r}
0.08 \\
\times\ \ 15 \\
\hline
1.2\cancel{0}
\end{array}
$$

PROOF

$$
\begin{array}{r}
0.45 \\
\times\ \ \ 7 \\
\hline
3.15
\end{array}
$$

RULE If the divisor has a *decimal,* you must make it a whole number by moving the decimal point to the right. Move the decimal point in the dividend the same number of places to the right and immediately place the decimal point directly above on the answer line. Then divide as with whole numbers. Prove your answer.

Example   10 ÷ 4.4

$$
\begin{array}{r}
2.27 \\
4.4\overline{)10.0\,00} \\
8\,8 \\
\hline
1\,20 \\
8\,8 \\
\hline
3\,20 \\
3\,08 \\
\hline
12\ \ \text{Remainder}
\end{array}
$$

PROOF

$$
\begin{array}{r}
2.27\ \ \text{(2 decimal places)} \\
\times\,4.\ \ \text{(1 decimal place)} \\
\hline
908 \\
908 \\
\hline
9988 \\
+\ \ \ 12\ \ \text{Remainder} \\
\hline
10.000 \\
3\,2\,1
\end{array}
$$

Example   30 ÷ 5.2

$$
\begin{array}{r}
5.7 \\
5.2\overline{)30.0\,0} \\
26\,0 \\
\hline
4\,0\,0 \\
3\,6\,4 \\
\hline
36\ \ \text{Remainder}
\end{array}
$$

PROOF

$$
\begin{array}{r}
5.2 \\
\times\,5.7 \\
\hline
36\,4 \\
260 \\
\hline
296\,4 \\
+\ \ 3\,6\ \ \text{Remainder} \\
\hline
30.00
\end{array}
$$

Note that, as with whole division, a remainder is not just added to the answer in decimal division. Additional division will allow the remainder to be converted to a decimal fraction.

Example   2.6 ÷ 4

$$
\begin{array}{r}
0.6 \\
4\overline{)2.6} \\
2\,4 \\
\hline
2\ \ \text{Remainder}
\end{array}
\qquad\qquad
\begin{array}{r}
0.65 \\
4\overline{)2.60} \\
2\,4 \\
\hline
20 \\
20
\end{array}
$$

REMEMBER   Keep all your decimals dark.

ANSWERS ON PAGE 366

WORKSHEET
1M

Division of Decimals

In the following problems, the divisor is a whole number. Place the decimal point on the answer line as illustrated in red in #1. Do NOT do the math in these problems.

1. $60\overline{)1.35}$

2. $20\overline{)15.6}$

3. $19\overline{)10.14}$

4. $7\overline{)60.5}$

5. $25\overline{)35.9}$

In the following problems, the divisor has a decimal. Make the divisor a whole number, move the decimal place in the dividend, and place the decimal point on the answer line as illustrated in red in #6. Calculate the answer to the *nearest tenth*. Add zeros to the dividend as necessary.

6. $0.85\overline{)1.35}$

7. $0.1\overline{)0.5}$

8. $4.8\overline{)2.04}$

9. $0.5\overline{)0.25}$

10. $0.12\overline{)0.44}$

ANSWERS ON PAGE 366

WORKSHEET 1N

More Division of Decimals

Divide the following and carry to the *third* decimal place if necessary, and prove your answers.

1. $200 \div 6 =$

2. $15.06 \div 6 =$

3. $79.4 \div 0.87 =$

4. $158.4 \div 48 =$

5. $670.8 \div 0.78 =$

6. $78.6 \div 2.43 =$

7. $26.78 \div 8.2 =$

8. $266.5 \div 5.78 =$

9. $10.80 \div 6.5 =$

10. $76.53 \div 10 =$

Changing Decimals to Fractions

RULE The numbers to the *right* of the decimal can be written as a fraction because they are only part of the whole number.

REMEMBER The first number past the decimal to the *right* is ten*ths*, the second is hundred*ths*, the third is thousand*ths*, the fourth is ten-thousand*ths*, and so on.

So if your problem has 3 numbers to the *right* of the decimal, just remove the decimal and put the number over 1000.

Examples

■ 0.376 has 3 numbers to the *right* of the decimal. To make a fraction out of 0.376 and also get rid of the decimal, place it over 1000.

0.376 written as a fraction is $\frac{376}{1000}$.

■ It's easy to remember: 3 numbers on top and 3 zeros on the bottom.

0.95 written as a fraction is $\frac{95}{100}$.

The idea is the same as above: 2 numbers on top and 2 zeros on the bottom. The fraction $\frac{90}{100}$ can be reduced to $\frac{9}{10}$ by dividing the numerator and the denominator by 10.

ANSWERS ON PAGE 367

WORKSHEET 10

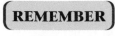

Changing Decimals to Fractions

Change the following decimals to fractions, and reduce to lowest terms.

1. 0.8 =   **2.** 0.4 =

3. 0.25 =   **4.** 1.32 =

5. 4.08 =   **6.** 0.5 =

7. 0.75 =   **8.** 0.2 =

9. 0.65 =   **10.** 0.7 =

Changing Common Fractions to Decimals

RULE   To change a common fraction to a decimal, divide the numerator by the denominator and place the decimal point in the proper position on the answer line.

Examples $\dfrac{2}{5} = 5\overline{)2.0}$ gives 0.4, with 20

$\dfrac{1}{8} = 8\overline{)1.000}$ gives 0.125, with 8, 20, 16, 40, 40

ANSWERS ON PAGE 368

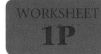

WORKSHEET 1P

Changing Common Fractions to Decimals

Carry out the following division problems to the *third* decimal place.

1. $\dfrac{1}{5} =$

2. $\dfrac{2}{3} =$

3. $5\dfrac{9}{16} =$

4. $\dfrac{19}{100} =$

5. $\dfrac{9}{7} =$

6. $\dfrac{1}{2} =$

7. $\dfrac{1}{12} =$

8. $\dfrac{6}{8} =$

9. $\dfrac{15}{200} =$

10. $\dfrac{20}{8} =$

Rounding Decimals

STEPS	Calculate *one* decimal place beyond the desired place.
	If the final digit is **4** or less, make no adjustment. If the final digit is **5** or more, *increase* the prior digit by one number.
	Drop the final digit.

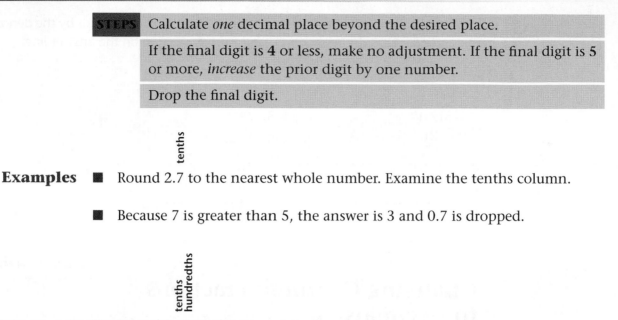

Examples

■ Round 2.7 to the nearest whole number. Examine the tenths column.

■ Because 7 is greater than 5, the answer is 3 and 0.7 is dropped.

■ Round 2.55 to the nearest tenth.
Examine the second decimal place (hundredths column).
Because the hundredths column is 5, the 2.5 is rounded up to 2.6 and the final 0.05 (hundredths) is dropped.

■ Round 3.762 to the nearest hundredth.
Examine the third decimal place (thousandths column).
Because 2 is less than 5, no adjustment will be made in the hundredths column and the 2 is dropped.
3.76 is the answer.

	Nearest Whole Number	Nearest Tenth	Nearest Hundredth
1.689	2	1.7	1.69
204.534	205	204.5	204.53
7.87	8	7.9	7.87
3.366	3	3.4	3.37
0.845*	1	0.8	0.85

*To reduce reading errors, maintain the habit of placing a zero (0) in front of the decimal when a whole number is absent.

CLINICAL ALERT

Do *not* round medication dosages to the nearest whole number. This could result in an overdose. Syringes are calibrated in tenths and hundredths of a milliliter; therefore rounding to a whole number could result in an overdose. For instructions on how to round medication doses, refer to Chapter 4 (page 89).

ANSWERS ON PAGE 368

WORKSHEET 1Q

Rounding Decimals

Round the decimal to the nearest whole number, the nearest tenth, and the nearest hundredth.

	Nearest Whole Number	Nearest Tenth	Nearest Hundredth
1. 93.489			
2. 25.43			
3. 38.1			
4. 57.8888			
5. 0.0092			
6. 3.144			
7. 8.999			
8. 77.788			
9. 12.959			
10. 5.7703			

ANSWERS ON PAGE 369

Rounding Decimal Products

Multiply or divide the following numbers. Round your answers to the nearest whole number, the nearest tenth, and the nearest hundredth.

	Nearest Whole Number	Nearest Tenth	Nearest Hundredth
1. $25.3 \times 4.2 =$	_____	_____	_____
2. $9.3 \times 2.86 =$	_____	_____	_____
3. $4.5 \times 7.57 =$	_____	_____	_____
4. $1.3 \times 9.69 =$	_____	_____	_____
5. $2.4 \times 5.88 =$	_____	_____	_____
6. $8 \div 5 =$	_____	_____	_____
7. $4.1 \div 3 =$	_____	_____	_____
8. $5 \div 1.2 =$	_____	_____	_____
9. $9 \div 2.2 =$	_____	_____	_____
10. $10.2 \div 3 =$	_____	_____	_____

Percentages, Decimals, and Fractions

The term "percent" and its symbol (%) means parts per hundred. A percent number is a fraction whose numerator is already known and whose denominator is always understood to be 100. 25% means 25 parts per hundred.

CHANGING A PERCENTAGE TO A DECIMAL

RULE To change a percentage to a decimal, divide the percentage by 100, moving the decimal point two places to the *left*. Remove the percent sign. (Remember that an implied decimal point immediately follows a whole number.)

Examples 5% ÷ 100 = 0.05 (5% has an implied decimal point after the 5)
0.5% = 0.005
10% = 0.1 (10% has an implied decimal point after the 10)

CHANGING A PERCENTAGE TO A FRACTION

RULE To change the percentage to a fraction, *first* change the percentage to a decimal by dividing the percentage by 100, moving the decimal point two places to the *left*. Write the decimal as a fraction.

Examples 5% (÷ 100) = 0.05 = $\frac{5}{100}$
The fraction can then be further reduced to $\frac{1}{20}$
0.1% = 0.001 = $\frac{1}{1000}$
10% = 0.1 = $\frac{1}{10}$

CONVERTING A DECIMAL TO A PERCENTAGE

RULE To change a decimal to a percentage, multiply the decimal by 100 by moving the decimal point 2 places to the *right* and add the percent sign.

Examples 0.1 (× 100) = 10%
0.01 = 1%
0.5 = 50%

ANSWERS ON PAGE 369

WORKSHEET
1S

Percentages, Decimals, and Fractions

Fill in the following blanks with the appropriate equivalents.

	Fraction	Decimal	Percentage
1.	$\frac{1}{2}$		
2.			50%
3.		0.05	
4.	$\frac{1}{12}$		
5.	$\frac{3}{1000}$		
6.		0.10	
7.			250%
8.		0.35	
9.	$\frac{4}{5}$		
10.			75%

FINDING THE PERCENTAGE

STEPS	Change the percentage to a decimal or common fraction.
	Multiply the number by this decimal.

Examples   50% of 120 = 0.5 × 120 = 60

10% of 120 = 0.1 × 120 = 12

In the hospital you might be asked to prepare a baby formula diluted to 50% ($\frac{1}{2}$) strength from a full-strength formula. If the baby was to receive 120 mL (4 oz) at each feeding, the nurse would multiply 0.5% (or $\frac{1}{2}$) × 120 for a result of 60 mL. 60 mL of full-strength formula would be measured and 60 mL of water added (120 mL − 60) for the total 120 mL to make a 50%-strength formula.

For 10% strength, the nurse would multiply 0.1 × 120 for a result of 12 mL full-strength formula. The nurse would measure 12 mL of full-strength formula and add 108 mL of water (120 mL total − 12 mL formula = 108 mL) for the total of 120 mL of 10%-strength formula.

Another way to do the math would be by ratio and proportion. This method will be introduced in Chapter 2. It is simpler to convert percentages, decimals, and fractions using basic arithmetic.

10 mL : 100 mL :: x mL : 120 mL

100 x = 10 × 120

x = 12 mL of full-strength formula

120 − 12 = 108 mL of water to be added

ANSWERS ON PAGE 369

ANSWERS ON PAGE 369

WORKSHEET 1T

Finding the Percentage

Solve the following problems.

1. 2% of 1500 =   **2.** 114% of 240 =

3. 28% of 50 =   **4.** 9% of 200 =

5. $\frac{1}{2}$% of 9328 =   **6.** $\frac{1}{3}$% of 930 =

7. 120% of 400 =   **8.** 5% of 105.80 =

9. 10% of 520 =   **10.** 3% of 40.80 =

ANSWERS ON PAGE 370

WORKSHEET 1U

Multiple-Choice Practice

Solve the following problems and select the correct answer. Estimate the correct answer before working the problem.

1. $\frac{30}{9}$ can be converted to which whole and mixed number?

   a. $3\frac{3}{9} = 3\frac{1}{3}$

   b. $2\frac{1}{30}$

   c. $2\frac{1}{8}$

   d. $4\frac{2}{9}$

2. Select the *improper fraction* equivalent for $3\frac{5}{6}$.

   a. $\frac{15}{6}$

   b. $\frac{23}{6}$

   c. $4\frac{1}{6}$

   d. $\frac{8}{6}$

3. $\frac{7}{8}$ and $\frac{3}{5}$ have which lowest common denominator?

   a. 8

   b. 10

   c. 13

   d. 40

4. $5\frac{1}{8} + 1\frac{1}{4} + 4\frac{1}{2} =$

   a. $10\frac{7}{8}$

   b. $9\frac{1}{6}$

   c. $12\frac{1}{2}$

   d. $10\frac{3}{4}$

5. $6\frac{3}{4} - 5\frac{1}{3} =$

   a. $\frac{1}{2}$

   b. $1\frac{1}{2}$

   c. $1\frac{5}{12}$

   d. $1\frac{5}{8}$

6. $\frac{5}{6} \times \frac{2}{8} =$

   a. $\frac{1}{12}$

   b. $\frac{5}{24}$

   c. $\frac{7}{14}$

   d. $\frac{10}{44}$

7. Divide the following fraction and reduce the lowest term: $\frac{1}{6} \div \frac{1}{3}$

   a. $\frac{2}{12}$

   b. $\frac{1}{2}$

   c. $\frac{1}{6}$

   d. $\frac{1}{3}$

8. Divide the following fraction and reduce the lowest term: $\frac{5}{6} \div \frac{1}{3}$

   a. $\frac{1}{6}$

   b. $\frac{5}{18}$

   c. $1\frac{1}{6}$

   d. $2\frac{1}{2}$

ANSWERS ON PAGE 370

WORKSHEET 1U

Multiple-Choice Practice (Continued)

9. Two and eighteen thousandths can be written in decimal form as:

    a. 2.0018

    b. 2.018

    c. 2.18

    d. 2.118

10. $0.41 - 0.2538 =$

    a. 0.1562

    b. 0.2503

    c. 0.4138

    d. 0.6638

11. $5 \times 0.9 =$

    a. 0.45

    b. 4.5

    c. 5.09

    d. 45

12. $79.4 \div 0.87 =$

    a. 12.024

    b. 21.084

    c. 80.276

    d. 91.264

13. Change $\frac{1}{6}$ to a decimal and round the answer to the nearest *hundredth*.

    a. 0.02

    b. 0.0625

    c. 0.166

    d. 0.17

14. 20% of 450 =

    a. 90

    b. 135

    c. 150

    d. 185

15. $6\frac{1}{4}$% of 9328 =

    a. 0.56

    b. 540

    c. 583

    d. 5596

16. Change 0.285 to a fraction.

    a. $\frac{285}{1000}$

    b. $\frac{28}{100}$

    c. $\frac{285}{100}$

    d. $\frac{29}{1000}$

17. Change $\frac{2}{5}$ to a decimal to the nearest *tenth*.

    a. 0.4

    b. 0.25

    c. 0.04

    d. 0.025

Continued

ANSWERS ON PAGE 370

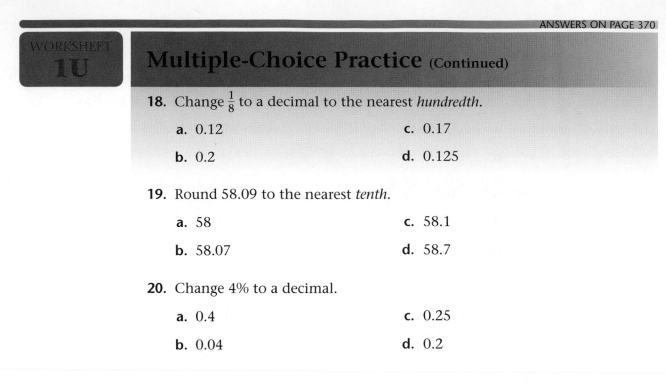

WORKSHEET
1U

Multiple-Choice Practice (Continued)

18. Change $\frac{1}{8}$ to a decimal to the nearest *hundredth*.

   a. 0.12   **c.** 0.17

   b. 0.2   **d.** 0.125

19. Round 58.09 to the nearest *tenth*.

   a. 58   **c.** 58.1

   b. 58.07   **d.** 58.7

20. Change 4% to a decimal.

   a. 0.4   **c.** 0.25

   b. 0.04   **d.** 0.2

ANSWERS ON PAGE 370

CHAPTER 1 Final

Change to whole or mixed numbers.

1. $\frac{25}{4}$

2. $\frac{32}{8}$

Change to an improper fraction.

3. $10\frac{1}{5}$

4. $3\frac{5}{6}$

Find the lowest common denominator in the following pairs of fractions.

5. $\frac{17}{20}$ and $\frac{4}{5}$

6. $\frac{7}{8}$ and $\frac{3}{5}$

Add the following.

7. $\frac{1}{18} + \frac{1}{4} + \frac{2}{9}$

8. $5\frac{1}{8} + 1\frac{1}{4} + 4\frac{1}{2}$

Subtract the following.

9. $\frac{7}{8} - \frac{2}{3}$

10. $6\frac{2}{4} - 5\frac{1}{2}$

Multiply the following.

11. $\frac{1}{5} \times \frac{1}{6}$

12. $\frac{5}{6} \times \frac{2}{8}$

Divide the following.

13. $\frac{3}{4} \div \frac{1}{8}$

14. $3\frac{3}{8} \div 4\frac{1}{2}$

Reduce the following fractions to lowest terms (numbers).

15. $\frac{2}{500}$

16. $\frac{9}{27}$

Write the following as decimals.

17. Five one hundredths

18. Two and seventeen thousandths

Add the following.

19. $5.01 + 2.999$

20. $36.87 + 8.26 + 15.84$

Subtract the following.

21. $4 - 0.176$

22. $0.41 - 0.2538$

Multiply the following.

23. 0.0005×0.02

24. 5×0.7

Divide the following and carry to the third decimal place.

25. $158.4 \div 48$

26. $79.4 \div 0.87$

Change the following to decimals.

27. $\frac{57}{48}$

28. $8\frac{1}{16}$

Find the following percentages.

29. 24% of 52

30. $6\frac{1}{4}$% of 9328

Change the following decimals to fractions.

31. 0.4

32. 0.285

Fill in the following blanks with the appropriate equivalents.

	Fraction	Decimal to Nearest Tenth	Decimal to Nearest Hundredth	Percentage
33.	$\frac{1}{3}$			
34.				5%
35.	$\frac{2}{5}$			
36.				22%
37.	$\frac{3}{8}$			
38.				10%
39.	$\frac{1}{12}$			
40.				$\frac{1}{2}$%
41.	$\frac{5}{16}$			
42.				15%
43.	$\frac{1}{4}$			
44.				12%
45.	$\frac{7}{9}$			
46.				80%
47.	$\frac{1}{6}$			
48.				33%
49.	$\frac{1}{250}$			
50.				75%

Refer to the Mathematics Review section of the enclosed student CD-ROM for additional practice problems.

Ratio and Proportion

Objectives

- Express ratios as fractions.
- Reduce fractions to lowest numerical terms.
- Solve verbal and numerical ratio/proportion problems for x.
- Solve one-step ratio/proportion problems.
- Estimate answers.
- Prove answers.

2 3 4 5 mL 6 7 8 9 10 mL

1/2 tsp 1 tsp 1 1/2 tsp 2 tsp

INTRODUCTION

Ratio and proportion is the easiest provable method of drug dose calculation for most students. The setup of problems is logical and systematic. Answers can be proven if the setup is correct.*

Ratio

A ratio indicates the relationship of one quantity to another. It indicates *division* and may be expressed in fraction form.

Example $\frac{1}{3}$ may be expressed as the ratio 1:3.

ANSWERS ON PAGE 372

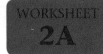

Expressing Ratios as Fractions

Express the following ratios as fractions reduced to lowest terms.

1. 2:4	**2.** 6:8	**3.** 2:500
4. 6:1000	**5.** 43:86	**6.** 2:13
7. 8:10	**8.** 1:10	**9.** 1:150
10. 4:100		

Proportion

A proportion shows the relationship between two equal ratios. A proportion may be expressed as 3 : 5 :: 6 : 10 or 3 : 5 = 6 : 10.

To solve the ratio and proportion problems, do the following:

STEPS	Multiply the two inside numbers.
	Multiply the two outside numbers.
	Check to see that the answers are the same.

Example 3 : 5::6 : 10

multiply

Multiply the two *inside* numbers: 5 × 6 = 30.
Multiply the two *outside* numbers: 3 × 10 = 30.

---

*Students who are familiar with dimensional analysis and prefer to use this method of solving problems are referred to Chapter 12.

SOLVING PROPORTION PROBLEMS WHEN ONE OF THE NUMBERS IS *UNKNOWN*, OR *x*

Example $2 : 8 :: x : 24$

multiply

Multiply the two *inside* numbers (means).

$$8 \times x = 8x$$

Multiply the two *outside* numbers (extremes).

$$2 \times 24 = 48$$

Place the $8x$ on the **left** side of the equation. It will now look like this:

$$8x = 48$$

| **HINT** | Placing the x product on the left side of the equation simplifies the work for many. |

Now you must get x to stand alone.

RULES   To get x alone, *divide* both sides of the equation by the number *next* to x. Those numbers will cancel each other. The result will be that x will stand alone.

....

What you do to one side of the equation, you must do to the other to keep the sides equal.

....

Example continued $\dfrac{\cancel{8}}{\cancel{8}}x = \dfrac{48}{8}$ This means $48 \div 8$ or $8\overline{)48}$ → $\dfrac{6}{}$

$$\begin{array}{r} 6 \\ 8\overline{)48} \\ \underline{48} \\ 0 \end{array}$$

$x = 6$
How do you know your answer is correct?

RULE   To check your answer, substitute the answer for the x in the problem, multiply the inside numbers together, and then multiply the outside numbers together. The products should be equal.

....

PROOF $8 \times 6 = 48$ (product of inside numbers, or means)
$2 \times 24 = 48$ (product of outside numbers, or extremes)

Another way to view this example is:

$\dfrac{2}{8} \overset{\times}{=} \dfrac{x}{24}$

Cross-multiplication solves this equation: $8x = 48$

$$x = 6$$

Example $2:3::6:x$ 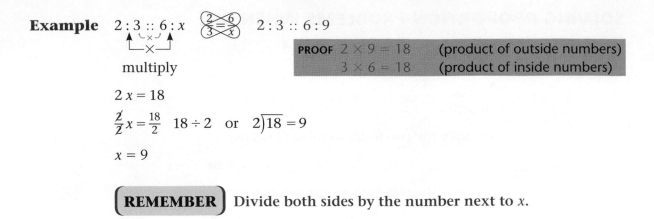 $2:3::6:9$

multiply

$$2x = 18$$

$$\frac{\cancel{2}}{\cancel{2}}x = \frac{18}{2} \quad 18 \div 2 \quad \text{or} \quad 2\overline{)18} = 9$$

$$x = 9$$

$\boxed{\textbf{REMEMBER}}$ Divide both sides by the number next to x.

ANSWERS ON PAGE 372

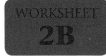

Solving Proportion Practice Problems for the Value of x

Multipy the two inside numbers, multiply the two outside numbers, and put x on the *left*. Solve for x.

1. $9 : x :: 5 : 300$

2. $9 : 27 :: 300 : x$

3. $\frac{1}{2} : x :: 1 : 8$

4. $\frac{1}{4} : 500 :: x : 1000$

5. $6 : 24 :: 0.75 : x$

6. $36 : 12 :: \frac{1}{100} : x$

7. $x : 600 :: 4 : 120$

8. $0.7 : 70 :: x : 1000$

9. $\frac{1}{1000} : \frac{1}{100} :: x : 60$

10. $6 : 12 :: \frac{1}{4} : x$

ANSWERS ON PAGE 373

WORKSHEET
2C

Solving Proportion Practice Problems for the Value of *x*

Solve the following proportions for *x*, and prove your answers.

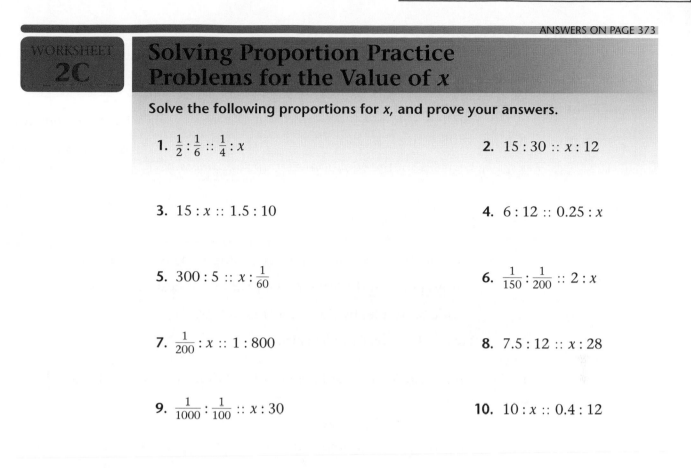

1. $\frac{1}{2} : \frac{1}{6} :: \frac{1}{4} : x$

2. $15 : 30 :: x : 12$

3. $15 : x :: 1.5 : 10$

4. $6 : 12 :: 0.25 : x$

5. $300 : 5 :: x : \frac{1}{60}$

6. $\frac{1}{150} : \frac{1}{200} :: 2 : x$

7. $\frac{1}{200} : x :: 1 : 800$

8. $7.5 : 12 :: x : 28$

9. $\frac{1}{1000} : \frac{1}{100} :: x : 30$

10. $10 : x :: 0.4 : 12$

ANSWERS ON PAGE 374

WORKSHEET
2D

Solving Proportion Practice Problems for the Value of *x*

Solve the following proportions for *x*, and prove your answers.

1. $3 : x :: 6 : 100$

2. $3 : 24 :: 0.25 : x$

3. $8 : 16 :: x : 24$

4. $x : 600 :: 4 : 120$

5. $5 : 3000 :: 15 : x$

6. $0.5 : 50 :: x : 1000$

7. $9 : 27 :: 300 : x$

8. $3 : 12 :: \frac{1}{4} : x$

9. $25 : x :: 75 : 3000$

10. $0.6 : 10 :: 0.5 : x$

Setting Up Ratios and Proportions

HINTS | To set up a ratio and proportion, you must always put on the *left*-hand side what you already *have*, or what you already *know*.

On the *right*-hand side, you will put your *x*, or what you *want* to know.

Each side of the equation is set up the *same way*.

Example Apples : *Pears* :: Apples : *x Pears*

STEPS | Multiply the two inside numbers. Multiply the two outside numbers.

Always put *x* on the left for your *final* multiplication.

Divide both sides by the number next to *x*.

Prove all answers and label them.

Examples ■ You wish to make a floral bouquet of 6 daffodils for every 4 roses. How many daffodils will you use for 30 roses?

KNOW   WANT TO KNOW

6 daffodils : 4 roses :: *x* daffodils : 30 roses

⌣ × ⌣

└─────── multiply ───────┘

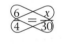

PROOF $4 \times 45 = 180$
$6 \times 30 = 180$

$\dfrac{\cancel{4}}{\cancel{4}} x = \dfrac{180}{4} = 180 \div 4 = 45$ daffodils

(REMEMBER) Place *x* on the left side of the equation to solve:

$4x = 180$
$x = 45$ daffodils

■ Make a necklace that has 19 blue beads for every yellow bead. How many blue beads are needed if you have 8 yellow beads?
(Prove your answer.)

KNOW   WANT TO KNOW

19 blue beads : 1 yellow bead :: *x* blue beads : 8 yellow beads

⌣ × ⌣

└─────────── multiply ───────────┘

$x = 152$ blue beads needed

PROOF $19 \times 8 = 152$
$1 \times 152 = 152$

ANSWERS ON PAGE 375

WORKSHEET
2E

Setting Up Ratios and Proportions

Set up a proportion for each of the following problems, and label and prove your answers.

1. You have to make a fruit basket with 6 bananas for every 9 apples. How many bananas will there be for 72 apples?

2. You are making coffee, and 7 scoops make 8 cups. How many scoops make 40 cups?

3. You have a recipe for cocoa: 4 scoops make 6 cups of cocoa. You want to make 18 cups for a party. How many scoops of cocoa are needed? Set up a proportion.

4. Ordered: 4 pills each day. The patient will be taking the medication for 21 days. How many pills will you give the patient?

5. You wish to plant 8 bushes for every 2 trees in your yard. How many bushes will there be if there are 36 trees? (Estimate and prove.)

6. Ordered: 4 cups of bran every day. How many days would it take to consume 84 cups of bran? (Estimate and prove.)

7. It takes 4 cups of flour to make 3 loaves of bread. How many loaves of bread can be made from 24 cups of flour?

8. Your recipe for punch calls for 3 cups of soda for every $\frac{1}{2}$ cup of fruit juice. How many cups of soda will be needed for 2 cups of fruit juice?

9. You need 4 tablespoons of sugar for every glass of lemonade you prepare. How many tablespoons of sugar will be needed for 6 glasses of lemonade?

10. Ordered: 4 capsules every day. How many capsules would be needed for 14 days?

ANSWERS ON PAGE 377

WORKSHEET
2F

Setting Up Ratios and Proportions

Use ratio and proportion to solve the following problems, and label and prove your answers.

1. The office needs 4000 envelopes. The boxes on hand contain 200 envelopes per box. How many boxes will you send to the office?

2. The order is for 300 computer disks. The packages on hand contain 10 disks per package. How many packages will you send?

3. If one computer is allocated for every 18 students, how many computers will be needed for an enrollment of 1280 students?

4. Your doctor tells you to drink 3 glasses of water and eat 2 apples every day. How many apples will you have eaten when you have drunk 24 glasses of water?

5. If all the teachers were to receive 6 pens for every 8 pencils, how many pens would you give them if the teachers have 72 pencils?

6. The nurse is assigned 6 patients per shift. How many nurses will be needed for 36 patients?

7. If each baby formula calls for 4 tablespoons of powdered formula for every 8 ounces of water, how many tablespoons of powdered formula would be needed for 56 ounces of water?

8. The hospital requires 2 nurses for every unit for each 12-hour shift. How many nurses are needed for each unit for 72 hours?

9. If a patient takes 8 aspirin tablets per day, how many aspirin tablets will the patient need for a 2-week vacation?

10. If a multidose liquid medication contains 100 mL, and the patient takes 5 mL (1 teaspoon) per day, how many days will the medication last?

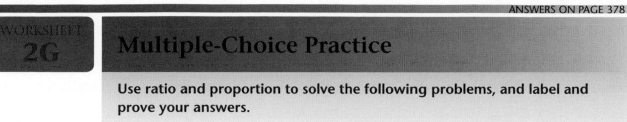

WORKSHEET
2G

Multiple-Choice Practice

Use ratio and proportion to solve the following problems, and label and prove your answers.

1. If you need 10 diapers a day, how many days will a package of 50 diapers last?
   a. 5 days   **c.** 15 days
   b. 10 days   **d.** 20 days

2. Ordered: 120 insulin syringes. They are delivered in units of 10 per package. How many packages will you receive?
   a. 10 packages   **c.** 15 packages
   b. 12 packages   **d.** 20 packages

3. You have to take 4 teaspoons of medicine every day. The bottle contains 80 teaspoons. How many days will the bottle last?
   a. 2 days   **c.** 10 days
   b. 5 days   **d.** 20 days

4. Ordered: 3 pills per day. How many pills will the patient need for 21 days?
   a. 12 pills   **c.** 31 pills
   b. 20 pills   **d.** 63 pills

5. You have a vial holding 30 mL of liquid. If the average dose given is 5 mL, how many doses are available?
   a. 5 doses   **c.** 8 doses
   b. 6 doses   **d.** 10 doses

6. The hospital has allotted 120 days of inservice for 15 departments. How many days of inservice can each department use?
   a. 4 days   **c.** 12 days
   b. 8 days   **d.** 15 days

7. The hospital staffs every 8 patients with one RN. How many RNs will be needed when the census is 240?
   a. 30 RNs   **c.** 90 RNs
   b. 60 RNs   **d.** 120 RNs

8. The directions state that for every $\frac{1}{2}$ cup portion of baby cereal you will need 4 ounces of milk. How many ounces of milk will you need to prepare 20 portions?
   a. 20 ounces   **c.** 80 ounces
   b. 40 ounces   **d.** 100 ounces

Continued

ANSWERS ON PAGE 378

WORKSHEET
2G

Multiple-Choice Practice (Continued)

9. If you receive $15 an hour overtime, how many hours would you need to work overtime to receive $450 in overtime earnings?
   a. 3 hours
   c. 30 hours
   b. 15 hours
   d. 45 hours

10. One nurse assistant is employed for every 20 beds. How many nurse assistants are employed for a 360-bed hospital?
    a. 18 assistants
    c. 25 assistants
    b. 20 assistants
    d. 30 assistants

CHAPTER 2 Final

ANSWERS ON PAGE 379

Solve each problem using ratio and proportion. Label and prove your answers.

1. The hospital assigns 5 nursing supervisors per shift. How many supervisors are needed for 3 shifts?

2. Each nurse is assigned 6 patients. How many nurses are needed for 150 patients in a hospital?

3. The hospital laundry provides 4 sheets per bed per day. How many sheets are needed per day for a 200-bed hospital?

4. The average number of discharges is 32 patients per day. How many patients are discharged each week?

5. A nurse earns $20 an hour extra pay for overtime hours. How much will the nurse earn for 24 hours of overtime in a pay period?

6. A CNA is hired for every 12 beds in the hospital. How many CNAs would be hired for a 360-bed hospital?

7. There is 1 nursing supervisor or administrator for every 30 nurses. How many supervisors or administrators would be needed for 150 nurses?

8. The hospital rents 25 portable oxygen canisters a week for $750. How much will a 4-week supply of canisters cost?

9. Approximately 1 resident and 2 interns are assigned for every 20 patients. How many interns are needed for 210 patients?

10. Some studies show that approximately 1 of every 6 medications involves an error. Approximately how many medication errors would occur for every 240 medications given?

11. If a patient has to take 1 pill every 6 hours, how many pills will he or she need for 3 days?

12. If a patient is discharged with a 1-week supply of pills and is to take 4 pills per day, how many pills will the patient need?

13. Ordered: 2 tablets, 3 times daily. How many days will a bottle of 60 tablets last?

14. The patient is to drink 4 ounces of water every $\frac{1}{2}$ hour. How much water will the patient have consumed in 8 hours?

15. The budget permits 96 inservice days per year. There are 12 units. How many inservice days could each unit receive?

16. A multidose vial contains 20 mL. If each dose is 2.5 mL, how many doses are in the vial?

17. If the average adult weight is 150 pounds and the elevator can hold 1800 pounds, how many people, on average, can ride the elevator?

18. If each orientation for an RN costs approximately $3000, how many RNs can the hospital plan to hire with an annual orientation budget of $96,000?

19. If a guest speaker is paid a $50 honorarium, how many guest speakers can be invited if the budget is $600?

20. If a patient needs a 30-day supply of tablets and takes 2 tablets four times a day, how many tablets will the patient need at discharge?

Refer to the Mathematics Review section of the enclosed student CD-ROM for additional practice problems.

CHAPTER 3

Safe Medication Administration

Objectives

- Identify the knowledge and skills needed for safe administration of medications.
- Describe safe nursing practices that reduce medication errors.
- Interpret medication-related abbreviations and medication labels.
- Identify equipment for oral medication administration.
- Identify oral and liquid forms of medications.
- Identify key characteristics of medication administration records (MARs).
- Convert time to military hours.
- Explain the need for incident reports.
- Analyze medication errors using critical thinking.

INTRODUCTION

Safe medication administration involves more than accurate dose measurement and calculations. Prior to calculation, the nurse must be able to interpret the medication-related documents that will be encountered. This interpretation includes knowledge of medical terminology, hospital forms and abbreviations used in medication orders, drug forms, drug label contents, medication-related patient records, and current drug references. Attention to detail and patient rights are necessary elements for the protection of each patient.

Patient Rights

There are seven basic patient rights related to safe medication administration. As you read through them, think about the implications should one of these rights be violated.

RIGHT PATIENT

The patient for whom the medication is ordered must be the patient who receives the medication. Similar names and lack of attention to patient identification when the medication is in hand can result in a medication being administered to the wrong patient. There are strict agency and The Joint Commission procedures for safe patient identification. They include using two separate written identifiers, such as the *patient name* and medical record number or *birth date*.

RIGHT DRUG

The nurse must be able to interpert orders for the drug, identify and clarify incomplete or unclear orders by conferring with the prescriber, and compare supplied drugs by matching them exactly to the order. There are many similar-sounding drugs on the market, and they must be distinguished from each other.

RIGHT DOSE

Knowledge of abbreviations and measurement systems commonly used in the preparation and administration of medications is essential. The nurse must ascertain that it is a safe dose for the intended patient and must calculate and measure the precise dose ordered. Attention to decimals and zeros is vital for the prevention of errors.

RIGHT TIME

If a medication is omitted, delayed, or given too early, there can be serious consequences. A nurse must be able to interpet the 24-hour clock as well as read traditional time. Prioritizing emergency and stat drugs and identifying drugs that have to be given before, with, or after a meal are abilities that must be acquired through clinical practice and supervision. Knowledge of each drug's purpose and action is required. It is important to ask for help if the workload is too heavy to allow for perfect attention to detail.

52

> ### CLINICAL ALERT
>
> Always document the medication promptly *after* it is administered. Never document *before* a medication is administered. Doing so may lead to double dosing a medication.

RIGHT ROUTE

The nurse must prepare the medication so it can be administered via the route ordered. Abbreviations are usually used for medication routes. Many medications are available in solid and liquid forms for oral, intramuscular, or intravenous routes of administration. If the patient refuses or is unable to tolerate the route ordered, the nurse must obtain an order for change from the prescriber.

RIGHT DOCUMENTATION

Accurate and timely reporting and documentation in the patient medical records is an essential protection for the patient and the nurse.

RIGHT TO REFUSE A MEDICATION

Patients are entitled to refuse medications (and treatments). The reason should be ascertained, reported, and documented in a timely fashion so that corrective action can be taken if necessary. Include a comment on mental status when reporting and recording refusals.

Several studies have shown that many medications are given in error; the rate ranges from 2% to well over 10% when underreporting and wrong time of administration are considered.

Errors may occur in the prescriber's order, in the interpretation of the order by the pharmacy or the nurse, in the copying of the order into a computer or onto a record, on the label supplied by the pharmacy, or during the preparation and administration of the medication.

There are many Internet references well worth reading that pertain to medication errors. The following is a sampling of on-line sources:

www.nlm.nih.gov/medlineplus/drugsafety.html
www.fda.gov/cder/drug/MedErrors
www.ismp.org
www.jointcommission.org/PatientSafety/DoNotUseList
www.medscape.com
www.nccmerp.org/aboutMedErrors.html

> ### CLINICAL ALERT
>
> The nurse who prepares and administers the medication offers the last protection to the patient.

Abbreviations

In order to interpret prescriber orders, drug literature, and drug labels, the nurse must learn treatment-related and medication-related abbreviations; they are listed on the inside front cover. The nurse must also avoid writing the abbreviations that are on The Joint Commission's Do Not Use list as of January 2004; they appear on the inside front cover. These abbreviations have been misinterpreted and have led to medication errors. Only approved abbreviations may be used, and they must be written precisely. You will have to review them several times in order to memorize them. Use these worksheets to help yourself remember them. Abbreviations for drugs have led to errors and are best avoided. The trend is to reduce the number of approved abbreviations.

ANSWERS ON PAGE 380

WORKSHEET 3A

Abbreviations for Time and Route

Study the approved and recommended abbreviations and their patterns of similarities and differences as well as The Joint Commission's Do Not Use list inside the front cover. Then enter the approved or recommended abbreviation in the space provided.

Time	Abbreviation (if Applicable)	Time	Abbreviation (if Applicable)
before		after	
before meals		after meals	
daily	Write out daily	three times a day	
twice a day		every other day	Write out every other day
every day	Write out every day	every 6 hours	
every 4 hours		every 12 hours	
whenever necessary		as desired, freely	
immediately, at once		bedtime	Write out bedtime
with		without	

Route	Abbreviation (if Applicable)	Route	Abbreviation (if Applicable)
by mouth		nothing by mouth	
intravenous		intramuscular	
sublingual		subcutaneous	
intradermal		suppository*	
left eye	Write out left eye	right ear	Write out right ear
nasogastric		per gastrostomy tube	

*Orders for suppositories require further route identification: per vagina, per rectum, or per urethra.

MEASUREMENT ABBREVIATIONS

Metric abbreviations are commonly used for medication orders.

Metric measurement abbreviations are *not* pluralized. Two kilograms would be written as 2 kg, not 2 kgs; 2 grams would be written as 2 g, not 2 gs. Insert a space between the number and the metric unit: 10 g (not 10g).

ANSWERS ON PAGE 380

WORKSHEET 3B

Abbreviations for Drug Measurements

Study the abbreviations on the inside front cover. Pay attention to upper and lower case letters when learning the abbreviations. There are only a few instances when upper case is employed. Then provide the approved abbreviations for the measurements.

Metric Measurement Term*	Abbreviation (if Applicable)
microgram(s)	
milligram(s)	
gram(s)	
kilogram(s)	
milliliter(s)	
milliequivalent(s)	
unit	Write out unit
international unit	Write out international unit
liter	
square meter	
Other Measurement Term	**Abbreviation (if Applicable)**
grain (apothecary term)	Write out grain
one half	Write out one half
teaspoon	
tablespoon	
pound	

*The metric abbreviations are the same for singular and plural measurements.

CLINICAL ALERT

mcg, micrograms, may also be encountered written as μg. Write mcg for micrograms because μg has been misread as mg (milligrams) when poorly written; that is a thousandfold error.

cc is sometimes written interchangeably with mL (milliliters). It means cubic centimeters and has been mistaken for aa (of each) and u (units). Write mL instead. Do *not* write cc. Do *not* make up your own abbreviations for metric terms.

ANSWERS ON PAGE 381

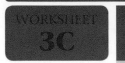

WORKSHEET
3C

Abbreviations for Drug Forms

Study the abbreviations on the inside front cover. Then provide the abbreviations in the spaces provided.

Term	Recommended Abbreviation
capsule	
tablet	
fluid	
solution	
suspension	
elixir	
teaspoon	
tablespoon	
liquid	
ounce	
double-strength	
extended release	
long acting	
sustained release	
controlled release	

CLINICAL ALERT

The following abbreviations are examples of other abbreviations that have caused errors and are best written out:

qid   Means four times a day but has been confused with the prohibited qd (daily).

HS   Is frequently encountered; usually refers to bedtime (hour of sleep) but has been mistaken for half strength when combined with a fluid or solution order. Write out "bedtime."

DC   Has been interpreted to mean discontinue and discharge. Write out the word.

$\overline{ss}$ Is an old English apothecary abbreviation meaning one half. Write out "one half."

gtt   Is an apothecary abbreviation meaning drop. Write out "drop."

gr   Is an apothecary abbreviation meaning grain. It has been confused with the metric term "gram." The measurements are not interchangeable. Use *metric measurements*. Call the pharmacy and consult current drug references and instructor if in doubt about any abbreviations. Further practice and explanations of measurements appear in the next chapter.

When you can translate the abbreviations into words, progress to the next sections in this chapter, which discuss orders and labels. Those sections and subsequent chapters will help you to transfer the abbreviations into your memory.

Medication Delivery

Many hospital pharmacies stock supply and resupply medication carts as shown in Figures 3-1 and 3-2. These carts are thought to provide greater security and reduce the chances of medication errors by replacing multidose stock bottles of oral medications with unit dose (single-serving) medications for one to three shifts at a time and one bottle at a time of multidose liquid medications (Figures 3-3, 3-4.

DRUG FORMS: SOLIDS AND LIQUIDS

As can be seen in the list and figures that follow, drugs can be provided in a variety of forms for both oral and other routes—tablets, capsules, suspensions, suppositories, and so forth. It is very important to distinguish among the forms and to ascertain the precise form intended by the prescriber. The form affects the rate of absorption of the drug and the route of administration.

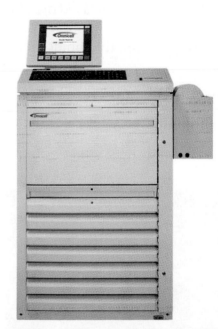

FIGURE 3-1   The OmniRx with OmniDispenser unit is an example of a computerized unit dose medication cabinet. Each dose is released individually, recorded automatically, and requires no counting when issued or at the end of a shift. The OmniRx is used for managing controlled substances, first doses, as-needed doses, floor stock, supplies, and other charge items. *(From Omnicell, Inc., Mountain View, CA.)*

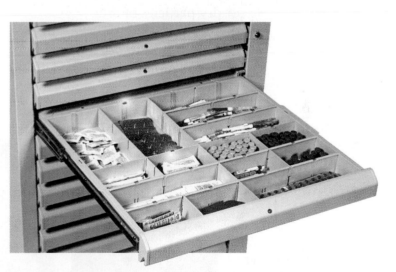

FIGURE 3-2   The Lighted Matrix Drawer is an example of a flexible medication and pharmacy supply drawer. *(From Omnicell, Inc., Mountain View, CA.)*

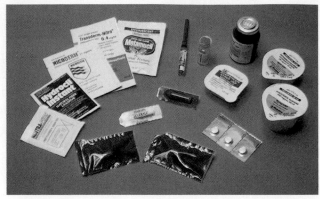

FIGURE 3-3   Unit dose packages. *(From Clayton BD, Stock YN, Harroun RD:* Basic pharmacology for nurses, *ed 14, St Louis, 2007, Mosby. Courtesy of Chuck Dresner.)*

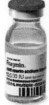

10,000 IU/mL
9.5 mL multidose vial
NDC 0013-2436-06

FIGURE 3-4   Multidose vial of Fragmin. *(Used with permission from Pfizer, Inc.)*

Solids

- Plain tablets (Figure 3-5, *A*): compressed powdered drugs
- Scored tablets (Figure 3-5, *B*): tablets with indentation; the only kind of tablet that may be broken
- Enteric-coated tablets (Figure 3-5, *C*): tablets with coating for delayed dissolution; should not be crushed or chewed
- Capsules (caps) (Figure 3-5, *D*): soluble case, usually gelatin, that holds liquid or dry particles of drug
- Extended-release capsules (S-R, slow-release) (Figure 3-5, *E*): capsules that contain beaded particles of drug for delayed absorption
- Powders/granules (Figure 3-5, *F*): loose or molded drug substance; usually to be dissolved in liquid or food

FIGURE 3-5   Various solid oral drug forms. **A,** Plain tablets. **B,** Scored tablets. **C,** Enteric-coated tablets. **D,** Capsules. **E,** Extended-release capsules. **F,** Granules. *(Courtesy Amanda Politte, St Louis, MO)*

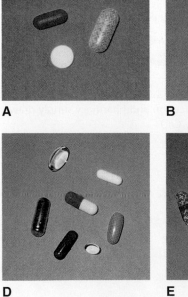

A

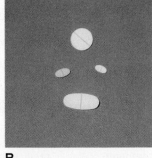

B

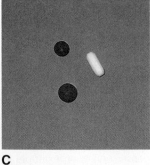

C

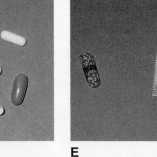

D

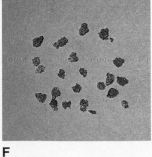

E

F

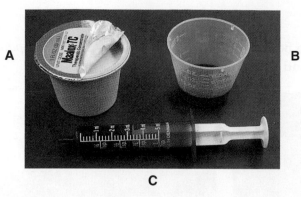

FIGURE 3-6   **A,** Liquid medication in a single-dose package. **B,** Liquid measured in medicine cup. **C,** Oral liquid medicine in syringe. *(From Potter PA, Perry AG: Fundamentals of nursing, ed 6, St Louis, 2005, Mosby.)*

Liquids

- Aqueous suspensions: solid particles suspended in liquid that must be mixed well before administration
- Elixirs: sweetened alcohol and water solutions
- Emulsions: fats or oils suspended in liquid by an emulsifier
- Extracts: syrups or derived forms of active drugs
- Fluid extracts: concentrated alcoholic liquid extracts of plants or vegetables

Liquids are administered in medicine cups, with medicine droppers, and sometimes with syringes (Figure 3-6). When pouring medicines into a cup, place the cup on a flat surface and pour the dose to the meniscus at your eye level. Note the equivalent household amounts for the metric system: Tbsp, oz, tsp.

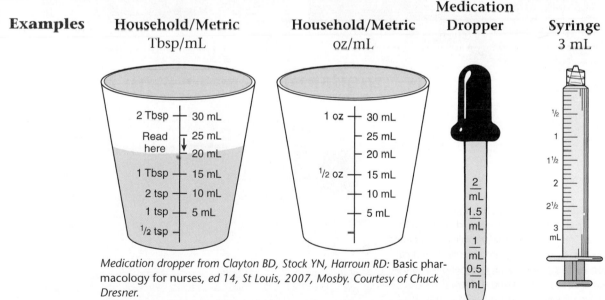

Examples

Household/Metric Tbsp/mL — Household/Metric oz/mL — Medication Dropper — Syringe 3 mL

Medication dropper from Clayton BD, Stock YN, Harroun RD: Basic pharmacology for nurses, ed 14, St Louis, 2007, Mosby. Courtesy of Chuck Dresner.
Syringe from Perry AG, Potter PA: Clinical nursing skills and techniques, ed 6, St Louis, 2006, Mosby.

CLINICAL ALERT

Do not substitute the ordered form of a drug for another form. Do not substitute household utensils, such as spoons, cups, and droppers, when measuring medications. Medication utensils are calibrated for exact doses according to the metric system of measurement.

LIQUID INJECTABLES

Liquids may also be supplied in injectable (also known as *parenteral*) forms in ampules, vials, and prefilled syringes (Figure 3-7).

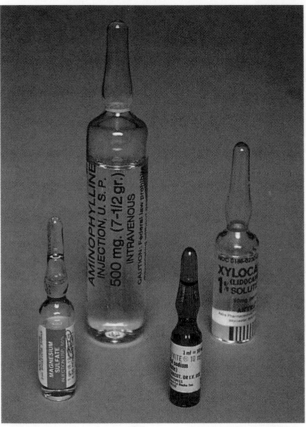

A

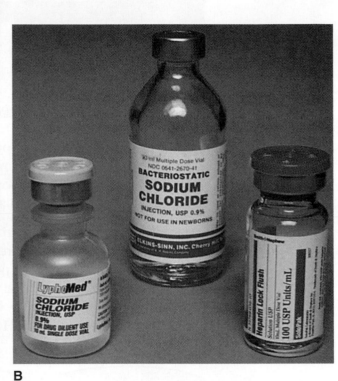

B

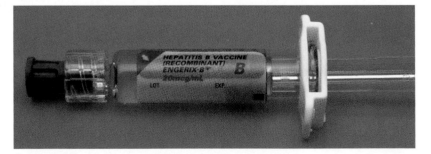

C

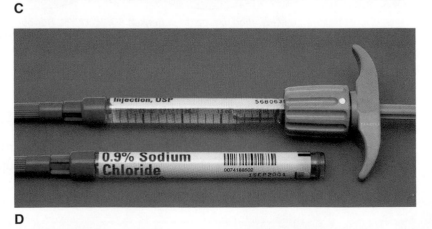

D

FIGURE 3-7 **A**, Injectable liquid supplied in ampules. **B**, Injectable liquid supplied in vials. **C**, Injectable liquid supplied in prefilled syringe. **D**, Tubex system: prefilled medication cartridge with attached needle and assembled system. *(A and B, From Perry AG, Potter PA: Clinical nursing skills and techniques, ed 6, St Louis, 2006, Mosby. C and D, From Macklin D, Chernecky C, Infortuna H: Math for clinical practice, St Louis, 2005, Mosby.)*

Medication Labels

It is helpful to study the information provided on medication labels so as to facilitate your interpretation of prescriber orders and of medication administration records. Some of the label information is already familiar because of personal experience with medication prescriptions and over-the-counter (OTC) products. The label must be read carefully to ensure that the medication is precisely what the prescriber ordered.

INTERPRETING MEDICATION LABELS

Medication labels can be confusing because of the vast amount of information they contain and the small print. Some labels are prepared in-house by pharmacists or pharmacy technicians. The most important information is as follows:

- Name, both generic (the first letter is usually lowercase) and proprietary, brand, or trade (the first letter is usually capitalized)
- Route
- Form
- *Unit dose* per milliliter, per tablet, or per capsule
- *Total* amount in the container
- Instructions for preparation (if applicable)
- Instructions for storage
- Expiration date (stamped by firm or pharmacist after manufacture)

Example

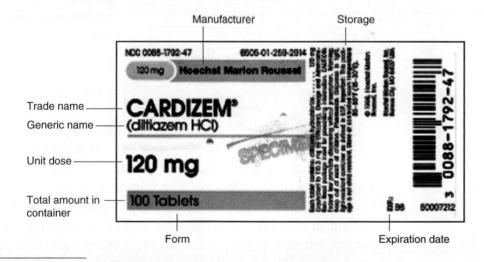

Note: The metric measurement mg is the abbreviation of milligrams.

Cardizem is the proprietary, or trade, name for this Hoechst Marion Roussel product. Diltiazem is the generic name used by all companies that produce this drug. There are 100 tablets total in the container; each tablet contains 120 mg (unit dose). Tablets are usually given by mouth. The route is not specified, but the storage directions are given and space is provided for an expiration date. When calculating a dose, place the 120 mg:1 tab on the left side of your ratio and proportion.

Example

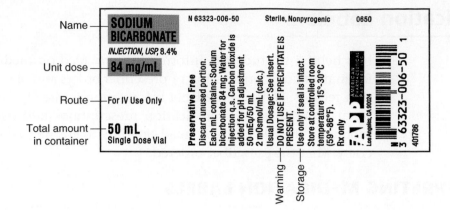

Name — SODIUM BICARBONATE
Unit dose — 84 mg/mL
Route — For IV Use Only
Total amount in container — 50 mL Single Dose Vial

Warning   Storage

This vial of sodium bicarbonate contains 50 mL of 84 mg/mL intravenous injection fluid. It is a single-dose vial. The directions state that the unused portion should be discarded. A multidose vial may be kept for a specified period and used for more than one patient or on more than one occasion. When calculating a dose, place the 84 mg : 1 mL on the left side of your ratio and proportion as your "have."

Example

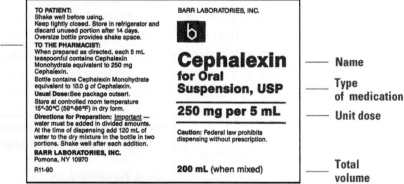

Directions and storage

Cephalexin for Oral Suspension, USP

250 mg per 5 mL

200 mL (when mixed)

Name

Type of medication

Unit dose

Total volume

This multidose preparation, cephalexin, is an aqueous suspension (solid particles suspended in liquid). Whether it is dispensed for hospital or home use, it is obvious that the directions for preparation, storage, and use are very important for distributing the medication properly throughout the suspension, for dispensing the correct strength, and for maintaining the strength of the drug during storage (in the refrigerator). When calculating a dose, use 250 mg : 5 mL for the left side of your ratio and proportion. Note that 200 mL would contain 40 doses of 250 mg each. Any dose other than 250 mg will require some metric mathematical skills!

Example

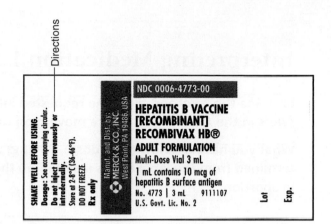

This hepatitis B vaccine label emphasizes that it is for adult use. The routes to be avoided are also emphasized. You would have to read the accompanying literature to determine whether it is to be given po or IM. (It is to be administered IM.) Also note the dose: 10 mcg : 1 mL. The nurse must be very aware of the difference between micrograms and milligrams (mg). This vaccine, like many medications, is also issued in other strengths. It is important to note that this is a *multidose* 3 mL vial, *not* a unit-dose vial.

◢ CLINICAL ALERT

A lethal error can be made if the *total* dose in a multidose container is mistaken for the *unit* dose or if an intramuscular preparation is given intravenously because the administrator failed to check the route.

ANSWERS ON PAGE 381

Interpreting Medication Labels

Examine the label and fill in the requested information. Check your answers in the Answer Key before moving on to the next problem.

What you have or know (unit dose), 100 mg : 1 tab or 50 mg : 1 mL, is determined from the label and is inserted on the left side of your ratio and proportion.

1.

NDC 0028-0051-10   FSC **3602**
6505-01-071-6557

Lopressor® 50 mg

metoprolol tartrate USP

EXP

LOT

1000 tablets

Keep this and all drugs out
of the reach of children.

Dispense in tight, light-resistant
container (USP).

Caution: Federal law prohibits
dispensing without prescription.

Geigy

PHARMACIST: Container closure is not child-resistant.
Dosage: See package insert.
Store between 59°- 86°F (15°- 30°C).
Protect from moisture.

Ciba-Geigy Corporation
Pharmaceuticals Division
Summit, NJ 07901

645120

N 3   0028-0051-10   6

a. Trade name (registered patent or brand name, capital first letter)
b. Generic name (common name, *usually* lowercase and in parentheses)
c. Unit dose and form (tab/cap/mL)
d. Total amount in container
e. Ratio for "what you have or know" (left side of your proportion)

2.

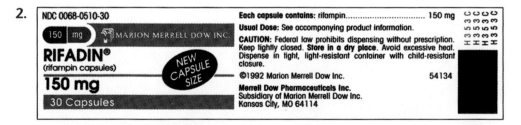

NDC 0068-0510-30

150 mg   MARION MERRELL DOW INC.

RIFADIN®
(rifampin capsules)

150 mg

30 Capsules

NEW
CAPSULE
SIZE

Each capsule contains: rifampin................................. 150 mg
Usual Dose: See accompanying product information.
CAUTION: Federal law prohibits dispensing without prescription.
Keep tightly closed. **Store in a dry place.** Avoid excessive heat.
Dispense in tight, light-resistant container with child-resistant
closure.
©1992 Marion Merrell Dow Inc.   54134

Merrell Dow Pharmaceuticals Inc.
Subsidiary of Marion Merrell Dow Inc.
Kansas City, MO 64114

H 3 5 3 C
H 3 5 3 C
H 3 5 3 C
H 3 5 3 C

a. Trade (brand) name
b. Generic (common) name
c. Unit dose and form
d. Total amount in container
e. Ratio for "what you have or know"

ANSWERS ON PAGE 381

WORKSHEET
3D

Interpreting Medication Labels (Continued)

3.

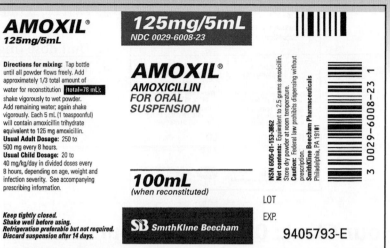

a. Trade name
b. Total amount (mL) of sterile water to add for reconstitution
c. Unit dose
d. Total amount (mL) in container after reconstitution
e. Ratio for "what you have"
f. Length of time permitted for storage

4.

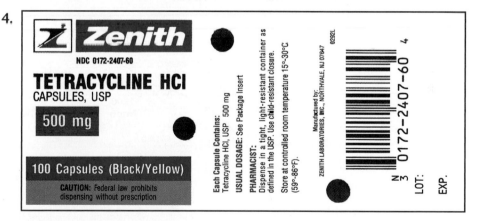

a. Generic name
b. Unit dose
c. Total amount in container
d. Ratio for "what you have"

⬡ **CLINICAL ALERT**

The unit dose is usually the average dose ordered for adults (*not* children or elderly patients). If your calculations call for more than one or two times the unit dose (more than 1 to 2 tab or 1 to 2 mL), double check the order and your math, and research the reason. This commonsense approach has saved many lives.

Continued

ANSWERS ON PAGE 381

Interpreting Medication Labels (Continued)

5.
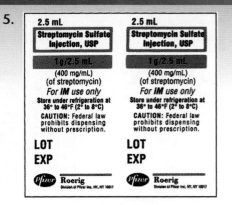

a. Generic name
b. Route
c. Unit dose (mg per mL)
d. Total amount in container
e. Storage directions

The 24-Hour Clock: 0000-2400 Hours

Interpreting time according to the 24-hour clock is important to understanding prescriber orders and patient medical records. Most agencies use a 24-hour computer-compatible clock, also known as *military* or *international* time (Figure 3-8).

All times are expressed in 4 digits, from 0001 to 2400, without colons and without reference to AM and PM.

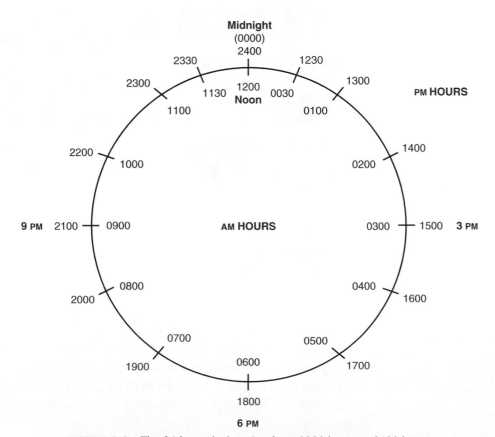

FIGURE 3-8 The 24-hour clock, going from 0000 hours to 2400 hours.

At 2400 (midnight, 12 AM), the clock changes to 0000 for counting purposes. Thus 0001 is 1 minute after midnight. The sequential numbering system helps to avoid AM/PM time confusion and potential errors.

The AM clock begins at midnight, 0000, and ends at noon, 1200 hours.

The PM clock begins at noon, 1200, and ends at midnight, 2400 hours.

Thus, midnight is noted two ways. It is most commonly written as 2400, but each minute after midnight is written as if midnight were 0000.

The afternoon hours begin at noon (12 PM) when the PM side of the clock is used. The major difference from traditional time is noted at 1300 (1 PM).

RULE   To convert *traditional* pm time to the *24-hour clock*, begin at 1:00 pm and add 1200 to the time. Delete colons and am/pm notation.

....

Examples   1:00 PM + 1200 = 1300 hours   or   1 + 12 = 13 and add 2 zeros
3:00 PM + 1200 = 1500 hours   or   3 + 12 = 15 and add 2 zeros

PM HOURS   AM HOURS

1200 = Noon (12 PM)   2400 = Midnight (12 AM) (0000)
1230 = Half past 12 noon   0030 = 1 half hour after midnight
1300 = 1 PM   0100 = 1 AM

RULE   To convert the *24-hour clock* pm hours to *traditional* time, subtract 1200 from the time starting with 1300 hours, insert a colon between the hour and minutes and add pm

....

Examples   1300 − 1200 = 100 = 1:00 PM or 13 − 12 = 1 and add colon, 2 zeros, and PM.
2020 − 1200 = 820 = 8:20 PM or 20 − 12 = 8 and add colon, minutes, and PM.

Learning the key times 0100 and 1300 to 2400 is helpful.

1159 = 1 minute before noon   2359 = 1 minute before midnight
1201 = 1 minute after noon   0001 = 1 minute after midnight

It is also helpful to study some key times in your daily schedule:

Your usual breakfast hour: _____

The time your shift begins: _____

The time your shift ends: _____

Your usual dinner hour: _____

Your usual bedtime hour: _____

Physician's Orders

Medication orders may be handwritten by the prescriber or entered into a computer by the prescriber or by the pharmacy and printed by the pharmacy.

All medication orders must contain the complete date and time, the name of the medication, the total dose and form (if supplied in more than one form) of each administration of the medication, the route, and the frequency schedule as well as any other comments.

Examples   12/01/08   1800   Aspirin tablets 650 mg PO at bedtime daily with a snack
OR
12/01/08   0900   Aspirin suppository 325 mg per rectum q6h for fever
over 38° C

Orders must be legible to avoid errors or misinterpretation. Questions pertaining to orders should be clarified with the prescriber and documented.

In most cases, the pharmacy provides a printed daily medication administration record (MAR) to the unit for the patient record. It is based on the prescriber's order and includes additional information for the nurse who will administer the medication (Figure 3-9).

CLINICAL ALERT

Consult The Joint Commission's and the hospital's policies and limitations pertaining to verbal and telephone orders.

Understanding Medication Administration Records

Every nursing institution has its own medication administration record (MAR) forms, and the trend is to record the medications on computer. Similar in content, most of these forms are self-explanatory. All contain places to record identifying patient data; allergies; medication orders, including the dose, route, and frequency and hour desired for administration; and full signature (with date) of the person administering the medication. Most MAR forms list suggested codes for data entry.

During orientation, a new employee must identify hospital policies that are not stated on the form. These include how to add a new order, how to indicate discontinuance of a medication, procedures for data entry and reporting of medication errors, and additional documentation required to support the MAR. Examples of MARs are shown in Figures 3-10 and 3-11.

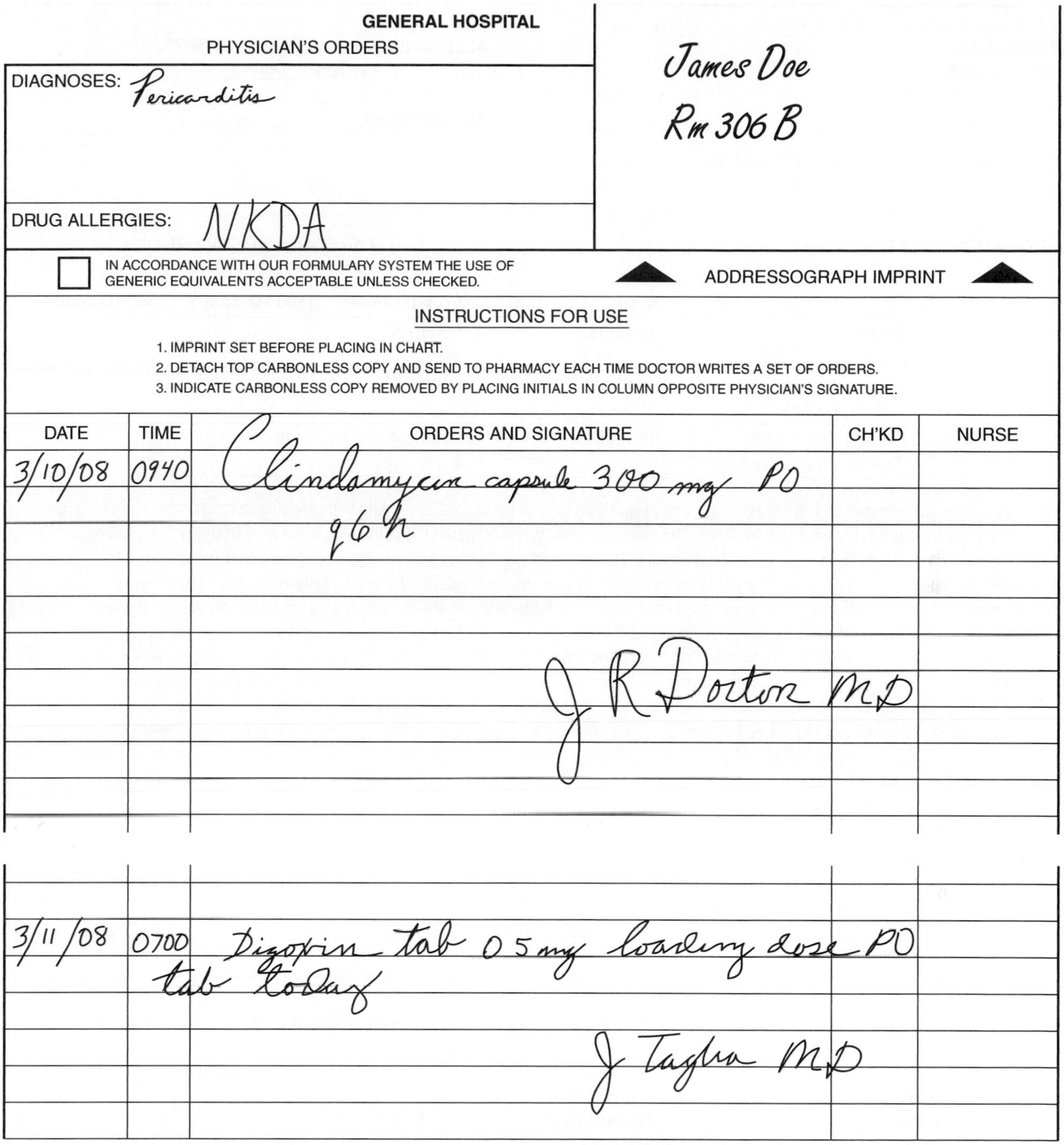

GENERAL HOSPITAL
PHYSICIAN'S ORDERS

DIAGNOSES: *Pericarditis*

James Doe
Rm 306 B

DRUG ALLERGIES: NKDA

☐ IN ACCORDANCE WITH OUR FORMULARY SYSTEM THE USE OF GENERIC EQUIVALENTS ACCEPTABLE UNLESS CHECKED.

▲ ADDRESSOGRAPH IMPRINT ▲

INSTRUCTIONS FOR USE

1. IMPRINT SET BEFORE PLACING IN CHART.
2. DETACH TOP CARBONLESS COPY AND SEND TO PHARMACY EACH TIME DOCTOR WRITES A SET OF ORDERS.
3. INDICATE CARBONLESS COPY REMOVED BY PLACING INITIALS IN COLUMN OPPOSITE PHYSICIAN'S SIGNATURE.

DATE	TIME	ORDERS AND SIGNATURE	CH'KD	NURSE
3/10/08	0940	Clindamycin capsule 300 mg PO q6h		
		J R Dorton MD		
3/11/08	0700	Digoxin tab 0.5 mg loading dose PO tab today		
		J Taylor MD		

FIGURE 3-9 Example of a handwritten order for an oral antibiotic and an oral cardiac medication.

Brown, John
ID# 45764304
Age: 50   Sex: M   Rm: 406A
Dr. Marin, Cruz

ALLERGIES: DRUGS: *IV iodine, Aspirin*
FOODS: Denies

RN Verification: *FD*

MAR Date: 05-07-08 0700 - 05-08-08 0659

MEDICATION: Dose Route Freq

Time of Administration, Site, and Initials

	START	**STOP**	**0700 TO 1459**	**1500 TO 2259**	**2300 TO 0659**
SCH	05-05-08 Digoxin 0.125 mg po Q AM	05-12-08	(0900) *JM* R		
SCH	05-05-08 Tylenol (acetaminophen) 500 mg po BID	05-12-08	0800 *JM*	2000	
SCH	05-05-08 Clotrimazole 1% CR TOP bid to affected area	05-12-08	0900 *JM* L	2100	

This is a pharmacy-generated MAR for a 24-hr period stated in military time beginning with the day shift, 5-7-08. The RN who signs the verification is verifying that the medication orders accurately match the provider orders and that the allergies have been noted. SCH means a regularly scheduled medication versus a PRN order. You must use the agency *code* for administration sites. A circled time denotes med NOT given. Additional documentation may need to be added elsewhere in the nurse's record. PRN meds and one time only meds have *separate* placeholders. You may add new orders by writing them in (refer to promethazine). This pharmacy prints instructions for diluting intravenous medications. The narcotic (meperidine) has an automatic 48-hr limit and then must have a written renewal order. This hospital policy calls for a yellow highlight to denote discontinued/expired orders. All discontinued orders, automatic or other must be renewed if it is necessary to continue them. On the SITE CODES note that if a medication is withheld other than for NPO or surgery, the reason must be documented on the patient record eg: "refused acetaminophen and states it 'doesn't do anything for him.' Dr. Marin notified."

ONE TIME ONLY AND PRN MEDS

	Start	**Stop**	**Time**	**Initials**	**Full Name/Title**
	05-07-08 Meperidine				
PRN	25 mg IV q6h PRN	05-09-08	*2300*	*FD*	*Florence Dane, RN*
	Dilute in 5 mL NS and give over 5 min	0700	C		
	05-07-08 promethazine 25 mg IM STAT	*5/7/08*	*1900 J*	*TR*	*T Robbins, RN*

Sign: *Joe Mack*   Initials: *JM*   Sign: *T Robbins*   Initials: *TR*   Sign: *Florence Dane*   Initials: *FD*

SITE CODES   **GENERAL HOSPITAL**

A	Abdomen (L)	J	Gluteus (LUQ)
B	Abdomen (R)	K	Gluteus (RUQ)
C	Arm (L)	L	Thigh (L)
D	Arm (R)	M	Thigh (R)
E	Eyes (both)	N	Ventrogluteal (L)
F	Eyes (left)	O	Ventrogluteal (R)
G	Eyes (right)	P	NPO: Lab
H	Deltoid (mid L)	Q	NPO: Surgery
I	Deltoid (mid R)	R	Withheld/See nurse's notes

Clinical Alert!	Verify pharmacy data on this sheet including dilution instructions. Remember this form is not a *copy* of the original orders. These data have been recopied into the computer.

FIGURE 3-10   Sample medication administration record (MAR).

			MEDICATION AMINISTRATION RECORD
Acct: Admitted: 10/05/08 1630 Att Phys: Diagnosis: Respiratory Allergies: Morphine/Beta-Adrenergic blocking agts	MR#: Age: 77Y Sex: F HT: 5'7.0" / 170.2 cm WT: 224 lbs / 101.606 kg		M A R

Start Date/Time	Stop Date/Time	RN/ LPN	Medication	0731-1530	1531-2330	2331-0730
			** ****************** **PRN** ******************* ***			
10/05/08 2143	10/12/08 2142		**Promethazine HCL** **(Phenergan Equiv)** **25 mg = 0.5 mL** IV #020 **Q6H PRN** **PRN N/V**			
			When administering IV: **Must be diluted to a** **final concentration of 25 mg/mL.** **IV administration to be at a rate** **not to exceed 25 mg/minute.**			
10/05/08 2100	10/08/08 2059		**Zolpidem Tartrate** **(Ambien)** **10 mg = 2 tablet** Oral #016 **At bedtime PRN** ****Narcotic sign-out****			Discontinue
10/05/08 2200	10/11/08 2159		**Alum-Mag Hydroxide-Simethicone** **(Maalox Plus/Mylanta Equiv)** **30 mL = 30 mL** Oral #022 **Q4H PRN** **Stagger one hr from other meds**			

This is an example of a computer-generated MAR for PRN orders only. There are many similarities to the MAR in Figure 3-10 and also some differences noted: this MAR states the medication unit dose supplied; the medication nurse must enter the exact time the medication was given. In addition to dilution instructions, scheduling instructions are given with the last medication. The site code is different and the dose omission code is amplified. Even if no medication is given to a patient, the MAR must be signed by the nurse responsible for the patient each shift. Medications which are refused, withheld, or mischarted must be circled, timed, and initialed—a standard procedure that may require additional entries on the patient record if the code is not self-explanatory.

Order Date	RN INIT.	Date/Time To Be Given	One Time Orders and Pre-Operatives Medication-Dose-Route	Actual Time Given	Site Codes			Dose Omission Code
					Arm	LA	RA	A = pt absent
					Deltoid	LD	RD	H = hold
					Ventrogluteal	LVG	RVG	M = med absent
					Gluteal	LG	RG	N = NPO
					Abdomen	LUQ	RUQ	O = other
					Abdomen	LLQ	RLQ	R = refused
								U = unable to tolerate
					INIT	Signature	INIT	Signature

60321 (8/98)A   CHART

FIGURE 3-11   Computer-generated MAR sample for PRN orders. *(From Scottsdale Healthcare, Scottsdale, AZ)*

Entering the time on the wrong MAR or entering the wrong date or wrong shift may result in time-consuming frustration. To avoid entry errors on MARs, it is recommended that you use the following order when checking or entering data concerning a patient:

1. Patient ID
2. Correct date on MAR
3. Correct medication
4. Time when the medication was last given
5. Correct shift column

If the last dose of a scheduled medication was given late, it may be necessary to delay the next dose that you are preparing. This is done to protect the patient from a drug-overload injury.

Many hospitals have policies for charting by "exception," meaning entering a narrative explanation of data that requires more explanation than is allowed for on a flow sheet.

If a medication is withheld, the time it was to be administered is entered on the MAR, usually circled and initialed. According to hospital policy, this is sometimes noted on the MAR with a word such as "refused" or "ref" and circled and initialed, with a brief narrative explanation in the nurse's notes section (see Figure 3-10).

Any time a nonscheduled medication is given, such as a stat or prn medication, it is necessary to document prompt follow-up assessments and the time. This can be recorded on the nurse's notes or flow sheet, according to hospital policy. For example, "1630 states nausea is relieved."

If an entry error is made, follow hospital policy for corrections; an example of a medication incident report is shown in Figure 3-12. The original data must be legible. It is *illegal* to discard a record or to erase or obscure any entry on medical records.

As with all medical records, the MAR is considered confidential information, and permission to make photocopies must be specifically obtained.

Some institutions preprint the *exact* times for administration on the MAR. Refer to the MAR if the medication is administered at a *different* time; the time printed should be *circled,* and the actual time written in next to it, with the nurse's initials.

Realistically, it is impossible to give five different patients their medications at, for instance, 0900. Some institutions allow the nurse to initial the printed time if the actual time is within 1 half hour. An experienced nurse knows which medications do not permit flexible administration times and *prioritizes* the medication administration order.

- -

MEDICATION INCIDENT REPORT

Patient name: _____   Date of incident: _____
                                                   Time of incident: _____

Where incident occurred: Hospital: _____   Unit: _____

Admitting diagnosis: _____

Type of incident: _____   Wrong drug
                                     _____   Wrong time
                                     _____   Wrong dose
                                     _____   Wrong patient
                                     _____   Wrong route

Medication order: _____

Account of incident and intervention taken: _____
_____
_____
_____

Was the physician notified? _____   Time: _____

Why do you feel the incident occurred? _____
_____

What were possible consequences to the patient as a result of this incident? _____
_____
_____

What can you do to prevent this type of incident from occurring again? _____
_____
_____

Persons familiar with incident or involved: _____
_____

_____   _____
Provider signature   Date   Supervisor signature   Date

- -

Incident reports are used to analyze errors and determine error patterns and methods of error prevention. They also assist agency insurers in assessing risk for liability for incidents. Each agency has its own forms and protocols for incidents.

FIGURE 3-12   Example of a medication incident report.

ANSWERS ON PAGE 382

Interpreting the MAR

Using the MAR in Figure 3-10, briefly answer the following questions.

1. Does the patient have a commonly seen surname? If so, why should the medication nurse take special note of this? _____

2. Does the patient have any medication allergies? If so, which? _____

3. This MAR indicates how many days of medication administration? _____

4. Which drug ordered was withheld or not given as scheduled? _____

5. By what route is Clotrimazole 1% to be administered? _____

6. Which order has expired? _____

7. Which drug was given at 11 PM and in which location? _____

8. When must the meperidine order be discontinued or reordered to continue administration? _____

9. When is the next time Tylenol may be given according to the 24-hour clock? According to traditional time? _____

10. Why do you think this form requires both the initials and the signature of the person giving the medications? _____

ANSWERS ON PAGE 382

Identifying Incomplete Medication Orders

Read the physician order and in a few words state why the order would have to be clarified.

1. Cozaar 25 mg daily in AM

2. Aspirin 2 tablets q4h po prn headache

3. Ampicillin 500 mg q6h × 3 days

4. Morphine sulfate 5 mg IV for pain

5. Tylenol 2 teaspoons q6h for fever over 100° F

Summary of Safe Medication Administration Practices

There are many measures a nurse can take to reduce the chances of a medication error. The following list includes a few of the many medication-related safety precautions. Study your hospital's policies pertaining to medication administration. As you read through these recommendations, think about the kinds of errors that can be prevented if the recommendations are followed.

INTERPRETING ORDERS

Know the standard approved and prohibited abbreviations.

Call the prescriber to clarify unclear orders. Do not guess.

Be aware of the patient's allergies when reading medication orders.

Phone orders are for emergencies only. Check hospital policy. If possible, have a second person listen to the orders also. Repeat the orders. Repeat doses numeral by numeral: "30 three zero milligrams."

PREPARATION

Keep your reading glasses handy if needed.

Clean and clear the area. Focus on the task. Try to avoid distractions.

Recheck allergies cited on the record.

Reconfirm when the medication was last given.

If the patient is a transfer or postoperative patient, check the operating and recovery room notes to see which medications were given and when, so that the patient does not receive a double dose or experience an interaction with new orders.

Assess recent relevant laboratory results.

Read and match the label very carefully to the order. If a liquid, check for dilution instructions.

Discard medications that have incomplete labels.

If the dose will exceed the basic unit supplied (e.g., 1 tablet or capsule per package or 1 mL ampule), recheck the original order and a pharmacology reference. If in doubt, call the prescriber.

Check for lack of sediment and presence of discoloration in liquids and for intact seals on controlled substances.

Recheck the label before returning or discarding medications from a multi-dose bottle. With single-dose medications, retain the container at least until the medication has been administered.

Read package inserts.

CALCULATIONS

Learn to do your own dose calculations accurately. Estimate your answers before calculating the dose. Do not rely on others.

Check with the prescriber or pharmacy if there is a question about the dose. Document the verification on the medical record.

Know the difference between a unit dose and a total dose in a multidose container.

Know the correct average and usual dose for the weight and age of your patient.

Have a current pharmacology-drug reference on hand to verify usual dilution and administration timing techniques and appropriate or usual dose for your patient.

ADMINISTRATION

The Joint Commission requires that *two* methods be used to identify the patient. Check the wristband of each patient. *Ask* the patient his or her name. Avoid saying, "Are you Mr. Doe?" because a confused or hard-of-hearing patient might answer yes. Compare the hospital number on the wristband with the records or ask the patient for a birthdate. For a child, check the wristband for name and number and verify with a parent or other nurse. Do *not* use bed and room numbers for identification purposes. There is a trend toward scanning the wristband and the medication with a hand-held bar code scanner to ensure accurate patient and medication identification.

Last but not least, document premedication administration assessments. Document administration promptly after the patient receives the medication. Follow-up with the patient for responses to the medication.

ANSWERS ON PAGE 382

WORKSHEET 3G

Multiple-Choice Practice

1. When administering a medication at the bedside, which should be the *first* priority?
   a. Make appropriate assessments.
   b. Identify the patient.
   c. Document the administration of the medication.
   d. Recheck the medication label.

2. If a medication-related problem is identified, which should be the *first* measure the nurse takes:
   a. Assess the patient for side effects.
   b. Notify the supervisor.
   c. Call the physician.
   d. Document the problem in detail on an incident report.

3. Which is the *unit dose* for the medication shown below?
   a. 50 mg/5 mL
   b. 1 pint
   c. 473 mL
   d. 200 mg

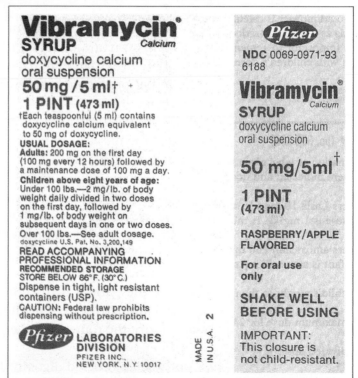

4. If a hand-written medication order is illegible or unclear, which would be the best nursing decision?
   a. Check with pharmacy.
   b. Rewrite the order to make it more legible.
   c. Give the usual unit dose and clarify.
   d. Clarify with the physician who wrote it.

Continued

ANSWERS ON PAGE 382

WORKSHEET
3G

Multiple-Choice Practice (Continued)

5. The nurse gives a medication at 1 PM. The correct equivalent international or military time on the 24-hour clock would be:
   a. 1000
   b. 1300
   c. 1500
   d. 0100

6. Which of the following statements regarding medications is *true?*
   a. Each nurse must be able to perform accurate simple and complex medication calculations.
   b. The unit dose and the total dose in a vial are one and the same.
   c. It is wise to rely on experienced colleagues to calculate drug doses.
   d. Medication errors rarely occur in the hospital setting.

7. Which of the following statements regarding potential medication errors is *false?*
   a. Medications to which the patient is allergic must be documented on admission and verified each time a new medication is administered.
   b. Many drugs have similar-sounding names.
   c. Verbal orders are best reserved for emergencies and have potential for error.
   d. Memorized calculation formulas are the most helpful measures to protect the nurse from making medication calculation errors with complex dosage calculations.

8. A tablet is ordered for a patient with a nasogastric feeding tube who is NPO. Which is the most appropriate action for the nurse to take?
   a. Crush the tablet, dilute with water, and administer via the tube.
   b. Consult with the charge nurse about the medication routine for NPO patients.
   c. Ask the patient if there have been any problems with swallowing the pill and then give it by mouth.
   d. Clarify the route with the physician who wrote the order.

9. A physician ordered digoxin (Lanoxin) 0.1 mg PO daily in the AM for a patient with cardiac failure. Available were digitoxin 0.05 mg tablets. The nurse administered two tablets of digitoxin in the morning with a glass of water. Which patient right was violated?
   a. Right drug
   b. Right dose
   c. Right route
   d. Right time

ANSWERS ON PAGE 382

WORKSHEET
3G

Multiple-Choice Practice (Continued)

10. An order for meperidine 50 mg IM q4h prn for pain expired after 48 hours, during the previous shift. The patient continues to complain of postoperative pain and requests another pain injection. Which action is an *inappropriate* nursing action?

   a. Attempt alternative measures for pain relief such as repositioning and other comfort measures.

   b. Administer the medication because the patient has had no untoward side effects as the result of any of the prior doses.

   c. Assess the patient for unexplained sources of continued pain.

   d. Explain that the medication order has expired but that you will call for a renewed order.

CRITICAL THINKING EXERCISES

Analyze the following examples of medication errors with your peers and/or instructor and discuss the issues suggested in the left-side guidelines, using this chapter and pharmacology references. As you study the error, consider which patient rights on pages 52 and 53 have been violated. What suggestions might you have for procedural changes at the hospital to prevent this from happening again? Include those that might involve pharmacy staff, providers, nurses, and patients.

1. **Ordered:**   Tylenol #2, stat

   Supplied: Tylenol in patient medication drawer and Tylenol #2 (in locked cabinet)

   Given: Two Tylenol tablets

   Error(s):   The wrong medication was given. Two tablets of plain Tylenol were given instead of one tablet of Tylenol #2, which contains a narcotic. (If an incident report must be filed, this is the way the incident should be described in the space provided for a description of the incident.)

   Potential injuries: Lack of comfort and its physiologic and emotional effects; lack of security; need for an alternative medication, perhaps to avoid acetaminophen (Tylenol) overdose.

   Nursing actions: Report to supervisor and provider.

   Obtain orders to give additional pain medication.

   Document on medical record and file incident report per hospital policy.

   Assess patient periodically for side effects and document the results.

   Preventive measures: Familiarize oneself with the medications ordered and commonly used in the unit, as well as with all controlled medications supplied, including those used in emergencies.

If this common medication was known to the giver, and a lack of attention or focus was a contributing cause, techniques to avoid distractions must be addressed. If this medication was not known to the giver, a pharmacology review of commonly used medications is in order. Nurses should always look up unfamiliar medications in current pharmacology references or check with the pharmacy before administering them. Nursing students should check with an instructor or supervisor after the reference check if they are unfamiliar with a medication. It is also wise to inform the patient at the bedside exactly which medications are to be given, because the patient may question the order. An informed patient presents the last line of defense in error prevention.

2. **Ordered:**   Aspirin 650 mg, two tablets at bedtime

   Supplied: Aspirin 325 mg per tablet

   Given: Aspirin 650 mg, two tablets by one nurse; aspirin 325 mg, two tablets by another nurse

   Error(s):

   Potential injuries:

   Nursing actions:

   Preventive measures:

3. **Ordered:**   Narcotic for pain q3h prn, last noted on record as given by recovery room nurse at 1445 hours

   Given: Narcotic for pain at 1545 hours by nurse who just started evening shift and admitted patient to unit

   Error(s):

   Potential injuries:

   Nursing actions:

   Preventive actions:

4. **Ordered:**   Prednisone 10 mg tid

   Given: Prednisone 100 mg tid

   Error(s):

   Potential injuries:

   Nursing actions:

   Preventive measures:

5. **Ordered:**   Percocet (automatic discontinuation 8/10)

   Given: 8/11 Percodan recorded on the medical record; patient allergic to aspirin

   Error(s):

   Potential injuries:

   Nursing actions:

   Preventive measures:

ANSWERS ON PAGE 383

1. List the seven patient rights stated in the text.

   a. _____

   b. _____

   c. _____

   d. _____

   e. _____

   f. _____

   g. _____

2. Fill in the recommended term or abbreviation in the space provided.

Term/ Abbreviation	Meaning	Term/ Abbreviation	Meaning
c		s	
po		npo	
IV		IM	
supp		bid	
tid		q6h	
prn		ad lib	
ac		pc	
subcut		ID	
SL		NG	
stat		top	

3. Write the approved abbreviation in the space provided.

Term	Abbreviation
milligram	
microgram	
gram	
kilogram	
liter	
milliliter	

4. State the comparable times in the space provided.

Traditional Time	24-Hour Clock	24-Hour Clock	Traditional Time
12 Noon (12 PM)		2100 hours	
Midnight (12 AM)		1400 hours	
1 PM		0145 hours	
9 AM		0030 hours	
1:45 AM		1645 hours	

5. Study the label and supply the requested information.

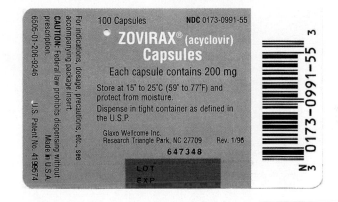

a. Generic name _____

b. Drug form _____

c. Unit dose per capsule _____

d. Unit dose or multidose container (circle one)

6. State 9 pieces of information that the medication label may contain:

a. _____

b. _____

c. _____

d. _____

e. _____

f. _____

g. _____

h. _____

i. _____

7. How would you write out this order? Aspirin tab 325 mg po q4h prn headache

8. What is the purpose of The Joint Commission's Do Not Use list?

9. What should the nurse do if an order is unclear?

10. How can decimal points lead to errors in medication orders?

Refer to the Safety in Medication Administration section on the enclosed student CD-ROM for additional information.

Drug Measurements and Dose Calculations

Objectives

- Convert milligrams, micrograms, grams, and kilograms.
- Memorize milliliter and liter conversions.
- Calculate gram and milligram conversion problems.
- Round medication doses to the nearest measurable amount.
- Identify metric and household liquid equivalents.
- Identify one- and two-step metric conversion problems.
- Distinguish unIt and milliequivalent labels.
- Calculate one- and two-step oral and parenteral metric conversion problems by the ratio-proportion method.
- Distinguish metric, household, and apothecary terms.
- Analyze medication errors using critical thinking.

2   3   4   5 mL   6   7   8   9   10 mL

1/2 tsp   1 tsp   11/2 tsp   2 tsp

INTRODUCTION

Medications are ordered and supplied primarily in the metric system of measurement. This chapter teaches the application of basic mathematics, ratio and proportion, nursing process and critical thinking used in safe medication preparation. Mastery of this chapter will provide the reader with an excellent foundation for all drug dose calculations.

Metric System

The International System of Units (SI), which is commonly known as *the metric system,* is now being used exclusively in the United States Pharmacopeia. SI is the abbreviation for the French *Système International d'Unités.* The metric system is the preferred system for weights, volume, and lengths and is used in computers. It is the preferred system for medication administration.

It is a decimal system based on the number 10 and all the math involved is done by moving decimals. The basic units are multiplied and divided by a multiple of 10 to form the entire system. Table 4-1 illustrates the relationships and values within the metric system. There are a few equivalents used frequently in medicine. These should be memorized and are as follows:

MEMORIZE ✶ **Weight**

1 mg (milligram)	= 1000 mcg (micrograms)
1 g (gram)	= 1000 mg (milligrams)
1 kg (kilogram)	= 1000 g (grams)

Volume

1 L (liter) = 1000 mL (milliliters)

> **REMEMBER** The abbreviation (such as g or mg) always *follows* the amount in the metric system. There is a space between the number and the abbreviation.

Examples 1000 mg
1 g

Examples

Weight	Volume	Length
microgram (mcg)	deciliter (dL)	kilometer (km)
kilogram (kg)	kiloliter (kL)	meter (m)
milligram (mg)	milliliter (mL)	centimeter (cm)

⬡ **CLINICAL ALERT**

The nurse may encounter the symbol mgm for mg (milligram), μg for mcg (microgram), gm for g (gram), lowercase l for L (liter), and cc for mL (milliliter). Use the preferred highlighted symbols. The others have led to medication errors.

TABLE 4-1   Metric Measurements, Prefixes, and Their Values

Prefix	Numerical Value	Power	Meaning	Example	Meaning
micro (mc)	0.000001	10^{-6}	**Millionth** (10 ÷ 10,000,000)	microgram	one millionth of a gram
milli (m)	0.001	10^{-3}	**Thousandth** (10 ÷ 10,000)	milliliter	one thousandth of a liter
centi (c)	0.01	10^{-2}	**Hundredth** (10 ÷ 1000)	centimeter	one hundredth of a meter
deci (d)	0.1	10^{-1}	**Tenth** (10 ÷ 100)	deciliter	one tenth of a liter
	1	10^{0}	**One** (10 ÷ 10)	gram	one gram
deka (da)	10	10^{1}	**Tens** (1 × 10)	dekagram	10 grams
hecto (h)	100	10^{2}	**Hundreds** (10 × 10)	hectogram	100 grams
kilo (k)	1000	10^{3}	**Thousands** (10 × 10 × 10)	kilogram	1000 grams

Note: The Numerical Value column illustrates that you are moving decimals to the right or the left, either multiplying by 10 or dividing by 10. The amount of decimal movement depends upon the exponent (power). These prefixes can be combined with any metric base unit such as liters, meters, and grams. They can be seen in medication and scientific literature as well as in laboratory reports.

Metric Conversions by Moving Decimals

The metric system is a *decimal system.*

> **REMEMBER**   1000 mg = 1 g
> 1000 mcg = 1 mg

RULE   To convert grams (large) to milligrams (small), multiply by 1000 or move the decimal point 3 places to the *right.*

Examples

5 g = 5.000. mg = 5000 mg

0.2 g = 0.200. mg = 200 mg

0.04 g = 0.040. mg = 40 mg

RULE   To convert milligrams (small) to grams (large), divide by 1000 or move the decimal point 3 places to the *left.*

Examples

250 mg = 0.250. g = 0.25 g

20 mg = 0.020. g = 0.02 g

5 mg = 0.005. g = 0.005 g

RULE To convert milligrams (large) to micrograms (small), multiply by 1000 or move the decimal point 3 places to the *right*.

Examples

5 mg = 5.000. mcg = 5000 mcg

0.8 mg = 0.800. mcg = 800 mcg

0.05 mg = 0.050. mcg = 50 mcg

RULE To convert micrograms (small) to milligrams (large), divide by 1000 or move the decimal point 3 places to the *left*. Figure 4-1 illustrates the decimal movement.

Examples

2500 mcg = 2.500. mg = 2.5 mg

400 mcg = 0.400. mg = 0.4 mg

10 mcg = 0.010. mg = 0.01 mg

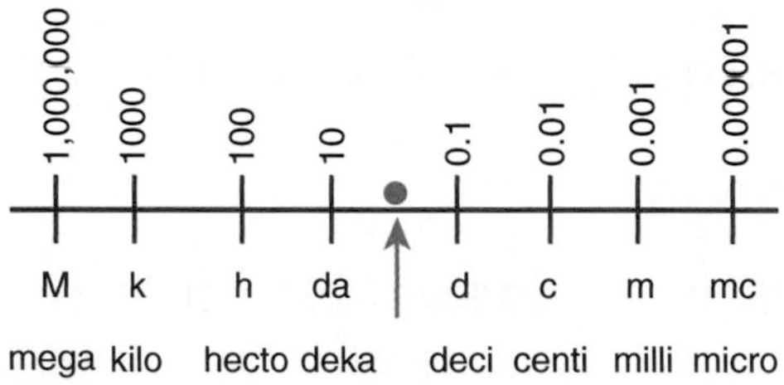

FIGURE 4-1   Metric units number line.

ANSWERS ON PAGE 385

WORKSHEET
4A

Metric Conversions by Moving Decimals

Make the following conversions by moving the decimals.

(**REMEMBER**) 1 g = 1000 mg. Move decimals.
1 mg = 1000 mcg

1. 1 g = _____ mg   **2.** 2 g = _____ mg

3. 0.5 g = _____ mg   **4.** 1.5 g = _____ mg

5. 0.25 g = _____ mg   **6.** 0.05 mg = _____ mcg

7. 0.05 g = _____ mg   **8.** 0.1 g = _____ mg

9. 0.3 g = _____ mg   **10.** 1.1 g = _____ mg

11. 25 mg = _____ g   **12.** 5 mg = _____ mcg

13. 3000 mg = _____ g   **14.** 1500 mg = _____ g

15. 15,000 mg = _____ g   **16.** 10 mg = _____ g

17. 100 mcg = _____ mg   **18.** 0.5 mg = _____ g

19. 7.5 mg = _____ g   **20.** 20.15 mg = _____ g

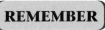

CLINICAL ALERT

The *microgram, milligram,* and *gram* are the most commonly used units of measurement in medication administration.

Medication tablets and capsules are most often supplied in milligrams. Antibiotics can be supplied in grams, milligrams, or units.* Micrograms are used in pediatrics and critical care cases for small doses and/or for powerful drugs, and the need to convert is frequent. You *must* be skilled in the measurement and conversion of all three units.

*Units must be written out. Refer to The Joint Commission's Do Not Use list on inside front cover.

Rounding Medication Doses

When the medication supplied is *not* the same strength as the *ordered dose,* recheck your order and calculations and check with the pharmacy to see if there is another strength available.

Example   You have to give 750 mg, and on hand is 200 mg. Call the pharmacy.

You have to give 50 mg, and on hand is 10 mg. Recheck the order, the usual dose, and your calculations, and then call the pharmacy and request a different strength. Pediatric forms of medications are often available in lower strengths than the adult forms, and the adult form may have been sent.

REMEMBER) Seldom should a patient receive more than one or two multiples of the unit dose supplied.

 Always round your answers to the nearest *measurable dose* after you verify that the dose is correct for that patient.

Example   Tablets: *scored*   Round to the nearest $\frac{1}{2}$ tablet

1.8 tabs	Give 2 tablets
1.5 tabs	Give 1.5 tablets
1.4 tabs	Give 1.5 tablets
1.2 tabs	Give 1 tablet

Tablets: *unscored*   Do not break unscored tablets. Verify order. Recheck if the dose is more than 1 or 2 tablets.

ROUNDING MILLILITERS

Examine the equipment you plan to use. On a syringe, the markings might be tenths or hundredths of a milliliter. On a larger syringe, markings might be in 0.2-mL increments. On an IV electronic infusion device, you would most likely use the nearest whole number in milliliters.

Rounding to the Nearest Tenth

 To round to the **nearest tenth,** examine the *hundredths* column. If it is 0.05 or greater, round up to the next tenth. If it is 0.04 or less, the tenths column remains the same.

....

Example   1.55 mL or 1.57 mL: Round to 1.6 mL
1.53 mL or 1.54 mL: Round to 1.5 mL

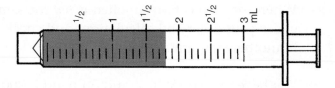

Ordered 1.75 mL. The 3-mL syringe shown above, the most commonly used syringe, is shaded to 1.8 mL, the nearest tenth, the nearest measurable dose.

Rounding to the Nearest Hundredth

 To round to the **nearest hundredth,** examine the thousandths column. If it is 0.005 or greater, round up to the next hundredth.

....

Example   0.756: Round to 0.76
0.754: Round to 0.75

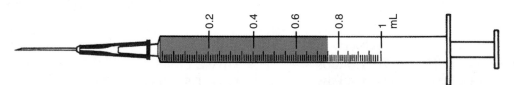

The 1-mL syringe is shaded to 0.75 mL, because the 1-mL syringe is calibrated in hundredths and permits more exact measurement of small doses.*

––––––––––

*For further discussion of syringe calibrations, refer to Figure 4-5.

DROPS

Drops are so small that it is impossible to divide them into parts.

If a specially calibrated dropper is provided to give drops of liquid medicines, you must use that calibrated dropper and measure exactly.

If an oral medication is to be administered, use the calibrated special spoon, prefilled syringe, or dropper provided (Figures 4-2 and 4-3) or draw it up in an appropriate syringe (without the needle) to the exact or nearest measurable amount (Figure 4-4). Then transfer it to a medication cup promptly.

RULE   Always round to the *nearest measurable calibration* on the equipment you are using.

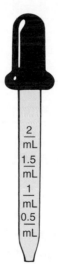

FIGURE 4-2
Medicine dropper.
(From Clayton BD, Stock YN, Harroun RD: Basic pharmacology for nurses, ed 14, St Louis, 2007, Mosby.)

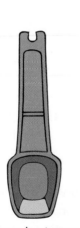

FIGURE 4-3   Measuring teaspoon. *(From Clayton BD, Stock YN, Harroun RD:* Basic pharmacology for nurses, *ed 14, St Louis, 2007, Mosby.)*

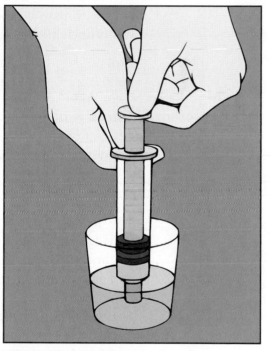

FIGURE 4-4   Withdrawing medicine from a cup with a syringe. *(Modified from Clayton BD, Stock YN, Harroun RD:* Basic pharmacology for nurses, *ed 14, St Louis, 2007, Mosby.)*

CLINICAL ALERT

To avoid overdosing the patient, never round up liquid medications to the nearest whole number. If the answer is 1.7 mL, DO NOT round up to 2 mL. Use a syringe with the appropriate calibrations to measure an exact dose.

One-Step Metric Ratio and Proportion Calculations

You learned how to move decimals 3 places to the left or right to calculate metric equivalents on pages 87 and 88. Ratio and proportion is a provable method of solving medication calculation problems. They can be used to calculate metric equivalents and medication doses with accuracy and logic. There are two types of metric one-step calculations: metric equivalent problems and metric dose problems.

Example   40 mg = ? g (metric equivalent problem)

RULE   Place the known metric equivalents from the metric tables on the **left**. Be sure to select the equivalents with the same terms as your problem (e.g., mg to g), and place the unknown on the **right** side of the equation in the same order as shown below.

Follow the same procedures as in Chapter 2 for ratio and proportion. Label all terms and prove your answer.

KNOW   WANT TO KNOW
1000 mg : 1 g :: 40 mg : x g
      (mg : g :: mg : g)

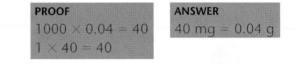

PROOF	ANSWER
$1000 \times 0.04 = 40$	40 mg = 0.04 g
$1 \times 40 = 40$	

$\frac{\cancel{1000}}{\cancel{1000}} \times \frac{\cancel{40}}{\cancel{1000}}$ or $100\overline{)4}$

$x = 0.04$ g (Always label problems and answers.)

Example   Ordered: 50 mg **unit dose on label:** 25 mg/tab (medication dose problem)

The second example of common metric one-step ratio and proportion problems is this: *Ordered: 50 mg. Label for the medicine: 25 mg/tab.* Since *both* the order and the label are in the same terms—milligrams—this involves only a *one-step* calculation.

RULE   Place what you have on hand or what you know (the label unit dose) on the **left** and what is ordered (want to have or know) on the right. Follow through with your math as shown in the ratio and proportion examples in Chapter 2.

KNOW   WANT TO KNOW
25 mg : 1 tab :: 50 mg : x tab

PROOF	ANSWER
$25 \times 2 = 50$	Give 2 tab
$1 \times 50 = 50$	

$\frac{\cancel{25}}{\cancel{25}} x = \frac{50}{25} = 2$

$x = 2$ tab

> ### CLINICAL ALERT
> Some of these problems can be easily solved without being written. However, it is safer to establish a routine using the **provable** ratio and proportion method (e.g., *Ordered: 0.3 mg—Label: 0.5 mg/2 mL*) so that you can solve more complex medication problems with ease when the need arises.

ANSWERS ON PAGE 385

WORKSHEET
4B

One-Step Metric Equivalents

Use ratio and proportion to solve the following one-step metric equivalent problems. Prove and label all answers.

REMEMBER
1000 mcg = 1 mg
1000 mg = 1 g
1000 g   = 1 kg (2.2 lb)
1000 mL = 1 L (liter)

Change milligrams to grams.

1. 4 mg   **2.** 200 mg   **3.** 0.3 mg

4. 25 mg   **5.** 15 mg

Change grams to milligrams.

6. 2.5 g   **7.** 4.6 g   **8.** 0.03 g

9. 0.5 g   **10.** 0.01 g

Change micrograms to milligrams.

11. 150 mcg   **12.** 500 mcg   **13.** 50 mcg

14. 2500 mcg   **15.** 3000 mcg

Change milligrams to micrograms.

16. 20 mg   **17.** 200 mg   **18.** 5 mg

19. 0.1 mg   **20.** 0.04 mg

Change kilograms to grams. (Both of these measurements are used for infant weights.)

21. 5.5 kg   **22.** 12 kg   **23.** 3 kg

24. 1.3 kg   **25.** 0.5 kg

Change liters to milliliters.

26. 0.5 L   **27.** 1.3 L   **28.** 1.5 L

29. 3 L   **30.** 2.8 L

Identifying Units and Milliequivalents in Medication Dosages

Measurements in addition to micrograms, milligrams, and grams may be seen in medication orders. They may also be seen in laboratory values.

Term	Abbreviation	Meaning
unit*	write out	Is a quantity that represents a laboratory standard of measurement. It is often used as unit of measure for products that have some or all animal or plant contents (e.g., heparin, insulin, antibiotics).
milliunit*	write out	Equals 1/1000 of a unit. Pitocin is an example of a medication ordered this way.
milliequivalent	mEq	Represents the number of grams of solute dissolved in a milliliter of solution. Electrolytes are commonly dissolved in solution and measured in milliequivalents (e.g., sodium, potassium, chlorides).
mEq/L		Equals one thousandth of 1 g of a specific substance dissolved in a liter of a solution. Electrolytes are frequently supplied in milliequivalents per liter for intravenous infusion (e.g., KCl 40 mEq/L).
mEq/mL		Equals one thousandth of 1 g of a specific substance dissolved in 1 mL. (The 1 is implied when a number is absent in front of mL.) 2 mEq/mL would equal two thousandths of a gram dissolved in 1 mL.

CLINICAL ALERT

"Unit" must be written out to avoid confusion with the number 0.

―――――――――

*Refer to The Joint Commission's Do Not Use list on the inside front cover.

ANSWERS ON PAGE 388

WORKSHEET
4C

Identifying Metric Unit Doses and Total Amounts on Medication Labels

Examine the following labels for unit and total dose in the containers and fill in the blanks as noted in problem 1. The unit dose is the individual dose supplied. Notice the similarities and differences in terms.

REMEMBER Distinguish mg for milligram ($\frac{1}{1000}$ of a gram) and mcg ($\frac{1}{1,000,000}$ of a gram). They look similar but are different symbols with different meanings.

1. a. Unit dose <u>300 mg</u>   **b.** Total amount in container <u>30 capsules</u>

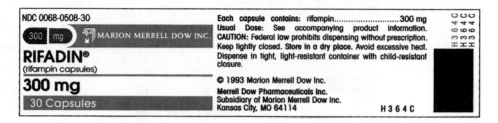

2. a. Unit dose _____   **b.** Alternative metric unit dose measurement _____

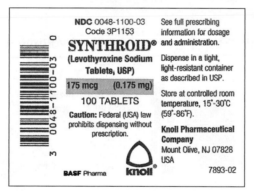

3. a. Unit dose _____   **b.** Total volume in container _____

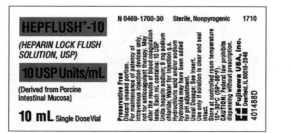

Continued

ANSWERS ON PAGE 388

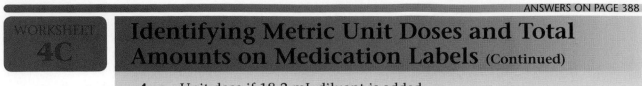

WORKSHEET 4C — Identifying Metric Unit Doses and Total Amounts on Medication Labels (Continued)

4. a. Unit dose if 18.2 mL diluent is added: _____

b. Average intramuscular dose _____

c. Total dose in container _____

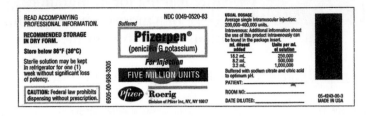

5. a. Unit dose _____   **b.** Total dose/total volume in container _____

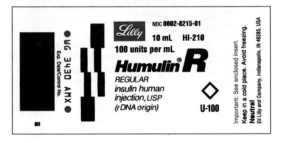

6. a. Unit dose _____   **b.** Total volume in vial _____

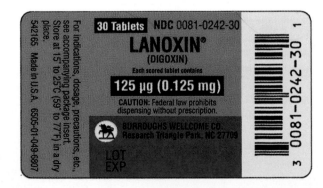

7. a. Unit dose _____   **b.** Alternative unit dose measurement _____

Note: The above label uses the abbreviation μg for micrograms. Use the preferred abbreviation mcg in patient records to avoid medication misreading errors.

ANSWERS ON PAGE 388

Identifying Metric Unit Doses and Total Amounts on Medication Labels (Continued)

Questions 8-10 pertain to the lactated Ringer's injection USP* IV contents label.

8. Total volume in milliliters in IV _____ mL

9. Milliequivalents per liter (mEq/L) of potassium in container _____ mEq/L
(Hint: Read label carefully.)

10. Milligrams of potassium chloride in container _____ mg

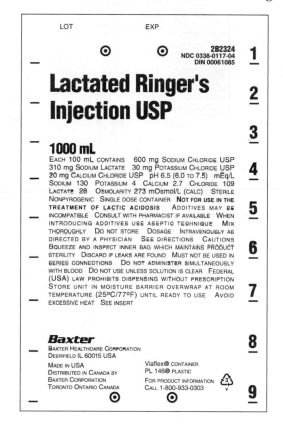

---

*USP refers to the United States Pharmacopoeia, a national listing of drugs.

ANSWERS ON PAGE 388

WORKSHEET
4D

One-Step Oral Medication Problems

Use ratio and proportion and metric conversions to solve the following problems, and prove all work.

1. Ordered: Amoxicillin 500 mg daily po. How many capsules will you administer?

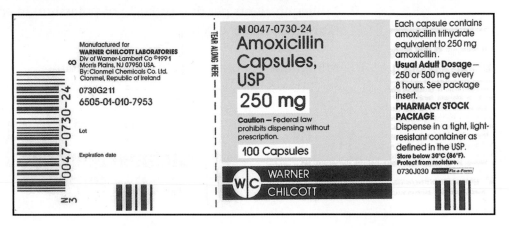

2. Ordered: Synthroid (levothyroxine sodium) 350 mcg daily po. How many *tablets* will you give?

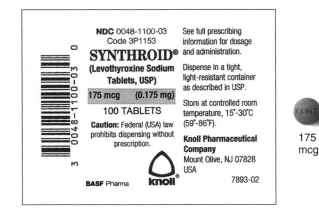

ANSWERS ON PAGE 388

WORKSHEET
4D

One-Step Oral Medication Problems (Continued)

3. Ordered: Lanoxin 0.0625 mg daily po. How many *tablets* will you give?

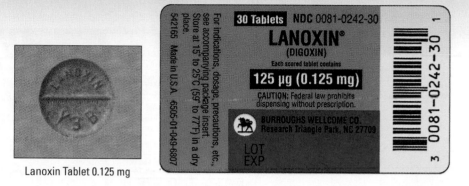

Lanoxin Tablet 0.125 mg

Note: This label uses the abbreviation µg for micrograms. Use the approved abbreviation mcg in patient records.

CLINICAL ALERT

If a tablet is scored, that is, has a line cut across it to denote a breaking point, you may break it. Unscored tablets may not be broken because they will not break evenly and because the medication is not distributed evenly in the tablet.

4. Ordered: Erythromycin ethylsuccinate suspension 300 mg po tid. How many milliliters will you administer?

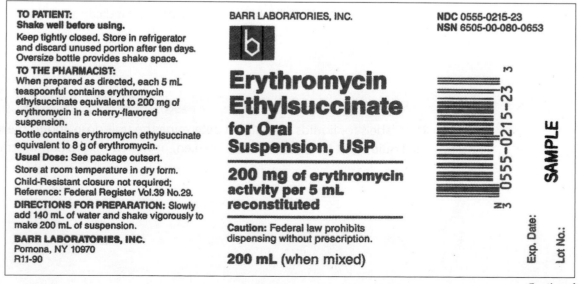

Continued

ANSWERS ON PAGE 388

WORKSHEET 4D

One-Step Oral Medication Problems (Continued)

5. Ordered: Infants' Tylenol (acetaminophen) Concentrated Drops 40 mg q4h po prn for pain/restlessness. How many milliliters will you give?

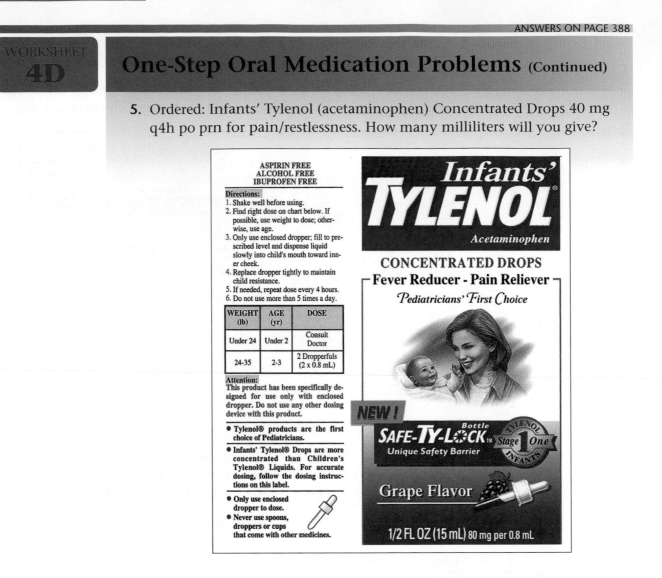

ASPIRIN FREE
ALCOHOL FREE
IBUPROFEN FREE

Directions:
1. Shake well before using.
2. Find right dose on chart below. If possible, use weight to dose; otherwise, use age.
3. Only use enclosed dropper; fill to prescribed level and dispense liquid slowly into child's mouth toward inner cheek.
4. Replace dropper tightly to maintain child resistance.
5. If needed, repeat dose every 4 hours.
6. Do not use more than 5 times a day.

WEIGHT (lb)	AGE (yr)	DOSE
Under 24	Under 2	Consult Doctor
24-35	2-3	2 Dropperfuls (2 x 0.8 mL)

Attention:
This product has been specifically designed for use only with enclosed dropper. Do not use any other dosing device with this product.

● Tylenol® products are the first choice of Pediatricians.

● Infants' Tylenol® Drops are more concentrated than Children's Tylenol® Liquids. For accurate dosing, follow the dosing instructions on this label.

● Only use enclosed dropper to dose.
● Never use spoons, droppers or cups that come with other medicines.

Infants' TYLENOL®
Acetaminophen
CONCENTRATED DROPS
Fever Reducer - Pain Reliever
Pediatricians' First Choice

NEW!
SAFE-TY-LOCK™ Bottle
Unique Safety Barrier
Tylenol Stage One Infants

Grape Flavor

1/2 FL OZ (15 mL) 80 mg per 0.8 mL

◆ CLINICAL ALERT

Distinguish infants' medications from children's medications.

◆ CLINICAL ALERT

Read labels for liquids carefully to determine the unit dose and to see whether the liquid must be diluted, rolled, shaken, or mixed before administration.

ANSWERS ON PAGE 389

WORKSHEET
4E

Metric Oral One-Step Practice Problems

Use ratio and proportion and metric conversion to solve the following problems. Label and prove all work.

1. Ordered: Desyrel 75 mg. Label: Desyrel 50 mg scored tablets. How many tablet(s) will you give?

2. Ordered: Phenobarbital 30 mg. Label: 15 mg/tab. How many tablet(s) will you give?

3. Ordered: Theo-Dur 450 mg. Label: 300 mg scored tablets. How many tablet(s) will you give?

4. Ordered: Lanoxin 0.25 mg. Label: 0.125 mg/tab. How many tablet(s) will you give?

5. Ordered: Digitoxin 0.2 mg. Label: 0.1 mg tablets. How many tablet(s) will you give?

6. Ordered: KCl 20 mEq. Label: 8 mEq/5 mL. How many milliliters will you give?

7. Ordered: Synthroid 0.02 mg. Label: 0.01 mg tablets. How many tablet(s) will you give?

8. Ordered: Diazepam 5 mg. Label: Diazepam 10 mg scored tablets. How many tablet(s) will you give?

9. Ordered: Clinoril 800 mg. Label: Clinoril 400 mg tablets. How many tablet(s) will you give?

10. Ordered: Voltaren 450 mg. Label: Voltaren 150 mg tablets. How many tablet(s) will you give?

Two-Step Metric Ratio and Proportion Calculations

When a medication is ordered that is not in the same terms of measurement as the label—for example, grams ordered and milligrams on label, or micrograms ordered and milligrams on label—a two-step calculation must be completed.

Example   Ordered: 100 **mg**. You have 0.05 **g** tablets on hand. How many tablets will you give?

Step 1   Select the correct equivalents.
Have grams on hand. Need to change **mg** to the equivalent **g** on hand.

Equivalency tables: 1000 **mcg** = 1 mg
1000 **mg** = 1 g

KNOW   WANT TO KNOW
1000 mg : 1 g :: 100 mg : x g
(mg : g :: mg : g)

$\frac{\cancel{1000}}{\cancel{1000}} x = \frac{\cancel{100}}{1000} = 0.1$

$x = 0.1$ g

PROOF
$1000 \times 0.1 = 100$
$1 \times 100 = 100$

Step 2   Insert the equivalent measure from Step 1 into your ratio and proportion now that all terms of measurement are the same.

HAVE   WANT TO HAVE
0.05 g : 1 tab :: 0.1 g : x tab

$\frac{\cancel{0.05}}{\cancel{0.05}} x = \frac{0.1}{0.05}$ or $0.05\overline{)0.1}$

$x = 2$ tabs

PROOF
$0.05 \times 2 = 0.1$
$1 \times 0.1 = 0.1$

Tips on How to Avoid Errors

1. Analyze your problem. Is it a one-step or two-step calculation? (Are the terms the same or different?)
2. Always place a zero in front of a decimal when the number is less than one. It reminds you that the next figure is a decimal, not a number 1 (0.4).
3. Eliminate zeros at the end of a decimal (0.75$\cancel{0}$).
4. Write neatly; estimate and prove each step. Ask yourself whether this is a reasonable amount of medication. (Close to unit dose?)
5. If you doubt your math, recalculate without looking at your original work. If still in doubt, check reliable sources.

ANSWERS ON PAGE 390

WORKSHEET 4F

Metric Oral Two-Step Problems

Use ratio and proportion and metric equivalents to change the order to what is on hand for the first step, then use ratio and proportion to determine the correct dose for the second step. Prove all work. Remember to estimate your answer when you set up the second step. Refer to the metric equivalency table, page 87, and the two-step explanation, page 102.

1. Ordered: Procanbid (procainamide HCl) 0.5 g po daily. How many tablets will you give?

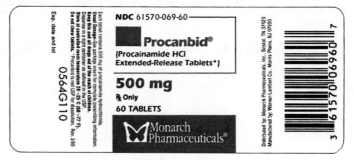

2. Ordered: Dilantin (extended phenytoin sodium) capsules 0.3 g tid po. How many capsules will you give?

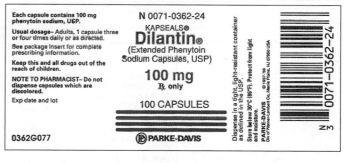

Step 1   Step 2

3. Ordered: Glucophage (metformin) 1 g po daily. How many tablets will you give?

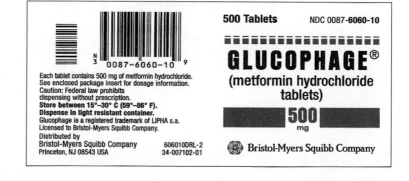

Step 1   Step 2

Continued

ANSWERS ON PAGE 390

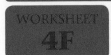

Metric Oral Two-Step Problems (Continued)

4. Ordered: Rifadin (rifampin) 0.3 g po daily. How many capsules will you give?

NDC 0068-0508-30

300 mg ⟪M⟫ MARION MERRELL DOW INC.

RIFADIN®
(rifampin capsules)

300 mg

30 Capsules

Each capsule contains: rifampin...........................300 mg
Usual Dose: See accompanying product information.
CAUTION: Federal law prohibits dispensing without prescription.
Keep tightly closed. Store in a dry place. Avoid excessive heat.
Dispense in tight, light-resistant container with child-resistant closure.

© 1993 Marion Merrell Dow Inc.
Merrell Dow Pharmaceuticals Inc.
Subsidiary of Marion Merrell Dow Inc.
Kansas City, MO 64114   H 3 6 4 C

Step 1   Step 2

5. Ordered: Lopid (gemfibrozil) 0.6 g po daily. How many tablets will you give?

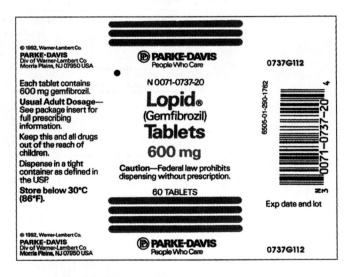

Step 1   Step 2

CLINICAL ALERT

Document all administered medications carefully and promptly according to hospital policy.

ANSWERS ON PAGE 391

WORKSHEET
4G

Metric One-Step and Two-Step
Problem Practice

Use ratio and proportion and metric conversions to solve the following problems. Observe the generic and trade names. Prove all work and label answers.

1. Ordered: alprazolam 0.5 mg po at bedtime nightly for a patient with anxiety. How many tablets will you give?

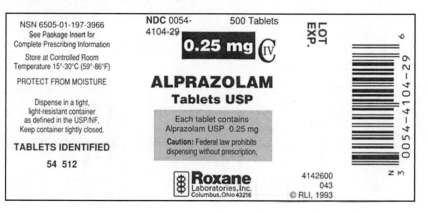

2. Ordered: zidovudine cap 0.2 g po tid for a patient with HIV infection. How many capsules will you give?

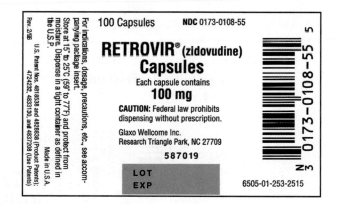

3. Ordered: Zofran 6 mg po 30 minutes before treatment for a patient receiving chemotherapy. How many mL will you give?

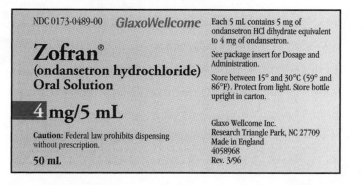

Continued

ANSWERS ON PAGE 391

Metric One-Step and Two-Step Problem Practice (Continued)

4. Ordered: levofloxacin tab 0.5 g po daily for 7 days for a patient with an infection. How many tablets will you give?

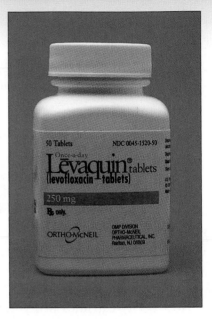

5. Ordered: fluoxetine hydrochloride sol. 25 mg po daily in the morning for a patient with depression. How many mL will you prepare, to the nearest tenth of a mL?

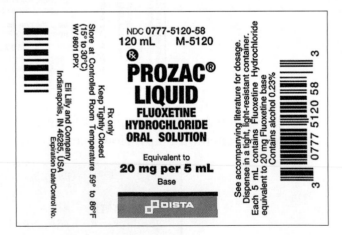

ANSWERS ON PAGE 392

WORKSHEET
4H

Additional Practice in Metric Oral Two-Step Problems

Solve the following two-step problems using ratio and proportion. First convert the order to the equivalent on hand, then calculate the amount of medication. Prove all work.

1. Ordered: Halcion (triazolam) 125 mcg po at bedtime for a patient with insomnia. Label: 0.125 mg tablets. How many tablets will you give?

   Step 1   Step 2

2. Ordered: Valium (diazepam) 0.01 g bid po for a patient with anxiety. Label: 5 mg tablets. How many tablets will you give?

   Step 1   Step 2

3. Ordered: Dilantin (phenytoin) 0.2 g bid po for a patient with seizures. Label: 100 mg capsules. How many capsules will you give?

   Step 1   Step 2

4. Ordered: Diuril (chlorothiazide) 0.05 g po daily for a patient with hypertension. Label: 25 mg tablets. How many tablets will you give?

   Step 1   Step 2

5. Ordered: Lanoxin (digoxin) 0.25 mg every other day po for congestive heart failure. Label: 125 mcg tablets. How many tablets will you give?

   Step 1   Step 2

CLINICAL ALERT

qd (daily) and qod (every other day) have been mistaken for each other and have been placed on The Joint Commission's Do Not Use list (see the inside front cover). qid (four times daily) has also resulted in medication errors. Write out these abbreviations.

ANSWERS ON PAGE 393

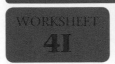

More Practice in Metric Oral Two-Step Problems

WORKSHEET
4I

1. Ordered: Biaxin (clarithromycin) 0.5 g po q12h for a patient with an infection. How many tablets will you give?

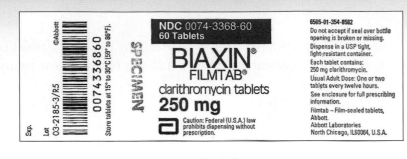

Step 1   Step 2

2. Ordered: CellCept (mycophenolate mofetil) 0.5 g po bid for a patient who received a transplant. How many capsules will you give?

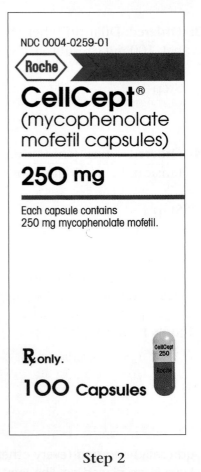

Step 1   Step 2

ANSWERS ON PAGE 393

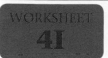

More Practice in Metric Oral Two-Step Problems (Continued)

3. Ordered: Depakene (valproic acid) syrup 0.3 g po four times daily for a patient with seizures. How many mL will you give?

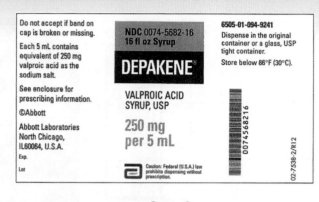

Step 1   Step 2

4. Ordered: Dynapen (dicloxacillin) 1 g po stat for a patient with an infection. How many capsules will you give?

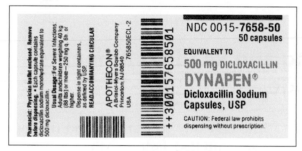

Step 1   Step 2

⬡ CLINICAL ALERT

Some medications ordered for elderly patients have a potential for adverse effects for physiological reasons, such as impaired renal or liver function, and so forth.

These effects include high risk for injury due to confusion, sedation, agitation, gastrointestinal problems, hypotension, potassium imbalances, dehydration, elevated and toxic serum levels of the medication, and medication interactions, to name a few. Dosages for elderly patients often are lower than those for average adults.

If a patient experiences a *new* problem after admission (confusion, constipation, diarrhea, or others from the above list), review the medication orders and drug serum levels, if applicable, and you may discover the source of the problem. Report and document problems promptly.

Continued

ANSWERS ON PAGE 393

WORKSHEET 4I

More Practice in Metric Oral Two-Step Problems (Continued)

5. Ordered: Cytotec (misoprostol) 0.2 mg daily with breakfast for a patient with an intermittent history of gastric ulcers. How many tablets will you give?

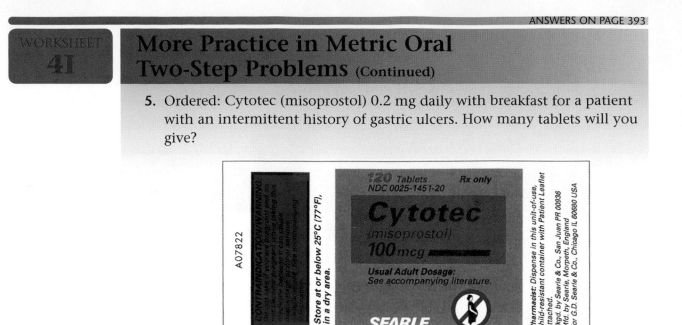

Step 1   **Step 2**

Measuring and Reading Amounts in a Syringe

The best way to learn to read the measurements on a syringe is to examine some unfilled syringes while you read this (Figure 4-5). Then examine some filled syringes, and verify the amounts with your instructor or lab partner.

STEPS Examine the *total amount* the syringe contains first. The 3 mL hypodermic syringe is most commonly used for intramuscular injections and also for subcutaneous injections. The 1 mL tuberculin syringe is used mainly for skin tests.

Locate the 1 mL markings on each syringe.

Examine the calibrations in 1 mL, 0.2 mL, 0.1 mL, or 0.01 mL, depending on the size of the syringe. The larger the syringe, the larger the calibration.

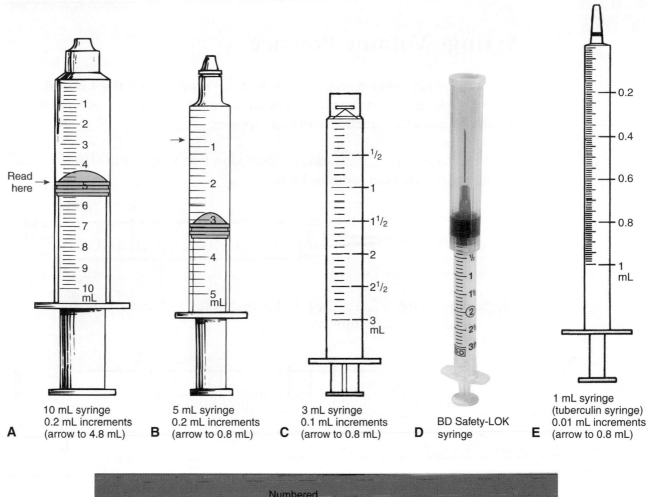

Read here →	→			
A 10 mL syringe 0.2 mL increments (arrow to 4.8 mL)	**B** 5 mL syringe 0.2 mL increments (arrow to 0.8 mL)	**C** 3 mL syringe 0.1 mL increments (arrow to 0.8 mL)	**D** BD Safety-LOK syringe	**E** 1 mL syringe (tuberculin syringe) 0.01 mL increments (arrow to 0.8 mL)

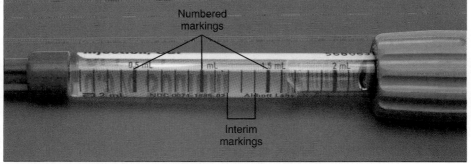

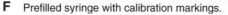

F   Prefilled syringe with calibration markings.

FIGURE 4-5   Comparison of syringe sizes and calibrations. Note where the dose is measured. There are two black rings on the plunger and a rounded or pointed tip. Ignore the rounded/pointed tip and read the uppermost ring, as shown in **A**. The rings are not shown in **C** and **E** so the dose and calibrations can be better visualized. **E**, 1 mL tuberculin syringe. **F**, Prefilled syringe with calibration markings. *(D, Courtesy Becton, Dickinson, and Company, Franklin Lakes, NJ. E, From Macklin D, Chernecky C, Infortuna H: Math for clinical practice, St Louis, 2005, Mosby.)*

ANSWERS ON PAGE 394

Syringe Volume Practice

Examine the following syringes. Note the total capacity and the 1 mL and 0.5 mL markings. Fill in the blanks and shade the syringe to the volume requested. If possible, practice with real syringes.

1. Total capacity: _____ mL. Calibrated in tenths or hundredths of a milliliter? (Circle one) Indicate 1.6 mL.

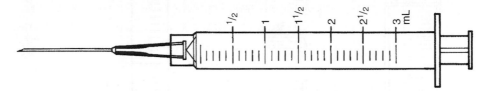

2. Total capacity: _____ mL. Calibrated in 0.1, 0.2, or 0.01 mL increments? (Circle one) Indicate 4.6 mL.

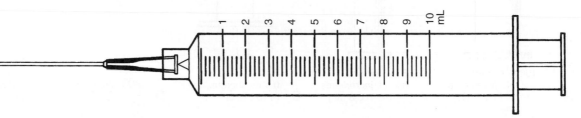

3. Total capacity: _____ mL. Calibrated in 0.1, 0.2, or 0.01 mL increments? (Circle one) Indicate 3.4 mL.

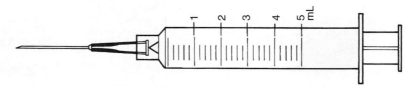

4. Total capacity: _____ mL. Calibrated in tenths or hundredths of a milliliter? (Circle one) Indicate 2.5 mL.

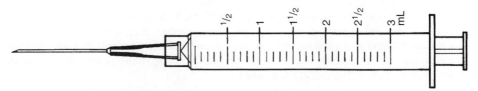

5. Total capacity: _____ mL. Calibrated in tenths or hundredths of a milliliter? (Circle one) Indicate 0.75 mL.

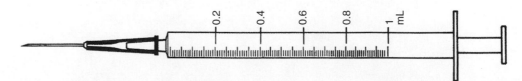

ANSWERS ON PAGE 395

Metric Parenteral Mixes

Combinations of the following narcotics and antiemetics, antihistamines, or anticholinergics are commonly ordered.

Calculate the amount to be given in milliliters *to the nearest tenth* for each of the two drugs ordered using the labels provided. Then *add* the results to find the total volume to be combined and administered in one syringe.* Estimate your answer. Round to the nearest tenth of a milliliter. Prove all work. Does your estimate match your answer? Shade in the total amount to be drawn on the 3 mL syringe illustration.

1. Ordered: Dilaudid 3 mg
   Prochlorperazine 2.5 mg $\Big\}$ IM stat for pain and nausea
   a. How many mg/mL of hydromorphone are available? (label)
   b. How many milliliters of hydromorphone will you prepare?
   c. How many mg/mL of Compazine will you prepare?
   d. Total volume in syringe? (Shade in syringe below.)

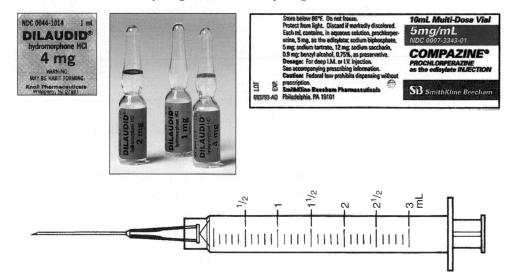

CLINICAL ALERT

Always consult a current, reliable compatibility reference before mixing parenteral medications. Consult a pharmacist if a reference is unavailable.

*Orders for mixes are usually bracketed in the medication administration record (MAR).

Continued

ANSWERS ON PAGE 395

Metric Parenteral Mixes (Continued)

2. Ordered: Morphine 6 mg ⎫
　　　　　 Promethazine HCl 25 mg ⎬ IM q4h prn for pain
　　　　　　　　　　　　　　 ⎭

　　a. How many mg/mL of morphine are available? (label)
　　b. How many milliliters of morphine will you prepare?
　　c. How many mg/mL of promethazine are available? (label)
　　d. How many milliliters of promethazine will you prepare?
　　e. Total volume in syringe (to nearest tenth)? (Shade in syringe below.)

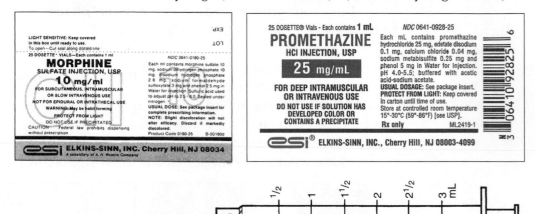

3. Ordered: Meperidine HCl 50 mg ⎫
　　　　　 Atropine sulfate 0.6 mg ⎬ IM preoperatively on call from OR
　　　　　　　　　　　　　　 ⎭

　　a. How many mg/mL of meperidine are available? (label)
　　b. How many milliliters of meperidine will you prepare?
　　c. How many mg/mL of atropine are available? (label)
　　d. How many milliliters of atropine will you prepare?
　　e. Total volume in syringe? (Shade in syringe.)

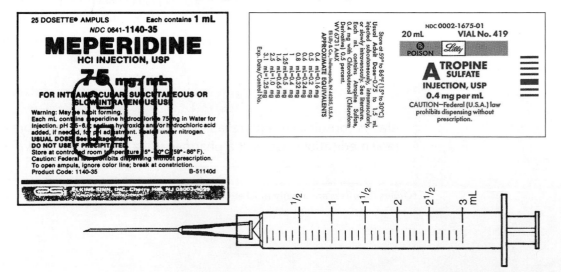

ANSWERS ON PAGE 395

WORKSHEET 4K

Metric Parenteral Mixes (Continued)

4. Ordered: Morphine 10 mg ⎱
         Vistaril 35 mg ⎰ IM q4-6h prn for pain

   a. How many milliliters of morphine will you prepare?
   b. How many milliliters of hydroxyzine will you prepare?
   c. Total volume in syringe? (Shade in syringe below.)

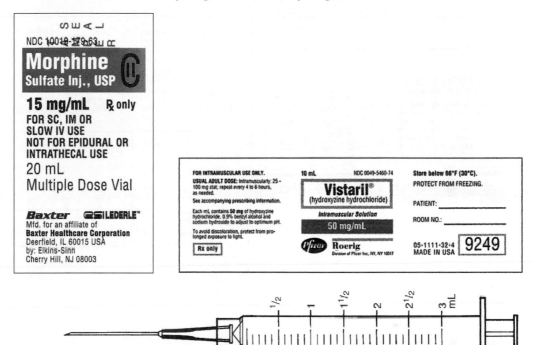

CLINICAL ALERT

To prepare the correct total volume, it is safer to prepare and verify the total for *each* medication separately and then combine the two in one syringe.

Beginning practitioners who prepare a mix using only one syringe risk making dose and vial contamination errors.

Continued

ANSWERS ON PAGE 395

WORKSHEET 4K

Metric Parenteral Mixes (Continued)

5. Ordered: Morphine sulfate 8 mg } IM stat postoperatively
   Vistaril 25 mg
   a. How many milliliters of morphine will you prepare?
   b. How many milliliters of Vistaril will you prepare?
   c. Total volume in syringe? (Shade in syringe below.)

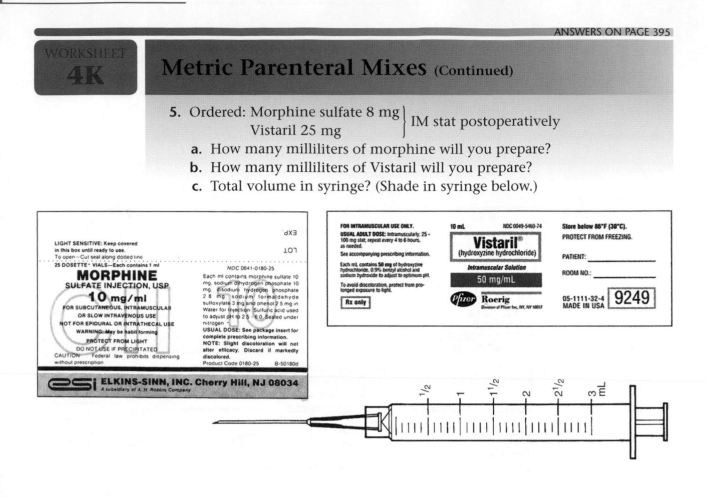

ANSWERS ON PAGE 398

WORKSHEET 4L

Metric One-Step and Two-Step Oral and Parenteral Problems

Examine the orders and labels below. Is the problem *one-step* or *two-step*? Before you perform the *final calculation,* determine whether you will give *more* or *less* of what you have on hand. Calculate the dose (to the nearest tenth of a milliliter if applicable). Prove your answers.

1. Ordered: Cleocin phosphate 0.2 g IM stat. (One-step or two-step?)

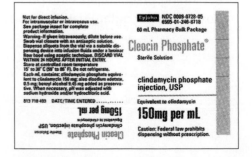

ANSWERS ON PAGE 398

WORKSHEET
4L

Metric One-Step and Two-Step Oral and Parenteral Problems (Continued)

2. Ordered: Xanax 500 mcg po at bedtime. (One-step or two-step?)

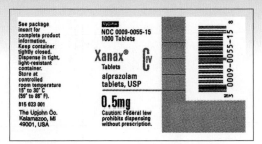

3. Ordered: Solu-Cortef 0.2 g IM daily in AM for 3 days. (One-step or two-step?)

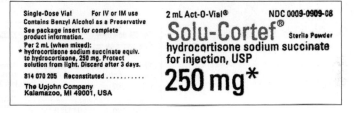

4. Ordered: Solu-Medrol 75 mg IM stat. (One-step or two-step?)

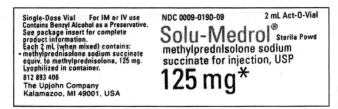

5. Ordered: Medrol 32 mg po daily. (One-step or two-step?)

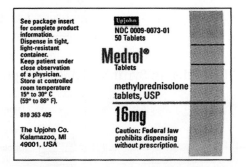

6. Ordered: Motrin 0.8 g po bid. (One-step or two-step?)

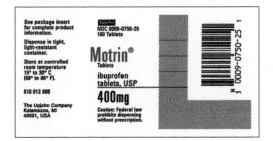

Continued

ANSWERS ON PAGE 398

Metric One-Step and Two-Step Oral and Parenteral Problems (Continued)

7. Ordered: Lincocin 250 mg IM daily. (One-step or two-step?)

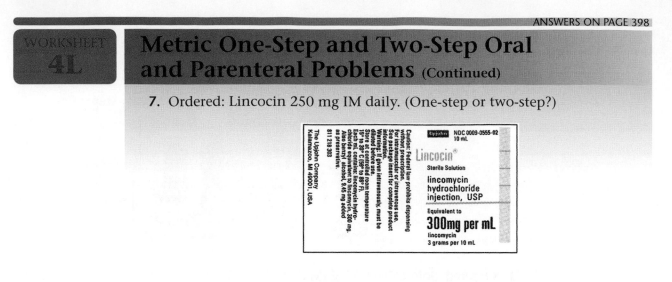

8. Ordered: Depo-Provera 0.3 g IM stat. (One-step or two-step?)

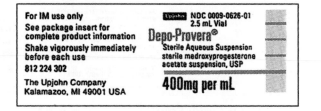

9. Ordered: Halcion 125 mcg po at bedtime. (One-step or two-step?)

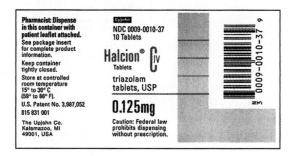

10. Ordered: Synthroid 350 mcg po daily. (One-step or two-step?)

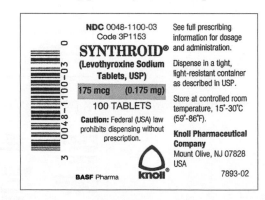

ANSWERS ON PAGE 399

WORKSHEET 4M

Comparing Metric, Household, and Apothecary Measurements

The metric decimal system is the preferred system for the measurement of medications. Household measures have become increasingly important with the trend toward home health care.

The apothecary system is an imprecise, old English system of measurement that has been mostly phased out of use. Even though it will rarely be encountered in a medication order, a nurse must be able to distinguish an apothecary term from metric measurements—particularly the difference between mg, g, and gr (grain).

You have learned that the metric system is written with Arabic numerals and decimals. The apothecary system is written in Roman numerals and fractions, lower case for numbers under 20.

Arabic numerals: 1, 2,   3,   4, 5,   6,   7,   8, 9, 10
Roman numerals: i, ii, iii, iv, v, vi, vii, viii, ix,   x (lower case)
                            I, II, III, IV, V, VI, VII, VIII, IX,   X (upper case)

Note the measurement terms in Tables 4-2 and 4-3. Some of the apothecary terms are also used in familiar household measures.

TABLE 4-2 Approximate Equivalents of Liquid Metric, Household, and Apothecary Measures

Metric	Household	Apothecary
5 mL*	1 teaspoon (tsp)	1 teaspoon (tsp)
15 mL	1 tablespoon (Tbsp)	1 tablespoon (Tbsp)
30 mL	2 tablespoons (Tbsp)	1 ounce
240 mL	1 measuring cup	8 ounces
500 mL	1 pint	16 ounces
1000 mL	1 quart	32 ounces

*The abbreviations mL and cc have been used interchangeably in the past. However, mL is preferred because cc has been misread and has led to medication errors.

Continued

ANSWERS ON PAGE 399

Comparing Metric, Household, and Apothecary Measurements (Continued)

Apothecary measurements are being considered for future inclusion in The Joint Commission's Do Not Use list. The grain (gr) has been confused with gram (g), a fifteen-fold error. The apothecary measurement for one half (ss) has also been misread and led to medication errors. Most agencies have already discontinued the use of apothecary abbreviations, but it is very important that a nurse be able to distinguish apothecary terms from metric terms if they appear in an occasional medication order. As can be seen on Table 4-3, there are considerable differences between the two systems.

TABLE 4-3   Volume and Weight Equivalents*

Metric Volume		Apothecary/Household Volume
4000 milliliters (mL)	=	1 gallon (gal) = 4 quarts (qt)
1000 milliliters =1 liter (L)	=	1 quart (qt) = 2 pints (pt) = 32 oz
500 mL = 0.5 L	=	1 pint (pt) = 16 oz
30 mL	=	1 ounce (oz) = 2 Tbsp (tbs)
5 mL	=	1 tsp
Metric Weight		**Apothecary/Household Weight**
1 kilogram (kg) = 1000 grams (g)	=	2.2 pounds (2.2 lb)
1000 mg = 1 g	=	gr $\overline{xv}$
500 mg = 0.5 g	=	gr $\overline{viiss}$
60-67 mg	=	gr $\overline{i}$
30 mg	=	gr $\overline{ss}$ = gr$\frac{1}{2}$
0.6 mg	=	gr$\frac{1}{100}$
0.4 mg	=	gr$\frac{1}{150}$
0.3 mg	=	gr$\frac{1}{200}$

The grain measurement for apothecary weight was originally derived from a grain of wheat; therefore the equivalents are all approximate, not precise. Use metric measurements, and recognize and clarify apothecary measurements according to agency policy.

*Apothecary/household equivalents are approximate, not exact. Refer to the inside back cover for the metric-apothecary conversion clock.

ANSWERS ON PAGE 399

WORKSHEET
4M

Comparing Metric, Household, and Apothecary Measurements (Continued)

The apothecary system does not convert exactly to the metric system, and neither the apothecary nor the metric system converts exactly to the household system. The patient at home must use special equipment for teaspoons and droppers if possible.

Discharge teaching must be scrupulous in explaining correct measurement to the patient and the family, taking into account that the equipment may not be provided and that the patient does not know that all droppers and teaspoons are not equal.

The apothecary system measurements have been, for the most part, phased out of use on labels. The following sample labels illustrate the differences in measurements between the apothecary and metric systems.

Examine the following labels and fill in the *unit dose* metric and apothecary equivalents in the spaces provided.

1.

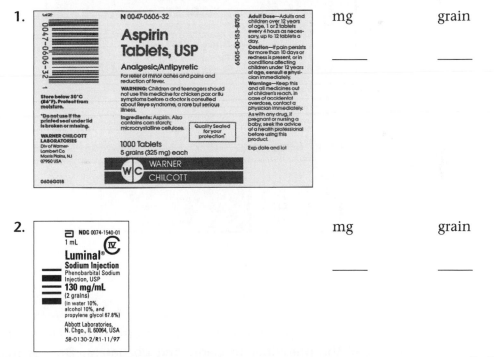

     mg   grain

     _____   _____

2.

     mg   grain

     _____   _____

Continued

ANSWERS ON PAGE 399

WORKSHEET 4M

Comparing Metric, Household, and Apothecary Measurements (Continued)

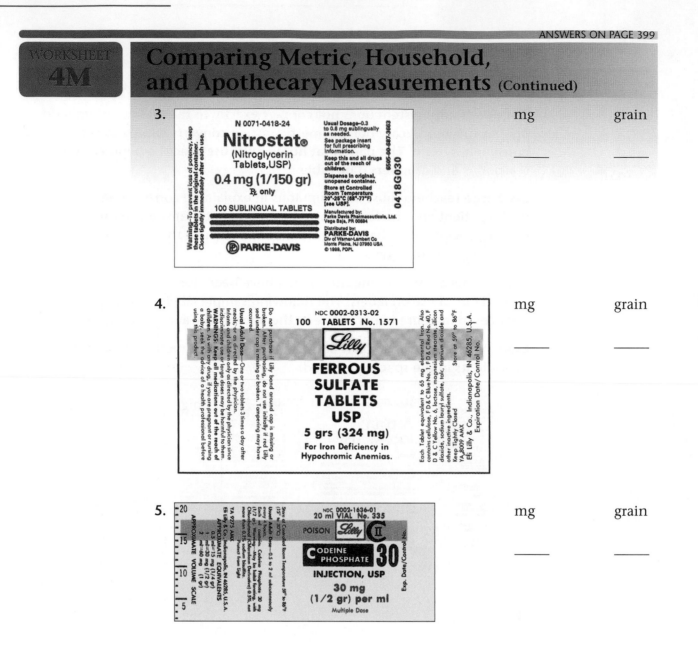

3.   mg   grain

               _____   _____

4.   mg   grain

               _____   _____

5.   mg   grain

               _____   _____

⬡ CLINICAL ALERT

Recognize apothecary terms. Use metric terms. Do not confuse g with gr. Call the prescriber to clarify and document. Do not make up your own abbreviations.

ANSWERS ON PAGE 399

WORKSHEET
4N

Multiple-Choice Practice

Solve the following problems and circle the correct answer. Use scrap paper, set up your ratio and proportion neatly, and *prove* your work. Remember to focus on whether the calculation is one-step or two-step and *estimate* your answer. If it does not seem right, recalculate the problem without looking at your original work.

1. Ordered: Stadol 1.8 mg IM stat postoperatively. Label: 2 mg/mL. How many milliliters will you give, to the nearest tenth of a mL?
   a. 0.5   **b.** 0.6   **c.** 0.7   **d.** 0.9

2. Ordered: Compazine (prochlorperazine maleate) 25 mg q4h IM prn for nausea. Label: 10 mg/mL. How many milliliters will you give?
   a. 1.5   **b.** 2.5   **c.** 3   **d.** 3.5

3. Ordered: Potassium chloride elixir 20 mEq bid po for a patient with potassium deficiency. Label: 8 mEq/5 mL. How many milliliters will you give?
   a. 12.5   **b.** 15   **c.** 32   **d.** 40

4. Ordered: Atropine 0.4 mg IM stat. Label: 0.3 mg/0.5 mL. How many milliliters will you give?
   a. 0.1   **b.** 0.5   **c.** 0.6   **d.** 0.7

5. Ordered: Quinidine sulfate 0.3 g bid po for a patient with an arrhythmia. Label: 150 mg tablets. How many tablets will you give?
   a. 0.5   **b.** 1   **c.** 2   **d.** 3

6. Ordered: L-Dopa (levodopa) 2 g bid po for a patient with Parkinson's disease. Label: 500 mg tablets. How many tablets will you give?
   a. 2   **b.** 3   **c.** 4   **d.** 5

7. Ordered: Vitamin B_{12} 1000 mcg deep IM once a month for a patient who has had a gastrectomy. Label: 0.5 mg/mL. How many milliliters will you give?
   a. 1   **b.** 1.5   **c.** 2   **d.** 2.5

8. Ordered: AZT (zidovudine) 0.2 g q4h po for symptomatic HIV infection. Label: 100 mg tablets. How many tablets will you give?
   a. 0.5   **b.** 1   **c.** 1.5   **d.** 2

9. Ordered: Lanoxin 0.25 mg daily po for a patient with CHF. Label: 0.125 mg tablets. How many tablets will you give?
   a. 0.5   **b.** 1   **c.** 1.5   **d.** 2

10. Ordered: Nembutal 0.1 g at bedtime po for sleep prn. Label: 50 mg capsules. How many capsules will you give?
    a. 1   **b.** 2   **c.** 3   **d.** 4

CRITICAL THINKING EXERCISES

Analyze these anecdotes.

Mr. R. is an alert, anxious-appearing, frail gentleman, 76 years old, weighing 65 kilograms. He was admitted two days before with complaints of chest pain. His medication orders included Lanoxin 0.125 mg daily every morning. This was the only medication ordered for the morning. On hand was digoxin 0.25 mg/tablet (scored).

After you provided care for him on the evening shift, he mentioned that his doctor must have changed his orders because for two days he had been taking only a half of a tablet in the morning, and yesterday and today, his new nurse had given him two tablets each day. His wife agreed. He wanted to know if this meant that his heart problem was getting worse.

Ordered:

Supplied:

Given:

Error(s):

Potential injuries:

Nursing actions:

Preventive measures: How could this have been avoided? If you were on a hospital committee that studies incidents, what sort of recommendations would you make for this specific incident, the nurse involved, and the pharmacy department, keeping in mind that you would not want to discourage the reporting of medication errors?

Mrs. D is a housewife who has been admitted to the hospital for surgery for a throat tumor. She has been taking fluoxetine (Prozac) tablets for the past year for depression. The prescriber changed her prescription to Prozac oral solution 60 mg daily because of postoperative throat discomfort. The nurse administered 60 mL (2 oz) of Prozac.

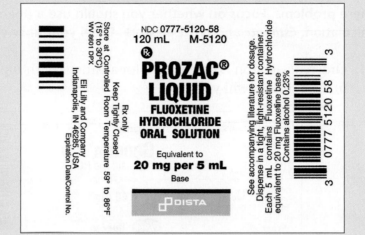

Ordered:

Supplied:

Given:

Error(s):

Potential Injuries:

Nursing actions:

Preventive measures (refer to the questions in the prior exercise):

CHAPTER 4 **Final**

ANSWERS ON PAGE 400

Use ratio and proportion and your knowledge of conversion tables to solve these problems. Focus on whether you should use a one-step or a two-step calculation. *Estimate* and *prove* all work. Label your answers.

1. Ordered: Geodon 80 mg po bid for a patient with bipolar disorder. How many capsules will you give?

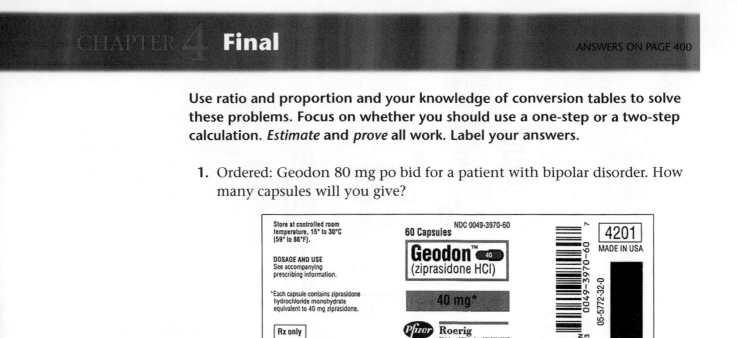

2. Ordered: Klonopin 1 mg tid po for a patient with panic disorder. How many tablets will you give?

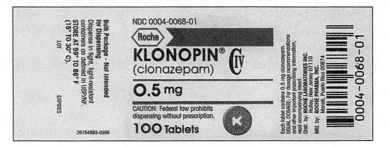

3. Ordered: Cipro 0.75 g po tab q12h for 10 days for a patient with an infection. How many tablets will you give?

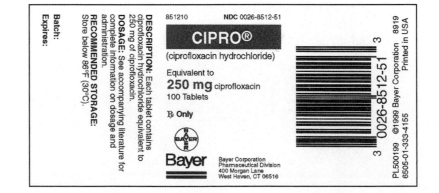

4. Ordered: Zyloprim 0.2 g po daily in AM. How many tablets will you give?

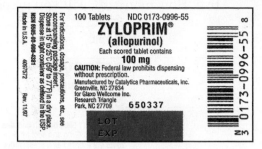

5. Ordered: Cytotec 0.1 mg po four times daily with meals and at bedtime for a patient with a history of gastric ulcers. How many tablets will you give?

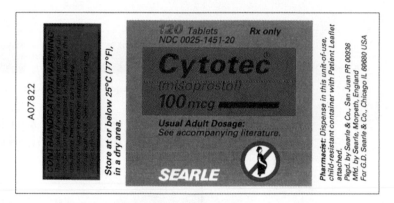

6. Ordered: fluoxetine oral solution 50 mg po daily in AM for a patient with obsessive-compulsive disorder (OCD) and anxiety. How many mL will you give?

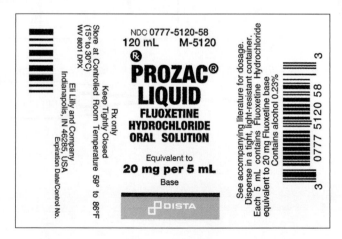

7. Ordered: zidovudine syrup 200 mg po bid for a patient who is HIV positive. How many mL will you prepare to the nearest tenth of a milliliter?

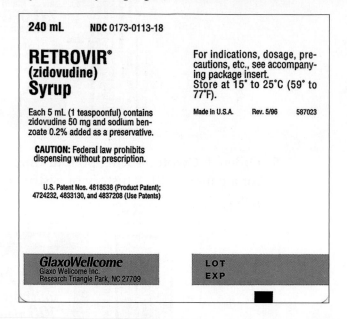

8. Ordered: morphine 10 mg IM stat for a patient experiencing pain. How many mL will you give? Indicate the nearest measurable dose on the syringe shown.

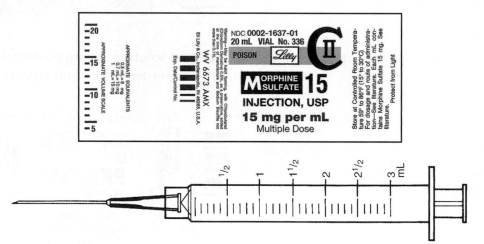

9. Ordered: Amikin 0.3 g IM q12h for a patient with an infection. How many mL will you give? Indicate the nearest measurable dose on the syringe shown.

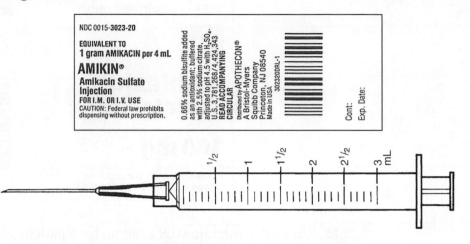

10. Ordered: Ativan 2 mg IM for a patient with agitation. How many mL will you give? Indicate the nearest measurable dose on the syringe shown.

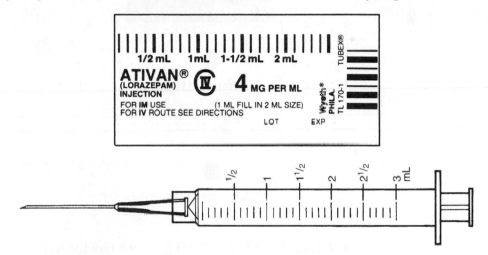

11. Ordered: promethazine HCl tablets 0.05 g po q6h prn nausea for a post-operative patient. How many tablets will you give?

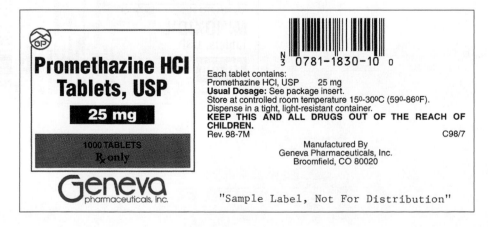

12. Ordered: isoniazid 0.3 g daily po as preventive therapy for a patient at high risk for tuberculosis. How many tablets will you give?

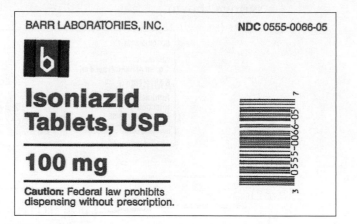

13. Ordered: cimetidine 0.8 g bid po for a patient with an ulcer. How many tablets will you give?

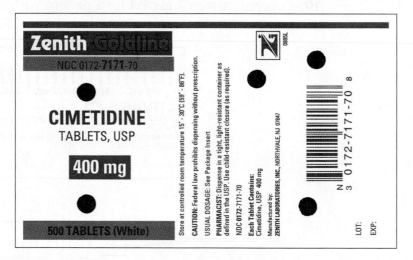

14. Ordered: minoxidil 0.04 g once a day for hypertension. How many tablets will you give?

15. Ordered: morphine sulfate 7 mg and atropine sulfate 0.3 IM preoperatively. How many milliliters (to the nearest tenth) each will you prepare of meperidine and atropine, and how many milliliters will there be in the combined dose (to the nearest tenth)?

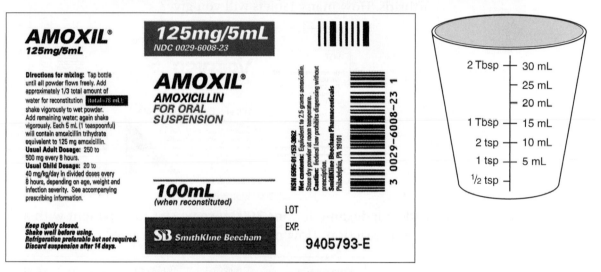

16. Ordered: Amoxil oral suspension 500 mg q6h for an elderly woman with influenza. How many milliliters will you prepare? Shade in the correct dose on the medication cup.

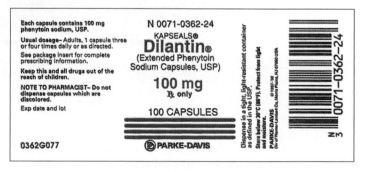

17. Ordered: Dilantin (phenytoin sodium) 0.2 g po daily for a patient with seizures. How many capsules will you give?

18. Ordered: Lanoxin (digoxin) 125 mcg IM daily.
    a. How many milliliters will you give?
    b. SDR is 0.125-0.5 mg daily for adults. Is the order safe?

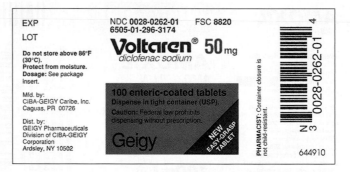

19. Ordered: Voltaren (diclofenac sodium) 0.05 g bid po for a patient with arthritis. How many tablets will you give?

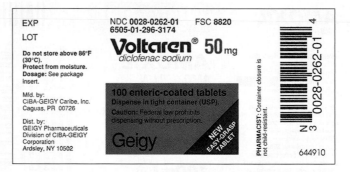

20. Ordered: dexamethasone 3000 mcg po stat for a patient with a severe allergic reaction. How many tablets will you give?

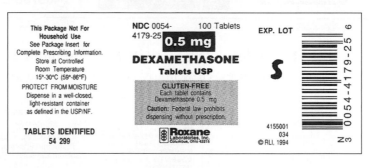

 Refer to the Drug Measures section of the enclosed student CD-ROM for additional information.

CHAPTER 5

Medications from Powders and Crystals: Oral and Intramuscular

Objectives

- Read reconstitution labels to determine specific diluents, diluent amounts, specific doses, conditions for storage, and expiration dates.
- State the importance of initialing and writing the date and time of reconstitution on the medication vial or bottle.
- Determine the best dilution strength to use for multiple-dosage strength vials.
- Calculate doses in milligrams, grams, and milliliters for oral and parenteral routes.
- Reconstitute and measure liquid medications.
- Reconstitute medications from powders and crystals.

INTRODUCTION

Preparation of reconstituted medications, mostly antibiotics, from powders and crystals is usually the nurse's responsibility. The medications are reconstituted by adding a diluent (liquid) recommended by the manufacturer as the vehicle for administration. The shelf life of reconstituted medications is usually short; therefore, careful consideration must be given to how they are stored, the date and time of reconstitution (initialed by the nurse), the expiration date, and the route of administration. This chapter teaches the steps for safely preparing medications from powders and crystals. The measurement of units will be spelled out in the physician's orders and is used in the problem setups.

Measuring Liquid Medications

When measuring a liquid medication, hold the transparent measuring device at eye level. The curved surface of the liquid is called *the meniscus* (Figure 5-1). All liquid medication is measured at the meniscus level.

Medications can be measured in a medicine cup and transferred to an oral syringe for ease in administration and accuracy (Figure 5-2).

However, liquid medications can be measured more accurately in a syringe than in a medicine cup (Figure 5-3).

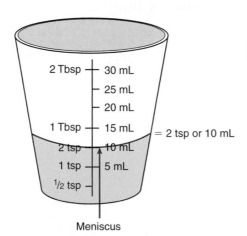

FIGURE 5-1 Measuring cup showing meniscus.

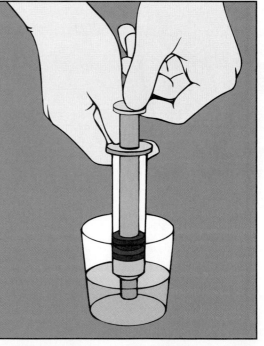

FIGURE 5-2 Filling a syringe directly from medicine cup. *(Modified from Clayton BD, Stock YN, Harroun RD:* Basic pharmacology for nurses, *ed 14, St Louis, 2007, Mosby.)*

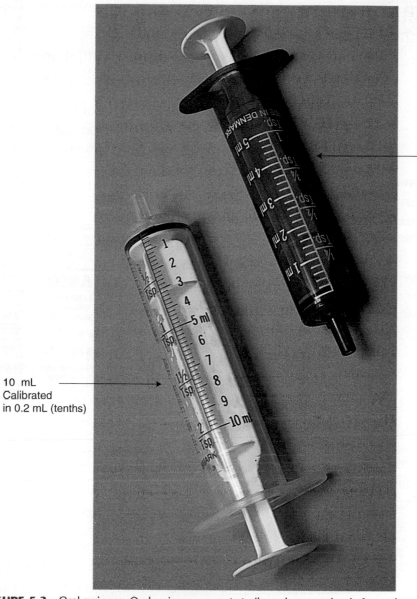

FIGURE 5-3   Oral syringes. Oral syringes are not sterile and are used only for oral medications. *(From Clayton BD, Stock YN, Harroun RD: Basic pharmacology for nurses, ed 14, St Louis, 2007, Mosby. Courtesy Chuck Dresner.)*

Reconstitution: Medication Labels

Labels for medications that require reconstitution contain information about the amount of diluent to use and the resulting concentration. The important information is as follows:

- Strength-reconstitution directions
- Usual dose
- Route

- Name—generic and proprietary
- Expiration date
- Storage conditions/shelf life

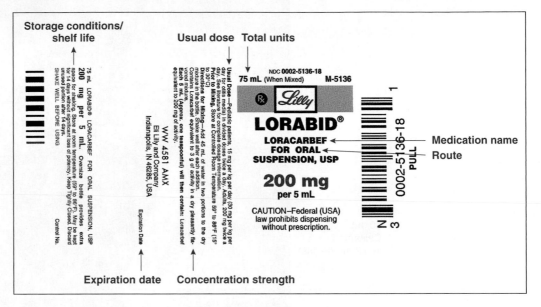

CLINICAL ALERT

If the vial is a multiple-dose vial, the nurse must note on the label the date, time, amount of diluent used, and his or her initials.

Many solutions are unstable after being reconstituted. Read labels carefully for directions on storing the solution in the refrigerator or in a dark place. There is usually a time limit or expiration date on the vial. It is important to date, label, and initial all reconstituted medications.

ANSWERS ON PAGE 401

WORKSHEET
5A

Practice in Reconstituting, Administering, and Measuring Liquid Medications

Show your calculations and proofs in the following problems. Shade in the correct dose on the medicine cup.

1. Ordered: Lorabid 150 mg po bid.

   Follow mixing directions on the label.
   a. How many total milliliters of water are needed?
   b. How many total milligrams of Lorabid are in the bottle?
   c. How many milliliters will provide 150 mg of Lorabid? Draw the amount you will give on the medicine cup.
   d. How many doses are in the bottle?

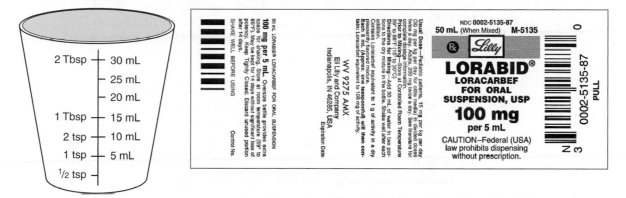

2. Ordered: erythromycin suspension 500 mg po bid.
   a. How many milliliters will you administer? Draw the amount you will give on the medicine cup.

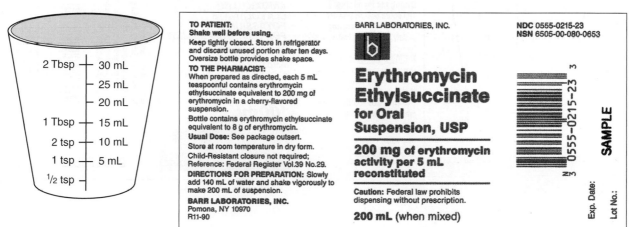

Continued

ANSWERS ON PAGE 401

WORKSHEET
5A

Practice in Reconstituting, Administering, and Measuring Liquid Medications (Continued)

3. Ordered: 500 mg of Vancocin suspension bid po.
   a. How many milligrams are in the bottle?
   b. How many milliliters will you administer? Draw the amount you will give on the medicine cup.

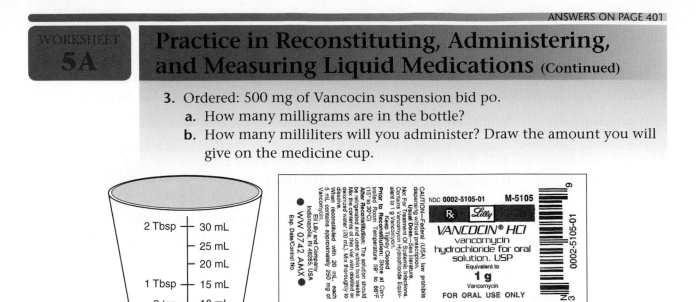

4. Ordered: Augmentin suspension 200 mg po q8h.
   a. How many milliliters of water will you add?
   b. How many total milliliters are in the bottle?
   c. How many milliliters of Augmentin will you administer? Draw the amount you will give on the medicine cup.

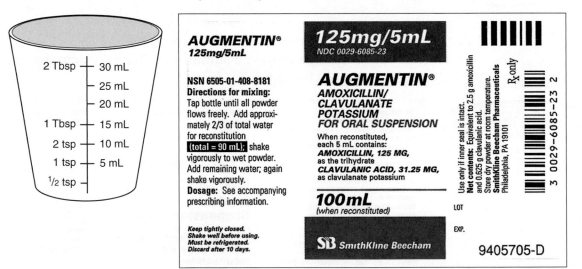

ANSWERS ON PAGE 401

WORKSHEET 5A

Practice in Reconstituting, Administering, and Measuring Liquid Medications (Continued)

5. Ordered: Lorabid 400 mg po q12h × 14 days 1 hour ac for pneumonia.

   Follow mixing directions on the label.
   a. How many total milliliters of water are needed?
   b. How many total milligrams of Lorabid are in the bottle?
   c. How many milliliters will provide 400 mg? Draw the amount you will give on the medicine cup.
   d. How many doses are in the bottle?

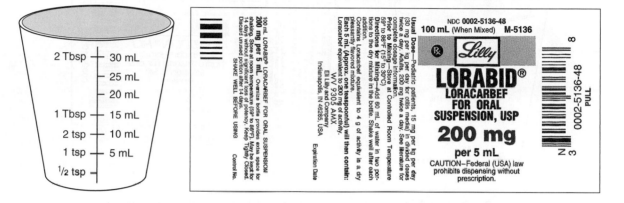

6. Ordered: erythromycin ethylsuccinate suspension 0.3 g po for intestinal amebiasis.
   a. How many milliliters of water will you add?
   b. How many total grams are in the 200 mL bottle?
   c. How many milliliters will you administer? Draw the amount you will give on the medicine cup.

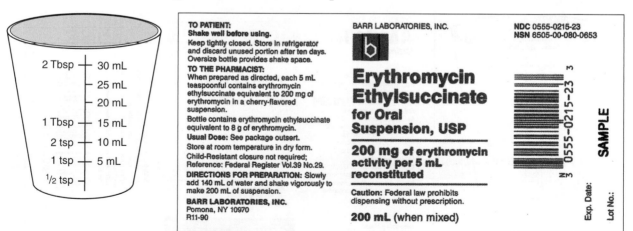

Continued

ANSWERS ON PAGE 401

Practice in Reconstituting, Administering, and Measuring Liquid Medications (Continued)

7. Ordered: Vancocin HCl 300 mg po bid for colitis.

   Follow mixing directions on the label.
   a. How many milliliters of distilled water are needed?
   b. How many total milligrams of Vancocin are in the bottle?
   c. How many milliliters of Vancocin HCl will provide 300 mg? Draw the amount you will give on the medicine cup.

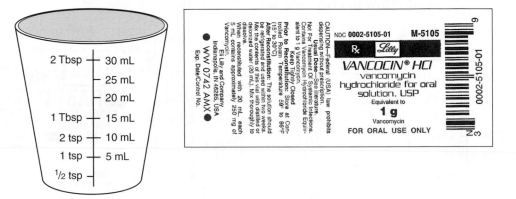

8. Ordered: Amoxil (amoxicillin) 500 mg po q8h for endocarditis prophylaxis.
   a. How many milliliters of diluent will you add?
   b. How many total milligrams are in the bottle?
   c. How many milliliters will you administer per dose? Draw the amount you will give on the medicine cup.
   d. How many doses are in the bottle?

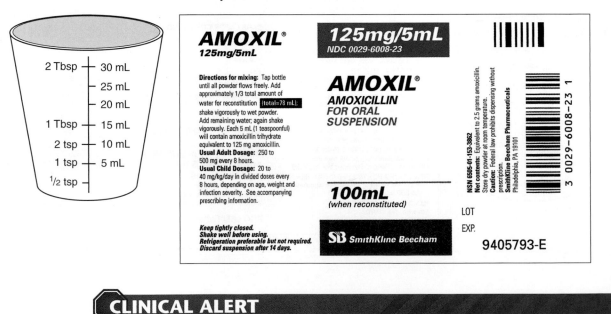

CLINICAL ALERT

For accuracy, read the medication's level at the meniscus.

ANSWERS ON PAGE 401

WORKSHEET
5A

Practice in Reconstituting, Administering, and Measuring Liquid Medications (Continued)

9. Ordered: 400 mg of Augmentin suspension po tid.
   a. How many milliliters will you administer per dose? Draw the amount you will give on the medicine cup.

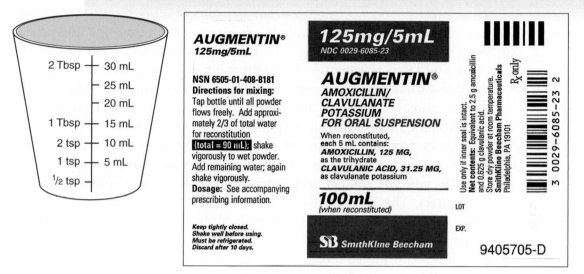

10. Ordered: Lorabid 200 mg po q12h 1 hour ac for bacterial bronchitis.

    Follow mixing directions on the label.
    a. How many total milliliters of water are needed?
    b. How many total milliliters of Lorabid are in the bottle?
    c. How many milliliters will the patient receive per dose? Draw the amount you will give on the medicine cup.
    d. How many doses are in the bottle?
    e. For how many days will the reconstituted medicine be effective?

Reconstituting Medications for Parenteral Use

Reconstituting medications is much like making a cup of soup out of dried soup mix from a package or using freeze-dried coffee crystals to make a cup of coffee. The concept is the same. When a lot of liquid, or diluent as it is referred to when mixing medications, is used, the soup or coffee becomes weaker. The less liquid or diluent used, the stronger the soup or coffee. For some medications that must be reconstituted, various amounts of diluent or liquid can be added to produce various strengths of the medicine. As an example, if you add 16 oz, or 1 quart, of water to 1 Tbsp of instant coffee, you will have very weak coffee. If you add 8 oz of water to 1 Tbsp of instant coffee, you will have stronger coffee and less total volume. The main point is that the amount of instant coffee remains constant; only the amount of liquid (diluent) changes to make stronger or weaker coffee. Reconstituting medications works in the same manner. There is always a certain amount of powder or crystals in the container before the diluent is added. The drug manufacturer tells you what the displacement factor is. This amount is added to the amount of diluent to give the total number of milliliters. The label on the medication vial states the strength (amount) of medication in the vial. That amount never changes. The only thing that can change is the amount of diluent (liquid) that is added.

Most reconstituted medications come in single-dose vials rather than multiple-dose vials, and various amounts of diluent can be added to make varying strengths of medication.

TYPES OF DILUENTS

It is important to use the type of diluent described in the directions for reconstitution. The diluents used to reconstitute powders vary based on the chemical properties of the powder. For example, erythromycin must be reconstituted with sterile water. If normal saline (NS) is used, the powder clumps and will not go into solution. The bacteriostatic agent used in bacteriostatic water is benzyl alcohol. If sterile water is used instead of bacteriostatic water, it may cause some products to clump instead of going into solution. The choice of diluent is based on the pH and the physical properties of the product (medication).

Dibasic sodium is added to some powders to correct the final pH of the product.

Lidocaine is added to ease pain during IM administration. The amount of lidocaine added to the medication would not affect vasoconstriction.

Diluting Powders or Crystals in Vials

Directions for dissolving medications in vials can be found in the accompanying literature. What will be given is the volume of the powder after it is dissolved in the diluent. For instance, the directions may read: *Add 1.4 mL NS to make 2 mL of reconstituted solution.* These directions tell the user that the powder takes up to 0.6 mL of space. The displacement factor is 0.6 mL.

1.4 mL + 0.6 mL = 2 mL of medication

Example Read the medication label to find out how many units, grams, milligrams, or micrograms are in each milliliter of the reconstituted drug.

Begin by adding 2.7 mL of air to the sterile water for injection (diluent) vial, and then invert the vial to withdraw the 2.7 mL of diluent. Add the 2.7 mL of diluent to the oxacillin sodium vial to make 500 mg of medication in 3 mL (Figure 5-4).

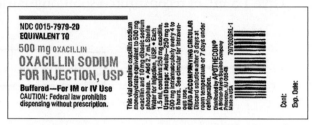

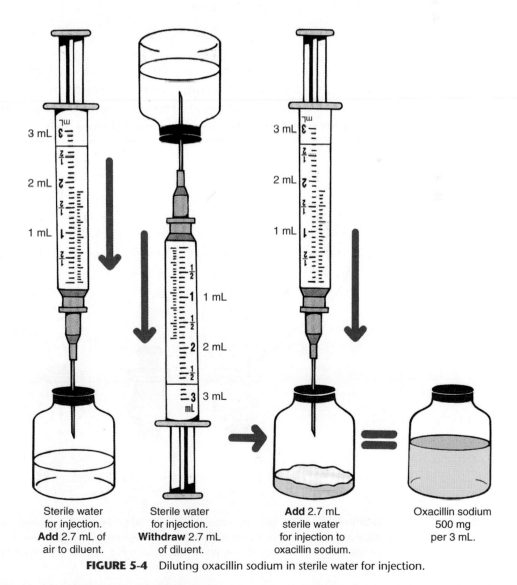

| Sterile water for injection. **Add** 2.7 mL of air to diluent. | Sterile water for injection. **Withdraw** 2.7 mL of diluent. | **Add** 2.7 mL sterile water for injection to oxacillin sodium. | Oxacillin sodium 500 mg per 3 mL. |

FIGURE 5-4 Diluting oxacillin sodium in sterile water for injection.

Ordered: 250 mg oxacillin sodium IM q6h.

KNOW   WANT TO KNOW

3 mL : 500 mg :: x mL : 250 mg

$500x = 3 \times 250 = 750$

$x = 1.5$ mL

PROOF

$500 \times 1.5 = 750$

$3 \times 250 = 750$

Give 1.5 mL of reconstituted solution for each 250 mg.

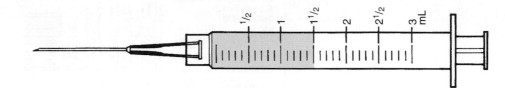

CLINICAL ALERT

When giving intramuscular injections, always aspirate before injecting. If blood is returned, discard the dose.

When medications to be reconstituted are packaged with the diluent attached, the sterility and accuracy of the reconstituted powder are ensured (Figure 5-5). Some medications are reconstituted by the manufacturer and are delivered in prefilled cartridges or syringes (Figure 5-6).

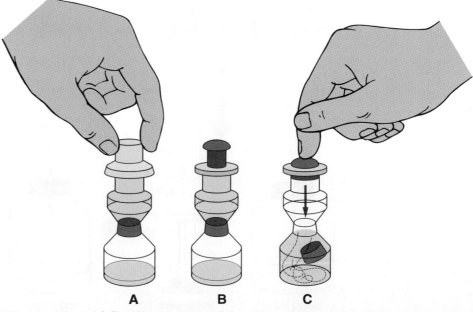

FIGURE 5-5   Mix-o-vial directions. **A,** Remove lid protector. **B,** Powdered medication is in lower half; diluent is in upper half. **C,** Push firmly on the diaphragm-plunger. Downward pressure dislodges the divider between the two chambers. *(From Clayton BD, Stock YN, Harroun RD: Basic pharmacology for nurses, ed 14, St Louis, 2007, Mosby.)*

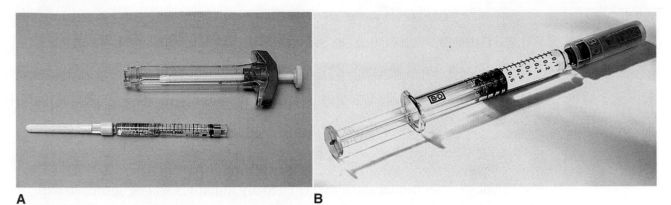

A   **B**

FIGURE 5-6   A, Carpuject syringe and prefilled sterile cartridge with needle. **B,** BD-Hypak prefilled syringe. (*A, From Potter PA, Perry AG: Fundamentals of nursing, ed 6, St Louis, 2005, Mosby. B, From Becton, Dickinson, and Company, Franklin Lakes, NJ.*)

This is a pharmacy generated MAR for 24 hours stated in military time for 8-hour shifts beginning at 0700. At the top, the orders must be signed by an RN indicating that the original order has been verified and is correct and allergies have been noted. SCH is a regularly scheduled medication. The start and stop dates are printed. PRN orders and One Time Only Meds are written in a separate space. Narcotic orders must be rewritten q48h. Discontinued orders are highlighted according to hospital policy and must be renewed if it is necessary to continue them. Site codes are in alpha order. Withheld meds use the code R circled with a nurse's note on the chart. The nurses giving the meds must initial each dose and sign the bottom of the MAR to identify their initials.

Doe, John   ALLERGIES: DRUGS: __Codeine__
ID# 45764304   FOODS: __none__
Age: 50 Sex: M Rm: 406A
Dr. Marin, Cruz   RN Verification: _Mary Smith_

Date: *11-09-08* **(Beg)**
        11-13-08 **(End)**

MEDICATION: Dose Route Freq   Time of Administration, Site, and Initials

	START	STOP	0700 TO 1459	1500 TO 2259	2300 TO 0659
SCH	*11-09-08 Kefzol*	*11-13-08*	*0700*	*1500*	*2300*
	300 mg IM q8h		*N MS*	*O IB*	*N JB*

Each health care agency will have a protocol for charting injection sites. This is one example

ONE TIME ONLY AND PRN MEDS					
Start		**Stop**	**Time**	**Initials**	**Full name/title**
Lasix 11-16-08			*2000*	*IB*	*Irene Butler, RN*
40 mg IV STAT					

Sign: *Mary Smith*   Initials: *MS*   Sign: *Irene Butler*   Initials: *IB*   Sign: *Jill Beck*   Initials: *JB*

SITE CODES   **GENERAL HOSPITAL**
A	Abdomen (L)	J	Gluteus (LUQ)
B	Abdomen (R)	K	Gluteus (RUQ)
C	Arm (L)	L	Thigh (L)
D	Arm (R)	M	Thigh (R)
E	Eyes (both)	N	Ventrogluteal (L)
F	Eyes (left)	O	Ventrogluteal (R)
G	Eyes (right)	P	NPO: Lab
H	Deltoid (mid L)	Q	NPO: Surgery
I	Deltoid (mid R)	R	Withheld/see nurse's notes

FIGURE 5-7   Medication administration record (MAR).

ANSWERS ON PAGE 404

WORKSHEET 5B

Practice in Reconstituting Parenteral Dosages with Multiple-Strength Decisions

Show your calculations and proofs in the following problems. Shade in the correct doses on the syringes.

1. Ordered: Cefobid 1000 mg IM q12h. Available: Cefobid 1 g. Reconstitute IM doses with 2.2 mL of bacteriostatic water for injection (taken from insert). The powder displaces 0.4 mL. How many milliliters will be administered?

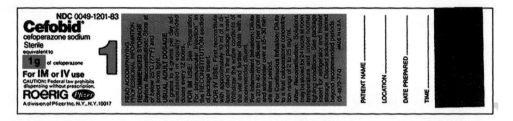

2. Ordered: Pfizerpen (penicillin G potassium) 400,000 units IM q12h. Available: 1 million units. Directions read:

mL Diluent Added	Units per mL of Solution
20	50,000
10	100,000
4	250,000
1.8	500,000

Select the most appropriate dilution for the ordered dose.
a. How many milliliters of diluent will you add?
b. How many milliliters will you administer?

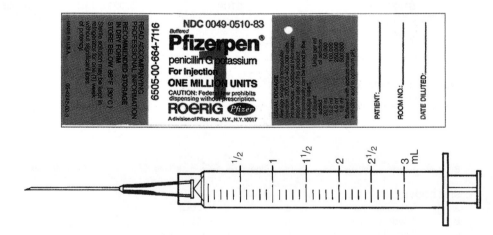

ANSWERS ON PAGE 404

WORKSHEET
5B

Practice in Reconstituting Parenteral Dosages with Multiple-Strength Decisions (Continued)

3. Ordered: Ampicillin 1000 mg q6h IM. Available: Ampicillin 1 g. Directions read: *Add 3.5 mL diluent. Each mL = 250 mg.*
   a. How many milliliters will you administer?
   b. How many milliliters will you give in each site?

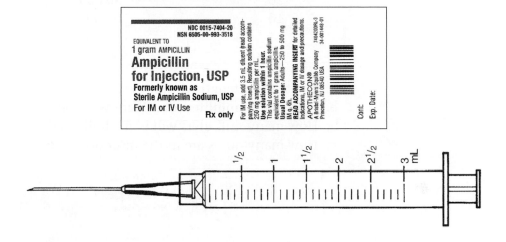

CLINICAL ALERT

The maximum single injection for adults is 3 to 4 mL. Not all patients can tolerate a 3 mL injection. Assess patient for muscle mass at the site of injection to ensure ability to tolerate medication amount.

4. Ordered: Oxacillin sodium 500 mg IV q6h. Available: A multidose vial that reads *Oxacillin sodium; add 5.7 mL sterile water for injection.* Each 1.5 mL of solution contains 0.25 g. How many milliliters will you administer?

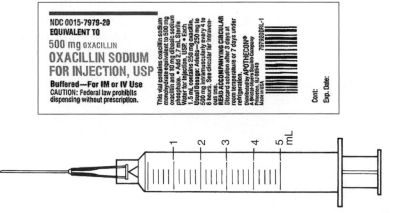

Continued

ANSWERS ON PAGE 404

WORKSHEET 5B

Practice in Reconstituting Parenteral Dosages with Multiple-Strength Decisions (Continued)

5. Ordered: Pfizerpen (penicillin G potassium) 300,000 units IM bid. Available: 1 million units. Directions read:

mL Diluent Added	Units per mL of Solution
20	50,000
10	100,000
4	250,000
1.8	500,000

Calculate the strength closest to the ordered amount.
   a. How many milliliters of diluent will you add?
   b. How many milliliters will you administer?
   c. How many doses are in the multidose vial?

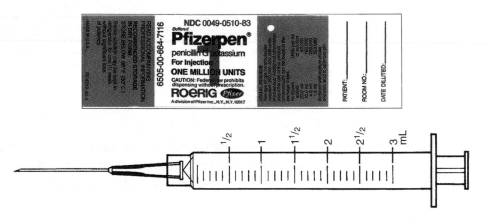

6. Ordered: Penicillin G potassium 300,000 units IM q4h. Available: A multidose vial containing 1 million units and the following directions:

Add Diluent	Concentration of Solution
9.6 mL	100,000 units/mL
4.6 mL	200,000 units/mL
1.6 mL	500,000 units/mL

ANSWERS ON PAGE 404

WORKSHEET 5B

Practice in Reconstituting Parenteral Dosages with Multiple-Strength Decisions (Continued)

Select the most appropriate dilution for the ordered dose. Work out all concentrations to determine the appropriate dose for the patient.

a. Which dilution will you make and label?

b. What amount will you administer?

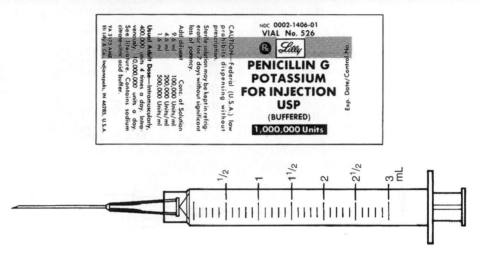

7. Ordered: Tazicef 250 mg IM q8h.
   Available: Tazicef 1 g for IM or IV use.
   Follow insert directions for reconstitution directions.

   a. How many mL of diluent will be added to the powder?

   b. How many mg/mL will this make?

   c. How many mL will you administer IM?

RECONSTITUTION

Single Dose Vials:
For I.M. injection, I.V. direct (bolus) injection, or I.V. infusion, reconstitute with Sterile Water for injection according to the following table. The vacuum may assist entry of the diluent. SHAKE WELL.

Table 5

Vial Size	Diluent to Be Added	Approx. Avail. Volume	Approx. Avg. Concentration
Intramuscular or Intravenous Direct (bolus) Injection			
1 gram	3.0 ml.	3.6 ml.	280 mg./ml.
Intravenous Infusion			
1 gram	10 ml.	10.6 ml.	95 mg./ml.
2 gram	10 ml.	11.2 ml.	180 mg./ml.

Withdraw the total volume of solution into the syringe (the pressure in the vial may aid withdrawal). The withdrawn solution may contain some bubbles of carbon dioxide.

NOTE: As with the administration of all parenteral products, accumulated gases should be expressed from the syringe immediately before injection of 'Tazicef'.

These solutions of 'Tazicef' are stable for 18 hours at room temperature or seven days if refrigerated (5°C.). Slight yellowing does not affect potency.

For I.V. infusion, dilute reconstituted solution in 50 to 100 ml. of one of the parenteral fluids listed under COMPATIBILITY AND STABILITY.

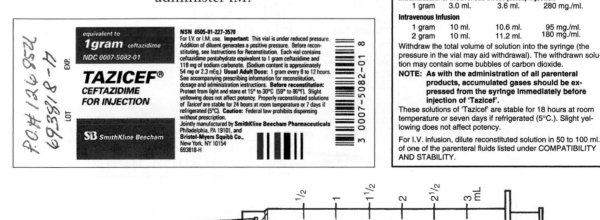

Continued

ANSWERS ON PAGE 404

Practice in Reconstituting Parenteral Dosages with Multiple-Strength Decisions (Continued)

8. Ordered: 100 mg ampicillin IM q12h.
   a. How many milliliters of diluent will be added?
   b. What is the shelf life after reconstitution?
   c. What is the total amount of medication in the vial?
   d. How many milliliters of ampicillin will you administer?

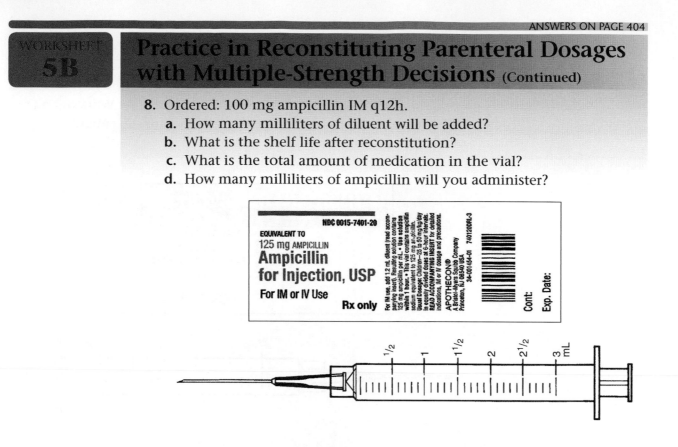

9. Ordered: Cefadyl 700 mg IM q6h. Available: Cefadyl 1 g. Directions read: *For IM use, add 2 mL sterile or bacteriostatic water for injection. USP. Each 1.2 mL contains 500 mg of cephapirin.*
   a. How many milliliters will you administer per injection?
   b. How many milligrams will the patient receive in 24 hours?
   c. How many vials will you need for a 24-hour period?

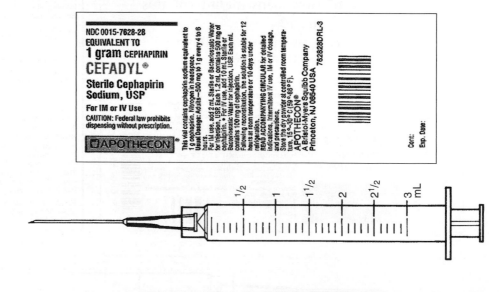

CLINICAL ALERT

Do not confuse units of medication with milligrams.

ANSWERS ON PAGE 404

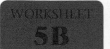

Practice in Reconstituting Parenteral Dosages with Multiple-Strength Decisions (Continued)

10. Ordered: Cefobid 2 g IM q12h. Available: Cefobid 2 g vial. Reconstitution for IM use is found on the package insert. Directions read: Add 3.4 mL of sterile water for injection. The Cefobid powder displaces 0.6 mL. Administer the entire dose.

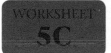

a. How many milliliters will you give for the first dose?

b. How many injections will you administer?

c. What sites will you select?

ANSWERS ON PAGE 408

Additional Practice in Reconstituting Parenteral Dosages with Multiple-Strength Decisions

Answer the questions in the following problems. Show your calculations and proofs; then shade in the correct dose on the syringes.

1. Ordered: Rocephin 500 mg IM bid

   Directions: For IM use, add sterile water for injection according to directions. Withdraw entire contents to yield 500 mg. Give deep in a large muscle. Aspirate before giving. Calculate both dosages to determine which amount is appropriate for your patient.

Vial Dose Size	Amount of Diluent to Be Added	
	1.8 mL ——— 250 mg/mL	
500 mg	1 mL ——— 350 mg/mL	

   Which concentration did you choose? Measure it on the syringe.

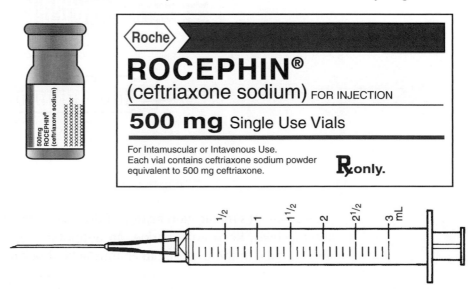

Continued

ANSWERS ON PAGE 408

WORKSHEET
5C

Additional Practice in Reconstituting Parenteral Dosages with Multiple-Strength Decisions (Continued)

2. Ordered: Cefadyl (cephapirin) 500 mg IM q6h.
   a. How many milliliters of sterile water will you add?
   b. How many mg/mL will you have?
   c. How many milliliters will you administer?

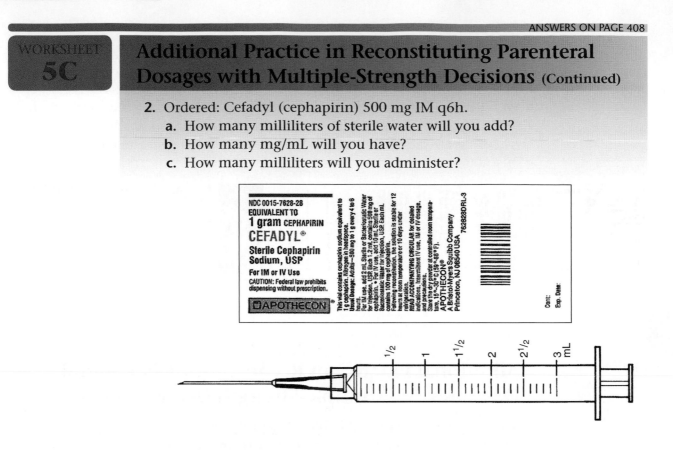

3. Ordered: Oxacillin sodium 300 mg IM q4h.
   a. How many milliliters of diluent should be used to reconstitute the medication?
   b. How many mg/mL will it make?
   c. What is the shelf life of the medication?
   d. How many milliliters will you administer?

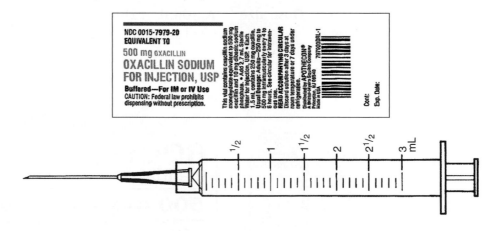

CLINICAL ALERT

Check patient's medication history of drug sensitivity before administration of antiinfectives. Keep epinephrine, an antihistamine, and resuscitation equipment nearby in the event of an anaphylactic shock reaction.

ANSWERS ON PAGE 408

WORKSHEET 5C

Additional Practice in Reconstituting Parenteral Dosages with Multiple-Strength Decisions (Continued)

4. Ordered: Ampicillin 500 mg IM q6h.
   a. How many milliliters of diluent are needed to reconstitute the medication?
   b. How many mg/mL will it make?
   c. What is the shelf life of the medication?
   d. How many milliliters will you administer?

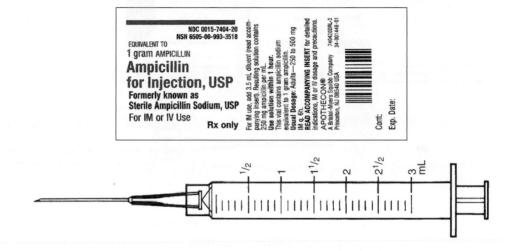

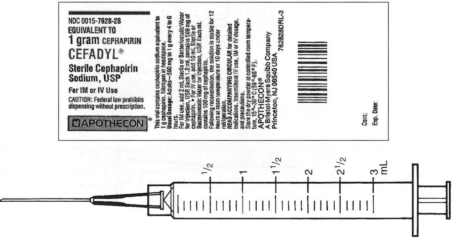

5. Ordered: Cefadyl 500 mg IM q4h for osteomyelitis. Follow directions on the label.
   a. How many milliliters of sterile water will be added?
   b. How many milliliters will be administered per dose?
   c. How many vials will be needed in 24 hours?

Continued

ANSWERS ON PAGE 408

WORKSHEET
5C

Additional Practice in Reconstituting Parenteral Dosages with Multiple-Strength Decisions (Continued)

6. Ordered: Pfizerpen 400,000 units IM q12h.
   a. Calculate all three strengths to decide the best dose amount for your patient.
   b. Fill in the amount you will administer on the syringe.

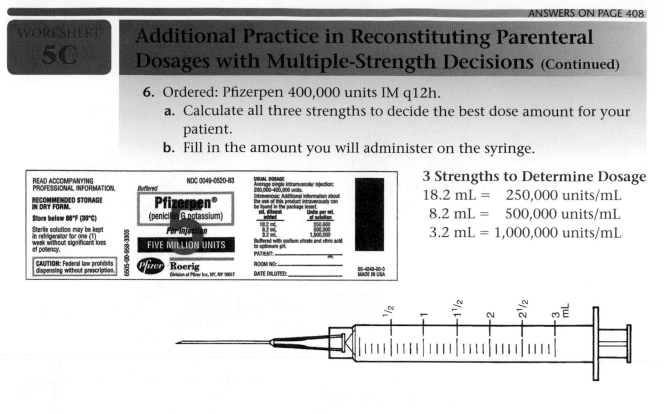

3 Strengths to Determine Dosage

18.2 mL =   250,000 units/mL
8.2 mL =   500,000 units/mL
3.2 mL = 1,000,000 units/mL

7. Ordered: Ticar 750 mg IM q8h.
   a. How many milliliters of diluent will be added?
   b. 2.6 mL of Ticar contains how many grams?
   c. What is the shelf life of the medication?
   d. What is the total amount of medication in the vial?
   e. How many milliliters will you administer?

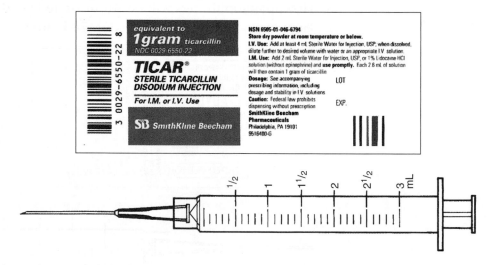

ANSWERS ON PAGE 408

WORKSHEET 5C

Additional Practice in Reconstituting Parenteral Dosages with Multiple-Strength Decisions (Continued)

8. Ordered: Penicillin G potassium 750,000 units IM q8h. Select the most appropriate dilution for the ordered dose. The directions read: *Sterile solution may be kept in refrigerator for 7 days without significant loss of potency. Add diluent 9.6 mL for 100,000 units/mL for concentration of solution; add diluent 4.6 mL for 200,000 units/mL; add diluent 1.6 mL for 500,000 units/mL.*
   a. Which strength will you use?
   b. How many milliliters of diluent will be used?
   c. How many milliliters of medication will you administer?
   d. What is the shelf life of the medication after reconstitution?

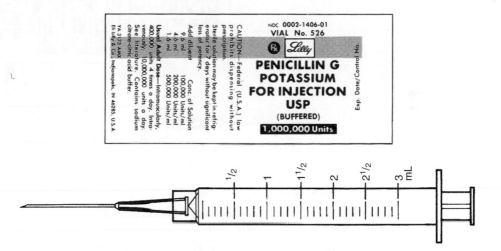

9. Ordered: 400,000 units Pfizerpen IM q6h.
   Available: Pfizerpen 1 million units with mixing options.
   Choose between adding 4 mL and adding 1.5 mL of diluent.
   a. How many units/mL will you administer if you use 4 mL of diluent? Mark the syringe.
   b. How many units/mL will you administer if you use 1.5 mL of diluent? Mark the syringe.

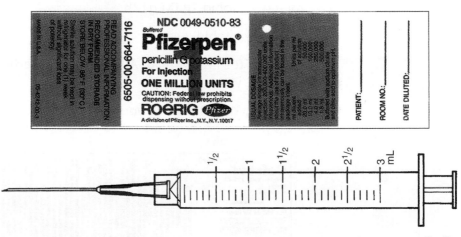

Continued

ANSWERS ON PAGE 408

WORKSHEET 5C

Additional Practice in Reconstituting Parenteral Dosages with Multiple-Strength Decisions (Continued)

10. Ordered: Oxacillin sodium 450 mg IM q6h.
    a. How many milliliters of sterile water will be used for the injection?
    b. How many mg/mL will it make?
    c. What is the shelf life of the medication after reconstitution?
    d. What is the total amount of medication in the vial?
    e. How many milliliters will you administer?

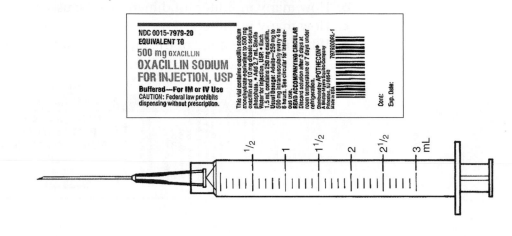

CLINICAL ALERT

Always make sure that the patient's body mass is adequate for the amount of medication, which will be given intramuscularly.

ANSWERS ON PAGE 411

WORKSHEET 5D

Multiple-Choice Practice

1. Ordered: Cefobid 1g IM q12h.

   Available: Cefobid 2 g vial.

   Directions for IM use read: Add 3.4 mL of sterile water for injection. Each 4 mL yields 2 g.

   How many milliliters will you administer?
   a. 3.5 mL   b. 4 mL   c. 2 mL   d. 2.5 mL

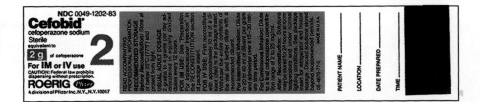

ANSWERS ON PAGE 411

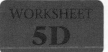

Multiple-Choice Practice (Continued)

2. Ordered: Ampicillin 250 mg IM q12h.

   Available: Ampicillin 125 mg.

   How many milliliters of diluent will you add?
   a. 2 mL   **b.** 1.2 mL   **c.** 3 mL   **d.** 1.5 mL

   How many vials will you need in 24 hours?
   a. 1 vial   **b.** 2 vials   **c.** 3 vials   **d.** 4 vials

> NDC 0015-7401-20
>
> EQUIVALENT TO
> 125 mg AMPICILLIN
> **Ampicillin**
> **for Injection, USP**
> For IM or IV Use
>   Rx only
>
> For IM use, add 1.2 mL diluent (read accompanying insert). Resulting solution contains 125 mg ampicillin per mL. • Use solution within 1 hour. • This vial contains ampicillin sodium equivalent to 125 mg ampicillin. Usual Dosage: Children—25 to 50 mg/kg/day in equally divided doses at 6-hour intervals. READ ACCOMPANYING INSERT for detailed indications, IM or IV dosage and precautions.
>
> APOTHECON®
> A Bristol-Myers Squibb Company
> Princeton, NJ 08540 USA   34-001464-01   7401200RL-3
>
> Cont:
> Exp. Date:

3. Ordered: Oxacillin sodium 500 mg IM q6h.

   Available: Oxacillin 1 gram

   How many milliliters of sterile water will you add?
   a. 3.7 mL   **b.** 5 mL   **c.** 3.1 mL   **d.** 5.7 mL

   How many milliliters will you administer?
   a. 1.5 mL   **b.** 3 mL   **c.** 2.5 mL   **d.** 2 mL

> NDC 0015-7981-20
> EQUIVALENT TO
> 1 gram OXACILLIN
> **OXACILLIN SODIUM**
> **FOR INJECTION, USP**
> Buffered—For IM or IV Use
> CAUTION: Federal law prohibits
> dispensing without prescription.
> APOTHECON®
>
> This vial contains oxacillin sodium monohydrate equivalent to 1 gram oxacillin and 20 mg dibasic sodium phosphate. Add 5.7 mL Sterile Water for Injection, USP. • Each 1.5 mL contains 250 mg oxacillin. • Usual Dosage: Adults and children—500 mg to 1 gram Intramuscularly—every 4 to 6 hours. See circular for intravenous use. READ ACCOMPANYING CIRCULAR. Discard solution after 3 days at room temperature or 7 days under refrigeration.
> APOTHECON®
> A Bristol-Myers Squibb Company
> Princeton, NJ 08540 USA   7981200RL-2
>
> Cont:
> Exp. Date:

4. Ordered: Cefobid 1.5 g IM q12h.

   Available: Cefobid 1 g vial.

   Directions read: Add 1.4 mL of sterile water for injection. Each 2 mL
   yields 1 g.

   How many milliliters will you administer?
   a. 2.5 mL   **b.** 3 mL   **c.** 2 mL   **d.** 1.5 mL

   How many vials will you need for 24 hours?
   a. 2 vials   **b.** 2.5 vials   **c.** 3.5 vials   **d.** 3 vials

> NDC 0049-1201-83
> **Cefobid**®
> cefoperazone sodium
> Sterile
> equivalent to
> **1g** of cefoperazone
> **For IM or IV use**
> CAUTION: Federal law prohibits
> dispensing without prescription.
> **ROERIG** *Pfizer*
> A division of Pfizer Inc. N.Y., N.Y. 10017
>
> PATIENT NAME
> LOCATION
> DATE PREPARED
> TIME

Continued

ANSWERS ON PAGE 411

WORKSHEET
5D

Multiple-Choice Practice (Continued)

5. Ordered: Lorabid 200 mg po bid.

   Available: Lorabid 100 mg for oral use.

   How many milliliters of water will you add?
   a. 60 mL   **b.** 30 mL   **c.** 50 mL   **d.** 100 mL

   How many milliliters of medication will you administer?
   a. 20 mL   **b.** 10 mL   **c.** 5 mL   **d.** 15 mL

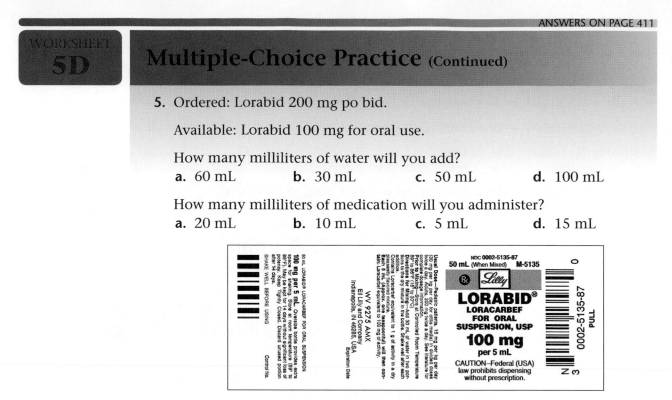

6. Ordered: Ticar 500 mg IM tid.

   Available: Ticar 1 gram.

   Directions read: Add 2 mL of sterile water for injection.

   How many milliliters will you administer?
   a. 2.6 mL   **b.** 2 mL   **c.** 1.3 mL   **d.** 3 mL

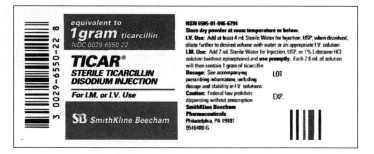

7. Refer to question 6.

   How many vials of Ticar will be needed in 24 hours?
   a. 3 vials   **b.** 4 vials   **c.** 2 vials   **d.** 5 vials

ANSWERS ON PAGE 411

WORKSHEET 5D

Multiple-Choice Practice (Continued)

8. Ordered: Pfizerpen 400,000 units IM bid.

   Available: Pfizerpen (penicillin G potassium) 1 million units.

   How many milliliters of diluent will you add?
   a. 5 mL   **b.** 10 mL   **c.** 1.5 mL   **d.** 20 mL

   How many milliliters will you administer?
   a. 2 mL   **b.** 2.5 mL   **c.** 1.6 mL   **d.** 0.8 mL

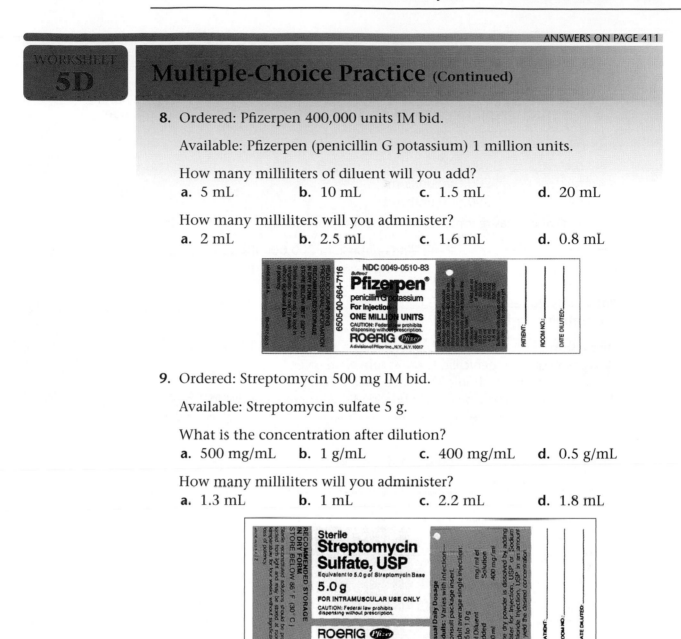

9. Ordered: Streptomycin 500 mg IM bid.

   Available: Streptomycin sulfate 5 g.

   What is the concentration after dilution?
   a. 500 mg/mL   **b.** 1 g/mL   **c.** 400 mg/mL   **d.** 0.5 g/mL

   How many milliliters will you administer?
   a. 1.3 mL   **b.** 1 mL   **c.** 2.2 mL   **d.** 1.8 mL

10. Ordered: Ancef 250 mg IM q6h.

    Available: Ancef 1 gram for reconstitution.

    How many mL will you administer?
    a. 2 mL   **b.** 0.5 mL   **c.** 0.8 mL   **d.** 4.5 mL

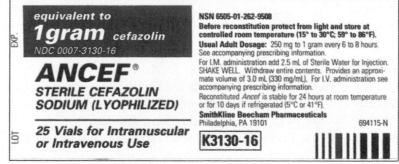

CRITICAL THINKING EXERCISES

1. A multiple-dose vial of penicillin G potassium has these directions for reconstitution:

Add Diluent	Concentration of Solution
9.6 mL	100,000 units/mL
4.6 mL	200,000 units/mL
1.6 mL	500,000 units/mL

The medication was reconstituted with 1.6 mL of diluent.

Ordered: Penicillin G potassium 200,000 IM q6h
Given: Penicillin G potassium 1 mL IM q6h
Error(s):
Potential injuries:
Preventive measures:

Discussion
How many units of penicillin G potassium were given?
How many milliliters should the nurse have given?
Which concentration would have provided the ordered amount in 1 mL?
Could the nurse use the 500,000 units/mL concentration and give the ordered dose of penicillin?

2. Ordered: Cefadyl 250 mg IM q12h × 4 doses

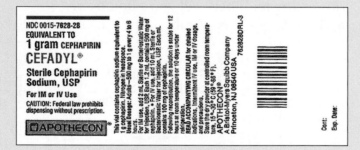

The Cefadyl (cephapirin) was reconstituted with 2 mL of sterile water for injection. The vial was labeled with the date, time, amount of diluent circled, and the nurse's initials. The nurse gave 0.6 mL of Cefadyl IM. The vial was returned to the medication drawer with the rest of the patient's medication. For the last injection, 48 hours later, the vial was taken from the patient's medicine drawer and discarded after giving the injection.

Ordered:
Given:
Error(s):
Preventive measures:
Potential injuries:

Discussion
Was the correct amount of diluent used?
Was the correct amount of medication injected?
What is the length of time needed to give 4 doses?
What should the nurse who gave the first injection have done?

1. Dilute a vial containing 100,000 units of Polycillin (ampicillin) so that each milliliter contains 50,000 units. Approximately how much distilled water will you need to add to the vial to get 50,000 units/mL?

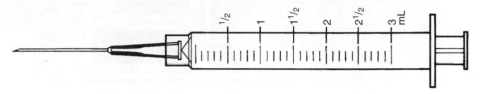

2. Ordered: Carbenicillin 200,000 units IM q6h.
   Available: a vial containing 500,000 units of carbenicillin. The directions read: *Add 4.8 mL of distilled water to make 5 mL of carbenicillin.* Each milliliter will contain 100,000 units. How many milliliters will you administer?

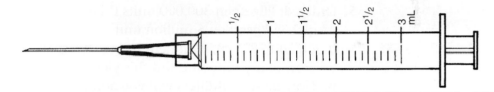

3. Ordered: Ampicillin 250 mg IM q4h for endocarditis prophylaxis.
   a. How much diluent will you add?
   b. How many milliliters will you administer? Shade in the amount on the syringe.

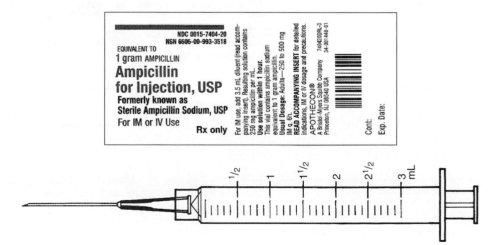

4. Ordered: Ticar 0.5 g IM q6h for salpingitis.
   a. How much diluent will you add?
   b. How many milliliters will you administer? Shade in the amount on the syringe.

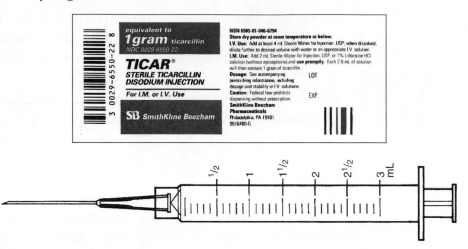

5. Ordered: Pfizerpen 300,000 units IM q12h.
   Available: Pfizerpen 5 million units.
   If you add 18.2 mL of diluent to the Pfizerpen:
   a. How many units/mL will this yield?
   b. How many milliliters will you administer?
   c. How many doses are in the multidose vial?

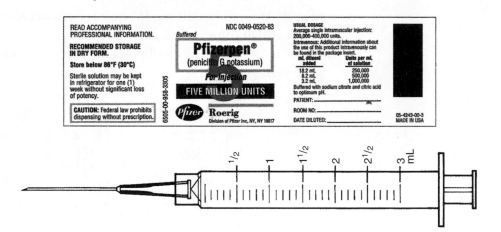

6. Ordered: Carbenicillin 750 mg IM q8h.

   Available: Geopen (carbenicillin) 5 gram for reconstitution.

   a. How many mL of diluent will you add?

   b. How many mL will you administer? Shade in the syringe.

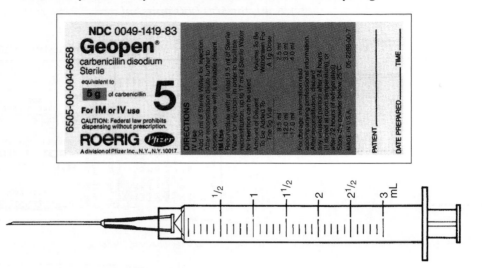

7. Ordered: Monocid 500 mg IM q12h.

   Available: Monocid 1 gram for reconstitution.

   a. How many mL of diluent will you add?

   b. How many mL will you administer? Shade in the syringe.

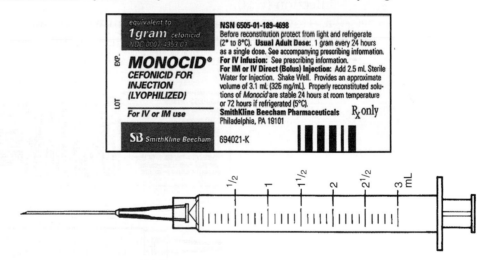

Refer to the Basic Calculations section of the enclosed student CD-ROM for additional practice problems.

8. Ordered: Penicillin G potassium 100,000 units IM q4h for pneumonia. The directions read: *Sterile solution may be kept in refrigerator for 7 days without significant loss of potency. Add diluent 9.6 mL for 100,000 units/mL concentration of solution; add diluent 4.6 mL for 200,000 units/mL; add diluent 1.6 mL for 500,000 units/mL.*

   a. Which dilution will you use? Why?

   b. How many milliliters will you administer? Shade in the amount on the syringe.

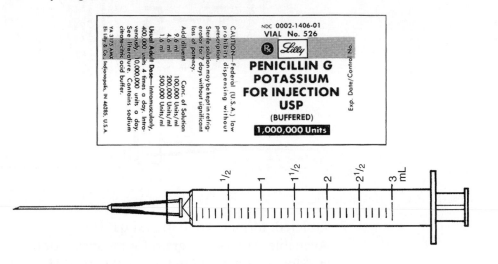

9. Ordered: Oxacillin sodium 250 mg IM q4h for a urinary tract infection (UTI).

   a. How many milliliters of diluent will you add?

   b. How many milliliters of oxacillin sodium will you administer? Shade in the amount on the syringe.

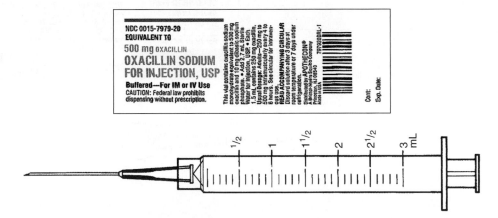

10. Ordered: Keflin 400,000 units IM q12h.
    Available: a vial with 600,000 units/mL. How many milliliters will you administer? Shade in the amount on the syringe.

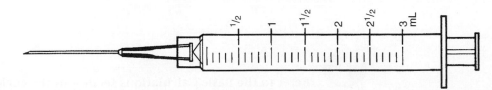

CHAPTER 6

Basic Intravenous Calculations

Objectives

- Calculate intravenous (IV) flow rates for gtt/min, mL/hr, mg/g/hr, and infusion time.
- Interpret IV labels.
- Identify various electronic IV infusion devices.
- Identify IV sets: primary, primary with a port, IVPB extension tubing, transfusion sets, and venous access devices for intermittent use.
- Calculate the amount of saline or heparin for use in keeping venous access patent.
- Calculate the grams of sodium chloride or dextrose in IV bags.
- Check physician's IV order for type of solution, amount, additives, and rate.
- Analyze IV orders for safe administration using critical thinking skills.

INTRODUCTION

It is the nurse's responsibility to calculate the milliliters per hour or drops per minute to regulate an intravenous infusion. Knowledge of electronic infusion devices is required as is knowledge of the basic hand-regulated primary sets. The nurse is responsible for calculating the intravenous piggyback (IVPB) infusions that are timed for shorter periods.

IV Infusions

Intravenous (IV) infusions are used more frequently today than intramuscular (IM) injections. Continuous medication therapy can be delivered via an IV route, minimizing multiple injections via the IM route. Intermittent medication therapy can be delivered through a saline/heparin lock (Figure 6-1), which allows the patient free movement until the next scheduled dose. The heparin lock is used for intermittent short-duration therapy in acute care, long-term care, and home care. Intermittent therapy can also be delivered as a piggyback with a continuous infusion.

Medications (additives) can be added to the IV by the manufacturer, pharmacist, or nurse. The physician orders the medication, strength, and amount, as well as the type and amount of diluent. It is important that the person responsible for the IV understand the actions of the medication, flow rate, adverse reactions, and antidotes. IV fluids flow directly into the vein, resulting in immediate action, and cannot be retrieved. Therefore, it is imperative that the correct calculations, medications, and flow rate be administered.

An intermittent IV lock is also known as a *saline lock, buff cap, PRN cap,* or *intermittent peripheral infusion device (IPID)*. All have needleless resealable valves (Figure 6-2).

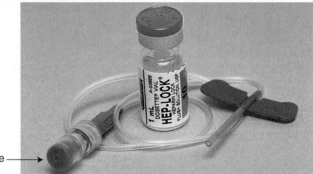

FIGURE 6-1   Saline/heparin lock. *(From Elkin MK, Perry AG, Potter PA:* Nursing interventions and clinical skills, *ed 2, St Louis, 2000, Mosby.)*

Resealable valve

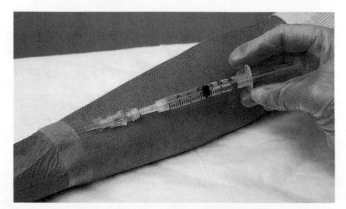

FIGURE 6-2   Saline/heparin lock with resealable port. The port is used to irrigate or flush the IV line to keep it patent. Lines can be flushed before and after medication administration according to hospital protocol. *(From Potter PA, Perry AG:* Fundamentals of nursing, *ed 6, St Louis, 2005, Mosby.)*

166

Types of IV Lines

There are many types of IV tubing used for temporary and long-term access to veins and arteries.

Peripheral A peripheral line is usually used for fluid replacement and temporary intermittent medication administration. The IV line is inserted in the hand, arm, or possibly leg if the hand or arm cannot be accessed. Foot and scalp sites are used for infants.

Peripheral inserted central catheter (PICC) A PICC line (Figure 6-3) is longer than a central catheter line (approximately 22 inches in length). The insertion point is usually the vein in the antecubital region of the arm, where the line is then advanced into the superior vena cava. It is inserted by a PICC-certified RN.

Central line A central line (Figure 6-4) is inserted by an MD directly into the jugular or subclavian vein and then into the superior vena cava. This type of line is for therapy requiring a longer period of time.

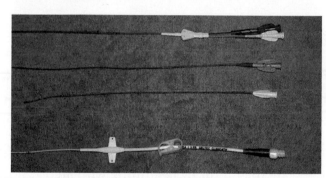

FIGURE 6-3 Peripheral inserted central catheter (PICC line). The double-lumen catheter is used to draw blood samples.

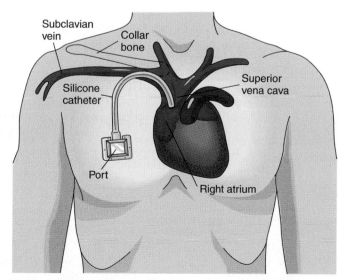

FIGURE 6-4 Central line with a medi-port. *(From Perry AG, Potter PA: Clinical nursing skills and techniques, ed 6, St Louis, 2006, Mosby.)*

Table 6-1 is a guide that can be used to maintain patency by flushing intermittent access locks. Always refer to hospital protocol for type of solution, volume, and frequency.

TABLE 6-1 **Intermittent Flushing Ranges**

Catheter	Flush Solution	Volume (mL)
Peripheral	Normal saline	1-3 mL
Central venous	Heparinized saline	2-5 mL
Peripherally inserted central catheter (PICC)	Normal saline	3-5 mL

CLINICAL ALERT

When flushing peripheral IV lines, a 10 mL syringe should be used. A smaller syringe creates greater pressure within the line, which may cause damage to the vein and be harmful to the patient.

IV Calculations

Check IV orders before beginning calculations. There are two steps in IV calculations. The first step is to find out how many *milliliters per hour* (volume) the IV is ordered to infuse. The second step is to calculate the *drops per minute* needed to infuse the ordered volume.

Analyze your problem. If the order says to infuse the IV for 24 hours, calculate the mL/hr by beginning with Step 1. If the order says to infuse the IV at 75 mL/hr, begin with Step 2.

STEP 1 mL/hr

RULE When the total volume is given, calculate the mL/hr.

$$\frac{\text{Total volume (TV)}}{\text{Total time (TT) in hours}} = \text{mL/hr}$$

Example Ordered: 2000 mL D5W (dextrose 5% in water) to be infused for 24 hours. The problem is to find out how many mL/hr the patient must receive for the 2000 mL to be infused in 24 hours.

Formula

$$\frac{\text{Total volume (TV)}}{\text{Total time (TT) in hours}} = \text{mL/hr}$$

Calculation

$$\frac{TV}{TT} = \frac{2000}{24} = 83 \text{ mL/hr}$$

We now know that to infuse 2000 mL of fluid in 24 hours, the patient must receive 83 mL/hr. Infusion devices are calibrated for mL/hr.

DROP FACTOR CALCULATIONS

STEP 2 gtt/min

The drop factor is needed to calculate gtt/min. The drop factor is the number of drops in 1 mL. The diameter of the needle where the drop enters the drip chamber varies from one manufacturer to another. The bigger the needle, the fatter the drop (Figure 6-5, *A*); it takes only 10 macrodrops to make a milliliter. The smallest unit is the microdrop (60 gtt/mL) (Figure 6-4, *B*). This is used for people who can tolerate only small amounts of fluid, such as pediatric and geriatric patients and patients who require fluid restrictions. Drop factors of 10, 15, 20, and 60 (microdrip) are the most common. The drop factor is determined by the manufacturer and is found on the IV tubing package.

RULE   When the mL/hr is given, calculate the gtt/min.

$$\frac{\text{Drop factor or gtt/mL (from IV package)}}{\text{Time in minutes}} \times \text{Total hourly volume (V/hr)} = \text{gtt/min}$$

Example   Ordered: D5W to infuse at 83 mL/hr. The drop factor (Df) is 10.

$$\frac{\text{Df}}{\text{Time (min)}} \times \text{V/hr} = \frac{10\ (\text{Df})}{60\ (\text{min})} = 83\ (\text{V/hr})$$

$$\frac{10}{60} \times \frac{83}{1} = \frac{1}{6} \times \frac{83}{1} = \frac{83}{6} = 13.8 \text{ or } 14 \text{ gtt/min}$$

Drops cannot be timed in tenths, only in whole numbers. If the decimal is greater than or equal to 0.5, round to the next higher number.

Example   Ordered: Antibiotic to infuse at 100 mL in 30 min. The drop factor is 15.

$$\frac{\text{Df}}{\text{Time (min)}} \times \text{V/hr} = \frac{15\ (\text{Df})}{30\ (\text{min})} = 100\ (\text{V/hr})$$

$$\frac{15}{30} \times \frac{100}{1} = \frac{1}{2} \times \frac{100}{1} = \frac{100}{2} = 50 \text{ gtt/min}$$

Summary   Two-step IV flow rate calculations

Step 1 $\frac{\text{TV}}{\text{TT in hr}} = \text{mL/hr}$

Step 2 $\frac{\text{Df}}{\text{Time in min}} \times \text{V/hr} = \text{gtt/min}$

REMEMBER   Reduce the fraction Df/min *before* multiplying by the volume.

Example   Which would you rather calculate?

$$\frac{12}{60} \times 60 \quad \text{or} \quad \frac{1}{5} \times 60$$

The reduced fraction is easier to calculate.

REMEMBER   When the IV tubing is microdrip, 60 gtt/mL, the gtt/min will be the same as the mL/hr.

Example   1000 mL to infuse in 8 hours with a microdrip set.

Step 1 $\dfrac{TV}{TT \text{ in hr}} = \dfrac{1000}{8} = 125 \text{ mL/hr}$

Step 2 $\dfrac{Df}{\text{Time in min}} \times V/hr = \dfrac{60}{60} \times 125 = 125 \text{ gtt/min}$

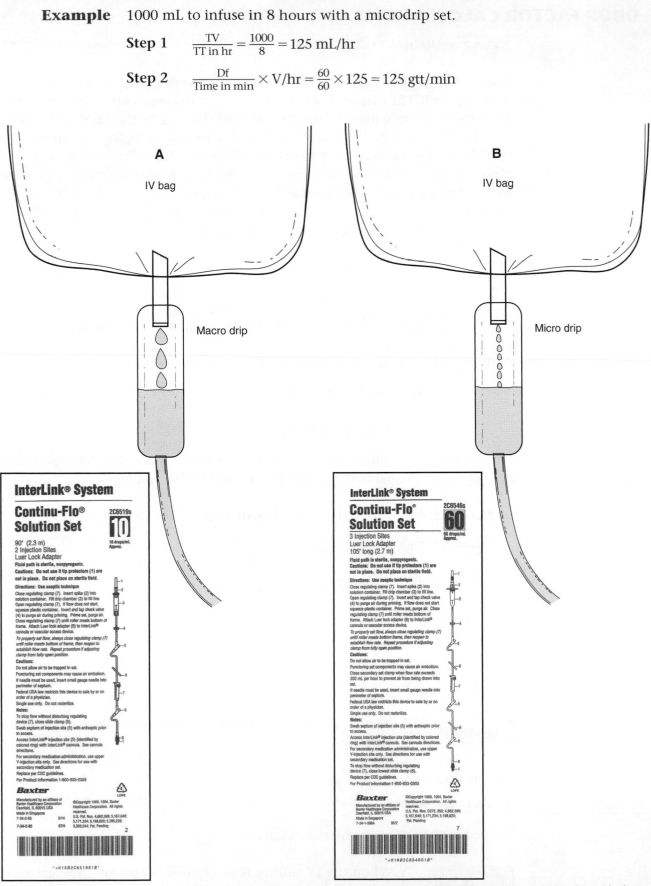

FIGURE 6-5 Drops per minute must be calibrated for gravity flow. **A,** InterLink® System Continu-Flo® Solution Set with drop factor of 10 (10 gtt = 1 mL). **B,** InterLink® System Continu-Flo® Solution Set with drop factor of 60 (60 gtt = 1 mL).

Drops per Minute by Manufacturer

A simple approach to calculate gtt/min after you have determined the mL/hr is to memorize the reduced fraction numbers. Manufacturers have established rates for their products. Below is an example.

Product Drip Rates	Minutes	Df	=	Reduced Number
60 gtt/mL	60	60	=	1
20 gtt/mL	60	20	=	3
15 gtt/mL	60	15	=	4
10 gtt/mL	60	10	=	6

You may have to memorize only one number because most facilities purchase equipment from a single company.

Example   If you know you are using a set that delivers 20 gtt/mL, divide 3 into the mL/hr.

$$\frac{125}{3} = 41.6 = 42 \text{ gtt/min}$$

As you already know, the formula for calculating gtt/min is:

$$\frac{Df}{\text{Time in min}} \times V/hr \quad \text{or} \quad \frac{20}{60} \times 125 = \frac{1}{3} \times 125 = 41.6 = 42 \text{ gtt/min}$$

Now you know two different methods for calculating gtt/min.

CLINICAL ALERT

Check the IV every hour, even if an infusion device is used. Recheck drops per minute rate frequently because the IV rate can vary with position.

ANSWERS ON PAGE 414

WORKSHEET
6A

IV Calculations

Use either the Step 1 or the Step 2 formula to calculate mL/hr or gtt/min to answer the following questions.

Step 1 $\dfrac{TV}{TT\ in\ hr} = mL/hr$

Step 2 $\dfrac{Df}{Time\ in\ min} \times V/hr = gtt/min$ or $\dfrac{mL/hr}{reduced\ gtt\ rate}$

1. Ordered: 1500 mL to be infused for 12 hr. If the drop factor is 15, how many drops/min is this?

2. Ordered: 50 mL to be infused for 1 hr. How many drops/min will be administered with microdrip?

3. Ordered: 100 mL to be infused for 30 min. How many drops/min is this if the drop factor is 10?

4. Ordered: 1000 mL to be infused for 8 hr. How many drops/min will be administered if the drop factor is 10?

5. Ordered: 200 mL to be infused for 1 hr. If the drop factor is 15, how many drops/min will be administered?

6. Ordered: 1000 mL to be infused at 150 mL/hr. The drop factor is 20. How many drops/min will be infused?

7. Ordered: 75 mL to be infused for 45 min. The drop factor is 10. How many drops/min will be administered?

8. Ordered: 250 mL to be infused for 90 min. The drop factor is microdrip. How many drops/min will be administered?

9. Ordered: 150 mL to be infused for 40 min. The drop factor is 15 gtt/mL. How many drops/min is this?

10. Ordered: 1500 mL to be infused for 8 hr. How many mL/hr will be administered?
    a. How many drops/min is this with a drop factor of 10?
    b. How many drops/min is this with a drop factor of 15?

ANSWERS ON PAGE 415

Additional Practice in IV Calculations

Use either the Step 1 or the Step 2 formula to calculate mL/hr or gtt/min to answer the following questions.

1. Ordered: 2000 mL for 24 hr. The drop factor is 15. How many drops/min will be administered?

2. You have 500 mL 0.45% NS infusing for 4 hr. The drop factor is 15. How many drops/min will be infused?

3. A solution of 3000 mL D5W is being infused for 24 hr with 1.5 g carbenicillin. The drop factor is 60 (microdrip).
   How many drops/min will be infused?

4. You have 1500 mL normal saline (NS). The drop factor is 15. The solution is to be given for an 8-hr period.
   a. How many mL/hr will be infused?
   b. How many gtt/min will be infused?

5. Ordered: 1000 mL to be infused for 12 hr on microdrip. At how many drops/min will you regulate the infusion?

6. Ordered: 100 mL gentamicin to be infused for 30 min. The drop factor is 20.
   a. With which step will you begin?
   b. How many drops/min will be infused?

7. You have 2000 mL D5W being infused for 24 hr. How many mL/hr will be infused?

8. Ordered: 250 mL D5W is to be infused for 10 hr on a microdrip. How many drops/min will be administered?

9. Ordered: 1500 mL of Ringer's lactate solution to be infused for 12 hr.
   a. How many mL/hr will be infused?
   b. The drop factor is 15. How many drops/min will be infused?

10. Write your two-step formula again.
    Step 1   **Step 2**

ANSWERS ON PAGE 416

WORKSHEET
6C

More Practice in IV Calculations

Use either the Step 1 or the Step 2 formula to calculate mL/hr or gtt/min to answer the following questions.

1. Ordered: 100 mL to be infused for 30 min. The drop factor is 15. At how many drops/min will you set the IV rate?

2. Ordered: 50 mL to be infused for 30 min. At how many drops/min will you set the IV rate if the drop factor is 10?

3. Ordered: 1000 mL to be infused for 6 hr. How many drops/min will be administered if the drop factor is 15?

4. Ordered: 100 mL to be infused for 60 min. At how many drops/min will you set the IV rate if a microdrip is used? Is this the same as mL/hr?

5. Ordered: D5W continuous infusion at 85 mL/hr. The drop factor is 20. At how many drops/min will you set the IV rate?

6. Ordered: 100 mL/hr. At how many drops/min will you set the IV rate if the drop factor is 10?

7. Ordered: 1500 mL 0.45% NS for 24 hr. The drop factor is 10. At how many drops/min will you set the IV rate?

8. Ordered: 500 mL for 8 hr by microdrip. How many drops/min is this?

9. Ordered: 1000 mL Ringer's lactate solution at 75 mL/hr. The drop factor is 15. How many drops/min will be administered?

10. Ordered: 2000 mL to be infused for 12 hr. The drop factor is 60.
    a. At how many mL/hr will you set the IV rate?
    b. How many drops/min will this be?

Abbreviations for Common IV Solutions

NS	Normal saline; 0.9% sodium chloride (Figure 6-6)
$\frac{1}{2}$ NS	Normal saline; 0.45% saline or $\frac{1}{2}$ strength sodium chloride (Figure 6-7)
D5W or 5% D/W	Dextrose 5% in water (Figure 6-8)
D5RL	Dextrose 5% in Ringer's lactate solution (Figure 6-9)
RL, LR, or RLS	Ringer's lactate solution (Figure 6-10)
D5NS	Dextrose 5% in 0.9% normal saline (Figure 6-11)
D5 and $\frac{1}{2}$ NS (0.45% NS)	Dextrose 5% in $\frac{1}{2}$ normal saline or 0.45% sodium chloride (Figure 6-12)

Percentage of Solute in IV Bags

The percentage numbers of the IV bags indicate the amount of dextrose, sodium chloride, or other constituents in the infusion. To determine the number of milliliters of dextrose or sodium chloride the percentage (%) represents, use the following formula. The dissolved substance or solute (dextrose, sodium chloride) is represented by a weight measurement (g). However, one mL of water weighs 1 g. Therefore, the solute is weighed in grams per 100 mL of solution. The percentage = g solute per 100 mL solution.

REMEMBER Percentage is based on 100.

Example How many g of dextrose are in 1000 mL of D5W?

KNOW   WANT TO KNOW

5 g (solute) : 100 mL :: x g (solute) : 1000 mL

$$\text{or} \quad \frac{5}{100} \times \frac{x}{1000} = \frac{10\cancel{0}x}{5 \times 10\cancel{00}} = \frac{1}{50} = 50 \text{ g or mL}$$

$100x = 5 \times 1000 = 5000$

$10\cancel{0}x = 500\cancel{0}$

$x = 50$ g (solute)

   or mL of dextrose in 1000 mL

PROOF
$100 \times 50 = 5000$
$5 \times 1000 = 5000$

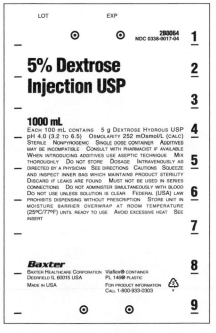

ANSWERS ON PAGE 417

WORKSHEET
6D

IV Solute Calculations

Calculate the g of NaCl and dextrose in the following intravenous fluids.

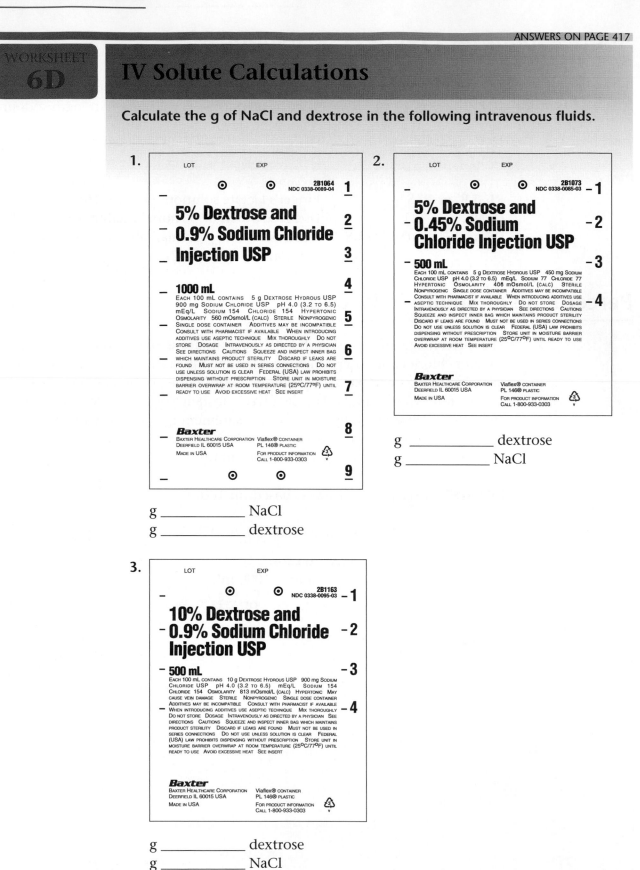

1.

LOT   EXP

2B1064
NDC 0338-0089-04

5% Dextrose and 0.9% Sodium Chloride Injection USP

1000 mL
EACH 100 mL CONTAINS   5 g DEXTROSE HYDROUS USP
900 mg SODIUM CHLORIDE USP   pH 4.0 (3.2 TO 6.5)
mEq/L   SODIUM 154   CHLORIDE 154   HYPERTONIC
OSMOLARITY 560 mOsmol/L (CALC) STERILE NONPYROGENIC
SINGLE DOSE CONTAINER   ADDITIVES MAY BE INCOMPATIBLE
CONSULT WITH PHARMACIST IF AVAILABLE   WHEN INTRODUCING
ADDITIVES USE ASEPTIC TECHNIQUE   MIX THOROUGHLY   DO NOT
STORE   DOSAGE   INTRAVENOUSLY AS DIRECTED BY A PHYSICIAN
SEE DIRECTIONS   CAUTIONS   SQUEEZE AND INSPECT INNER BAG
WHICH MAINTAINS PRODUCT STERILITY   DISCARD IF LEAKS ARE
FOUND   MUST NOT BE USED IN SERIES CONNECTIONS   DO NOT
USE UNLESS SOLUTION IS CLEAR   FEDERAL (USA) LAW PROHIBITS
DISPENSING WITHOUT PRESCRIPTION   STORE UNIT IN MOISTURE
BARRIER OVERWRAP AT ROOM TEMPERATURE (25°C/77°F) UNTIL
READY TO USE   AVOID EXCESSIVE HEAT   SEE INSERT

Baxter
BAXTER HEALTHCARE CORPORATION   Viaflex® CONTAINER
DEERFIELD IL 60015 USA   PL 146® PLASTIC
MADE IN USA   FOR PRODUCT INFORMATION
                                 CALL 1-800-933-0303

g _____ NaCl
g _____ dextrose

2.

LOT   EXP

2B1073
NDC 0338-0085-03

5% Dextrose and 0.45% Sodium Chloride Injection USP

500 mL
EACH 100 mL CONTAINS   5 g DEXTROSE HYDROUS USP   450 mg SODIUM
CHLORIDE USP   pH 4.0 (3.2 TO 6.5)   mEq/L   SODIUM 77   CHLORIDE 77
HYPERTONIC   OSMOLARITY   406 mOsmol/L (CALC)   STERILE
NONPYROGENIC   SINGLE DOSE CONTAINER   ADDITIVES MAY BE INCOMPATIBLE
CONSULT WITH PHARMACIST IF AVAILABLE   WHEN INTRODUCING ADDITIVES USE
ASEPTIC TECHNIQUE   MIX THOROUGHLY   DO NOT STORE   DOSAGE
INTRAVENOUSLY AS DIRECTED BY A PHYSICIAN   SEE DIRECTIONS   CAUTIONS
SQUEEZE AND INSPECT INNER BAG WHICH MAINTAINS PRODUCT STERILITY
DISCARD IF LEAKS ARE FOUND   MUST NOT BE USED IN SERIES CONNECTIONS
DO NOT USE UNLESS SOLUTION IS CLEAR   FEDERAL (USA) LAW PROHIBITS
DISPENSING WITHOUT PRESCRIPTION   STORE UNIT IN MOISTURE BARRIER
OVERWRAP AT ROOM TEMPERATURE (25°C/77°F) UNTIL READY TO USE
AVOID EXCESSIVE HEAT   SEE INSERT

Baxter
BAXTER HEALTHCARE CORPORATION   Viaflex® CONTAINER
DEERFIELD IL 60015 USA   PL 146® PLASTIC
MADE IN USA   FOR PRODUCT INFORMATION
                                 CALL 1-800-933-0303

g _____ dextrose
g _____ NaCl

3.

LOT   EXP

2B1163
NDC 0338-0095-03

10% Dextrose and 0.9% Sodium Chloride Injection USP

500 mL
EACH 100 mL CONTAINS   10 g DEXTROSE HYDROUS USP   900 mg SODIUM
CHLORIDE USP   pH 4.0 (3.2 TO 6.5)   mEq/L   SODIUM 154
CHLORIDE 154   OSMOLARITY 813 mOsmol/L (CALC)   HYPERTONIC   MAY
CAUSE VEIN DAMAGE   STERILE   NONPYROGENIC   SINGLE DOSE CONTAINER
ADDITIVES MAY BE INCOMPATIBLE   CONSULT WITH PHARMACIST IF AVAILABLE
WHEN INTRODUCING ADDITIVES USE ASEPTIC TECHNIQUE   MIX THOROUGHLY
DO NOT STORE   DOSAGE   INTRAVENOUSLY AS DIRECTED BY A PHYSICIAN   SEE
DIRECTIONS   CAUTIONS   SQUEEZE AND INSPECT INNER BAG WHICH MAINTAINS
PRODUCT STERILITY   DISCARD IF LEAKS ARE FOUND   MUST NOT BE USED IN
SERIES CONNECTIONS   DO NOT USE UNLESS SOLUTION IS CLEAR   FEDERAL
(USA) LAW PROHIBITS DISPENSING WITHOUT PRESCRIPTION   STORE UNIT IN
MOISTURE BARRIER OVERWRAP AT ROOM TEMPERATURE (25°C/77°F) UNTIL
READY TO USE   AVOID EXCESSIVE HEAT   SEE INSERT

Baxter
BAXTER HEALTHCARE CORPORATION   Viaflex® CONTAINER
DEERFIELD IL 60015 USA   PL 146® PLASTIC
MADE IN USA   FOR PRODUCT INFORMATION
                                 CALL 1-800-933-0303

g _____ dextrose
g _____ NaCl

ANSWERS ON PAGE 417

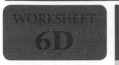

IV Solute Calculations (Continued)

Calculate the g of NaCl in the following intravenous fluids.

4. **FIGURE 6-6**
   Normal saline 0.9%
   (osmolarity range 280-308).

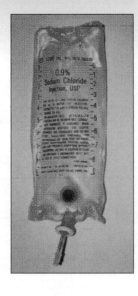

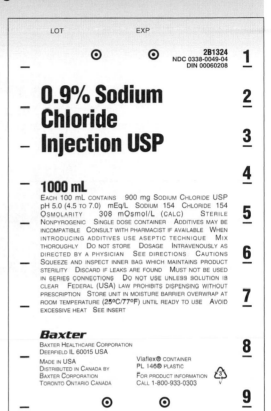

g _____ NaCl

5. **FIGURE 6-7**
   Normal saline 0.45%
   (osmolarity 154).

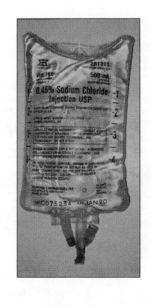

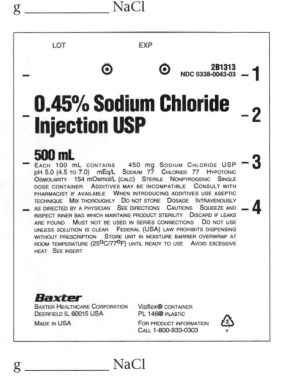

g _____ NaCl

Continued

WORKSHEET
6D

IV Solute Calculations (Continued)

Calculate the g of dextrose in the following intravenous fluids.

6. **FIGURE 6-8**
   5% dextrose.

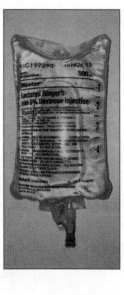

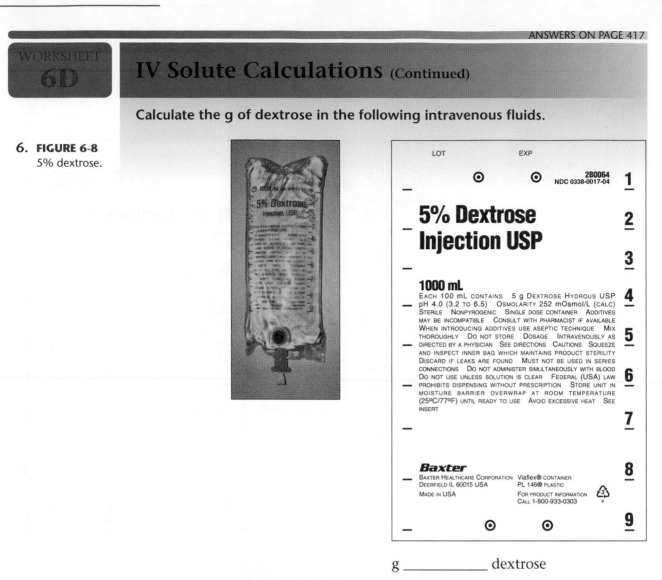

LOT   EXP

2B0064
NDC 0338-0017-04

5% Dextrose Injection USP

1000 mL
EACH 100 mL CONTAINS 5 g DEXTROSE HYDROUS USP
pH 4.0 (3.2 TO 6.5) OSMOLARITY 252 mOsmol/L (CALC)
STERILE NONPYROGENIC SINGLE DOSE CONTAINER ADDITIVES
MAY BE INCOMPATIBLE CONSULT WITH PHARMACIST IF AVAILABLE
WHEN INTRODUCING ADDITIVES USE ASEPTIC TECHNIQUE MIX
THOROUGHLY DO NOT STORE DOSAGE INTRAVENOUSLY AS
DIRECTED BY A PHYSICIAN SEE DIRECTIONS CAUTIONS SQUEEZE
AND INSPECT INNER BAG WHICH MAINTAINS PRODUCT STERILITY
DISCARD IF LEAKS ARE FOUND MUST NOT BE USED IN SERIES
CONNECTIONS DO NOT ADMINISTER SIMULTANEOUSLY WITH BLOOD
DO NOT USE UNLESS SOLUTION IS CLEAR FEDERAL (USA) LAW
PROHIBITS DISPENSING WITHOUT PRESCRIPTION STORE UNIT IN
MOISTURE BARRIER OVERWRAP AT ROOM TEMPERATURE
(25°C/77°F) UNTIL READY TO USE AVOID EXCESSIVE HEAT SEE
INSERT

Baxter
BAXTER HEALTHCARE CORPORATION Viaflex® CONTAINER
DEERFIELD IL 60015 USA PL 146® PLASTIC
MADE IN USA FOR PRODUCT INFORMATION
CALL 1-800-933-0303

g _____ dextrose

7. **FIGURE 6-9**
   Ringer's lactate solution and 5% dextrose.

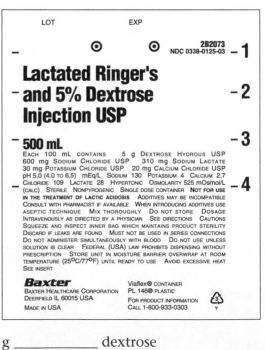

LOT   EXP

2B2073
NDC 0338-0125-03

Lactated Ringer's and 5% Dextrose Injection USP

500 mL
EACH 100 mL CONTAINS 5 g DEXTROSE HYDROUS USP
600 mg SODIUM CHLORIDE USP 310 mg SODIUM LACTATE
30 mg POTASSIUM CHLORIDE USP 20 mg CALCIUM CHLORIDE USP
pH 5.0 (4.0 TO 6.5) mEq/L SODIUM 130 POTASSIUM 4 CALCIUM 2.7
CHLORIDE 109 LACTATE 28 HYPERTONIC OSMOLARITY 525 mOsmol/L
(CALC) STERILE NONPYROGENIC SINGLE DOSE CONTAINER NOT FOR USE
IN THE TREATMENT OF LACTIC ACIDOSIS ADDITIVES MAY BE INCOMPATIBLE
CONSULT WITH PHARMACIST IF AVAILABLE WHEN INTRODUCING ADDITIVES USE
ASEPTIC TECHNIQUE MIX THOROUGHLY DO NOT STORE DOSAGE
INTRAVENOUSLY AS DIRECTED BY A PHYSICIAN SEE DIRECTIONS CAUTIONS
SQUEEZE AND INSPECT INNER BAG WHICH MAINTAINS PRODUCT STERILITY
DISCARD IF LEAKS ARE FOUND MUST NOT BE USED IN SERIES CONNECTIONS
DO NOT ADMINISTER SIMULTANEOUSLY WITH BLOOD DO NOT USE UNLESS
SOLUTION IS CLEAR FEDERAL (USA) LAW PROHIBITS DISPENSING WITHOUT
PRESCRIPTION STORE UNIT IN MOISTURE BARRIER OVERWRAP AT ROOM
TEMPERATURE (25°C/77°F) UNTIL READY TO USE AVOID EXCESSIVE HEAT
SEE INSERT

Baxter
BAXTER HEALTHCARE CORPORATION Viaflex® CONTAINER
DEERFIELD IL 60015 USA PL 146® PLASTIC
MADE IN USA FOR PRODUCT INFORMATION
CALL 1-800-933-0303

g _____ dextrose

ANSWERS ON PAGE 417

WORKSHEET 6D

IV Solute Calculations (Continued)

Calculate the g of NaCl in the following intravenous fluid.

8. **FIGURE 6-10**
   Ringer's lactate solution.

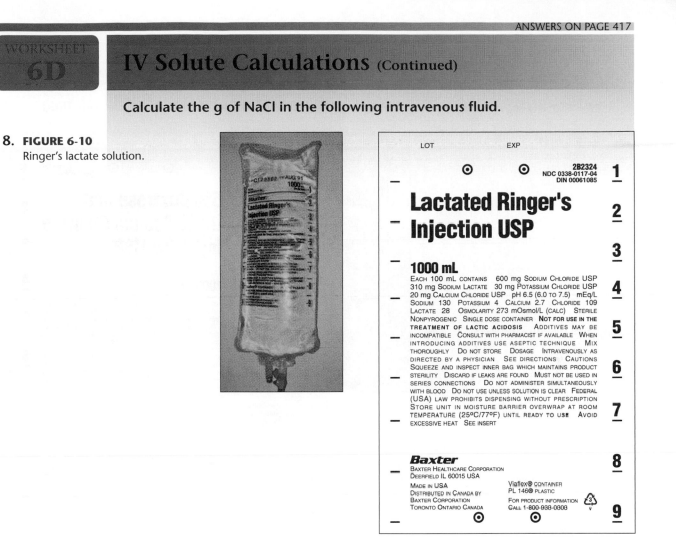

LOT   EXP

2B2324
NDC 0338-0117-04
DIN 00061085

1

Lactated Ringer's Injection USP

2

3

1000 mL

4

EACH 100 mL CONTAINS   600 mg SODIUM CHLORIDE USP
310 mg SODIUM LACTATE   30 mg POTASSIUM CHLORIDE USP
20 mg CALCIUM CHLORIDE USP   pH 6.5 (6.0 TO 7.5)   mEq/L
SODIUM 130   POTASSIUM 4   CALCIUM 2.7   CHLORIDE 109
LACTATE 28   OSMOLARITY 273 mOsmol/L (CALC)   STERILE

5

NONPYROGENIC   SINGLE DOSE CONTAINER   **NOT FOR USE IN THE
TREATMENT OF LACTIC ACIDOSIS**   ADDITIVES MAY BE
INCOMPATIBLE   CONSULT WITH PHARMACIST IF AVAILABLE   WHEN
INTRODUCING ADDITIVES USE ASEPTIC TECHNIQUE   MIX
THOROUGHLY   DO NOT STORE   DOSAGE   INTRAVENOUSLY AS
DIRECTED BY A PHYSICIAN   SEE DIRECTIONS   CAUTIONS
SQUEEZE AND INSPECT INNER BAG WHICH MAINTAINS PRODUCT

6

STERILITY   DISCARD IF LEAKS ARE FOUND   MUST NOT BE USED IN
SERIES CONNECTIONS   DO NOT ADMINISTER SIMULTANEOUSLY
WITH BLOOD   DO NOT USE UNLESS SOLUTION IS CLEAR   FEDERAL
(USA) LAW PROHIBITS DISPENSING WITHOUT PRESCRIPTION
STORE UNIT IN MOISTURE BARRIER OVERWRAP AT ROOM

7

TEMPERATURE (25°C/77°F) UNTIL READY TO USE   AVOID
EXCESSIVE HEAT   SEE INSERT

Baxter
BAXTER HEALTHCARE CORPORATION
DEERFIELD IL 60015 USA

8

MADE IN USA
DISTRIBUTED IN CANADA BY
BAXTER CORPORATION
TORONTO ONTARIO CANADA

Viaflex® CONTAINER
PL 146® PLASTIC

FOR PRODUCT INFORMATION
CALL 1-800-988-0808

9

g _____ sodium chloride

Continued

ANSWERS ON PAGE 417

IV Solute Calculations (Continued)

Calculate the g of NaCl and dextrose in the following intravenous fluids.

9. **FIGURE 6-11**
   5% dextrose in
   normal saline.

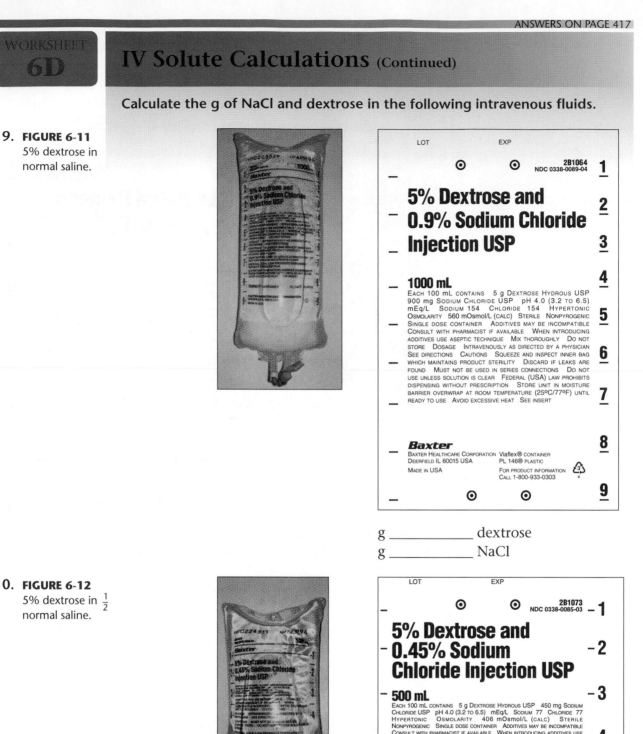

LOT   EXP

2B1064
NDC 0338-0089-04   **1**

5% Dextrose and 0.9% Sodium Chloride Injection USP

1000 mL
EACH 100 mL CONTAINS   5 g DEXTROSE HYDROUS USP
900 mg SODIUM CHLORIDE USP   pH 4.0 (3.2 TO 6.5)
mEq/L   SODIUM 154   CHLORIDE 154   HYPERTONIC
OSMOLARITY 560 mOsmol/L (CALC) STERILE NONPYROGENIC
SINGLE DOSE CONTAINER   ADDITIVES MAY BE INCOMPATIBLE
CONSULT WITH PHARMACIST IF AVAILABLE   WHEN INTRODUCING
ADDITIVES USE ASEPTIC TECHNIQUE   MIX THOROUGHLY   DO NOT
STORE   DOSAGE   INTRAVENOUSLY AS DIRECTED BY A PHYSICIAN
SEE DIRECTIONS   CAUTIONS   SQUEEZE AND INSPECT INNER BAG
WHICH MAINTAINS PRODUCT STERILITY   DISCARD IF LEAKS ARE
FOUND   MUST NOT BE USED IN SERIES CONNECTIONS   DO NOT
USE UNLESS SOLUTION IS CLEAR   FEDERAL (USA) LAW PROHIBITS
DISPENSING WITHOUT PRESCRIPTION   STORE UNIT IN MOISTURE
BARRIER OVERWRAP AT ROOM TEMPERATURE (25°C/77°F) UNTIL
READY TO USE   AVOID EXCESSIVE HEAT   SEE INSERT

Baxter
BAXTER HEALTHCARE CORPORATION   Viaflex® CONTAINER
DEERFIELD IL 60015 USA   PL 146® PLASTIC
MADE IN USA   FOR PRODUCT INFORMATION
CALL 1-800-933-0303

1 2 3 4 5 6 7 8 9

g _____ dextrose
g _____ NaCl

10. **FIGURE 6-12**
    5% dextrose in $\frac{1}{2}$
    normal saline.

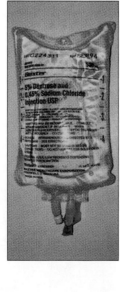

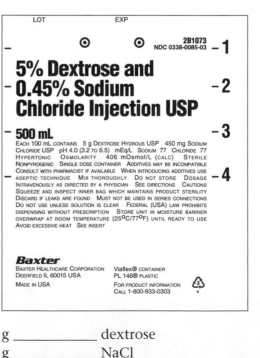

LOT   EXP

2B1073
NDC 0338-0085-03   **1**

5% Dextrose and 0.45% Sodium Chloride Injection USP

500 mL
EACH 100 mL CONTAINS   5 g DEXTROSE HYDROUS USP   450 mg SODIUM
CHLORIDE USP   pH 4.0 (3.2 TO 6.5)   mEq/L   SODIUM 77   CHLORIDE 77
HYPERTONIC   OSMOLARITY   406 mOsmol/L (CALC)   STERILE
NONPYROGENIC   SINGLE DOSE CONTAINER   ADDITIVES MAY BE INCOMPATIBLE
CONSULT WITH PHARMACIST IF AVAILABLE   WHEN INTRODUCING ADDITIVES USE
ASEPTIC TECHNIQUE   MIX THOROUGHLY   DO NOT STORE   DOSAGE
INTRAVENOUSLY AS DIRECTED BY A PHYSICIAN   SEE DIRECTIONS   CAUTIONS
SQUEEZE AND INSPECT INNER BAG WHICH MAINTAINS PRODUCT STERILITY
DISCARD IF LEAKS ARE FOUND   MUST NOT BE USED IN SERIES CONNECTIONS
DO NOT USE UNLESS SOLUTION IS CLEAR   FEDERAL (USA) LAW PROHIBITS
DISPENSING WITHOUT PRESCRIPTION   STORE UNIT IN MOISTURE BARRIER
OVERWRAP AT ROOM TEMPERATURE (25°C/77°F) UNTIL READY TO USE
AVOID EXCESSIVE HEAT   SEE INSERT

1 2 3 4

Baxter
BAXTER HEALTHCARE CORPORATION   Viaflex® CONTAINER
DEERFIELD IL 60015 USA   PL 146® PLASTIC
MADE IN USA   FOR PRODUCT INFORMATION
CALL 1-800-933-0303

g _____ dextrose
g _____ NaCl

ANSWERS ON PAGE 419

WORKSHEET
6E

IV Calculations

Directions: Calculate mL/hr, hours to infuse, and completion time.

1. Ordered: 1500 mL D5W to infuse in 4 hr. How many mL/hr should be delivered?

2. Ordered: 1000 mL of Ringer's lactate solution to infuse at 125 mL per hour. The IV was started at 0900. When will the infusion be completed?

3. Ordered: 5 g IV to infuse in 6 hr.
Available: 5 g Rocephin in 1000 mL of D5W.
How many mL per hour should infuse?

4. Ordered: 1000 mL normal saline with 500 mg erythromycin to infuse in 8 hr. The infusion was started at 0715 hours. When will the infusion be complete?

5. The patient is receiving an IV of D5W at 125 mL/hr. How many grams of dextrose per hour is the patient receiving?

6. Ordered: 500 mg aminophylline in 250 mL normal saline IVPB to infuse at 30 mL/hr. The IV started at 1330 hours. When will the infusion be complete?

7. Ordered: Magnesium sulfate/2 g over 4 hr.
Available: 500 mL D5W with 2 g of magnesium sulfate.
How many mL/hr should be infused?

8. Ordered: Aminophylline 1 g in 500 mL D5W to infuse at 40 mg/hr.
Available: 1 g of aminophylline in 500 mL of D5W. The IV was started at 2100 hours.
When will the infusion be complete?

9. Ordered: 2 g Keflin in 200 mL normal saline IVPB to infuse in 3 hr. How many mL per hour will the infusion device be set for?

10. Ordered: Rocephin 1 gm in 500 mL of normal saline to infuse in 4 hr. At what rate will you set the IV pump?

IV medications must be charted on a flow sheet called the medication administration record (MAR) (Figure 6-13).

NURSING CARE RECORD

HOSPITAL   Medical/Surgical

DATA FLOW RECORD   Date ___1-12-08___

TIME	0600	1600																
PULSE	84	80																
RESPIRATION	20	22																
BLOOD PRESSURE	150/92	152/90																
COUGH/ DEEP BREATH	✓	✓																
INITIALS	JG	CB																

The IV flow sheet may record the vital signs prior to initiating IV therapy and again on every shift. The IV site and location is recorded along with the time and date it was started. The catheter type and needle size are recorded next to the type and rate of the IV solution. Additional IV solutions are recorded in the date/time inserted column. When the IV is discontinued, the reason is recorded under the comments column.

IV THERAPY

SITE	DATE/TIME INSERTED	SITE LOCATION	CATH TYPE/ SIZE	IV SOLUTION	RATE	DEVICE	TUBING CHANGE	APPEARANCE 7-3	APPEARANCE 3-11	APPEARANCE 11-7	SITE D/C'd	COMMENTS
R	1-12-08 0600	LPF	22 angio	1000 D5W	75°			1				
R	1-12-08 1900	LPF	22 angio	1000 D5W	75°		△		1			
R	1-12-08 2200	LPF	22 angio						2		✓	Slight redness noted at site pt denies pain or tenderness.

HEALTH DEVIATION NEEDS

DCP ASSESSED: In Progress ☐   Revise Plan ☐

DCP Conference ☐ _____

_____

REFERRAL MADE: SS ☐   HHC ☐   Dietary ☐   Pharmacy ☐
Other _____

PATIENT/FAMILY TEACHING:
Pt/Other _____

_____

_____

PT/FAMILY TEACHING RESPONSE CODES
1 = Received Literature
2 = Communicates Understanding
3 = Requires Reinforcement
4 = Previous Experience
5 = Return Demonstration
6 = Objective Achieved
7 = Referral Initiated
8 = Refused
9 = Preprinted Teaching Protocol

IV CODES
Site Location
L = Left
R = Right
S = Scalp
Ft = Foot
F = Femoral
H = Hand
W = Wrist

AC = Antecubital
UA = Upper Arm
UPF = Upper Posterior Forearm
LPF = Lower Posterior Forearm

UAF = Upper Anterior Forearm
LAF = Lower Anterior Forearm
IJ = Internal Jugular
SC = Subclavian

Catheter
S.G. = Swan Ganz
H.D. = Hemodialysis
Hick = Hickman
G = Groshong
Port = Port-A-Cath or other implanted port
PP = Pace Port

Appearance
1 = Asymptomatic
2 = Red
3 = Swollen
4 = Ecchymotic
5 = Warm
6 = Cool
7 = Draining
8 = Leaking
Lumen
d = distal
m = middle
p = proximal

EMOTIONAL SUPPORT CODES
1 = Active Listening
2 = Reassurance/Comfort
3 = Relaxation
  A = Breathing
  B = Visualization/Imagery
4 = Coping Skills Review

△ = Change

PROCEDURES

TIME	DEPT.	MODE	TRANSPORTER	RETURN

INITIAL	SIGNATURE/TITLE	INITIAL	SIGNATURE/TITLE
mJ	J Jahle, RN		

FIGURE 6-13 Example of an IV therapy medication administration record (MAR).

IV Delivery Sets

Figure 6-14, *A*, shows a primary set. This is the basic set that delivers IV fluids for a short duration. It does not have a port for additions. This is a needleless connector.

Figure 6-14, *B*, shows a primary set with a port for adding piggyback medications. This set has a manual dial for the mL/hr rate.

SAFETY SYSTEMS FOR IV PORTS

Needleless IV systems (Figure 6-15) are designed to protect caregivers from accidental punctures by contaminated needles. The BD SafetyGlide™ needle (Figure 6-16) used to inject medication into IV ports is another measure to avoid accidental punctures.

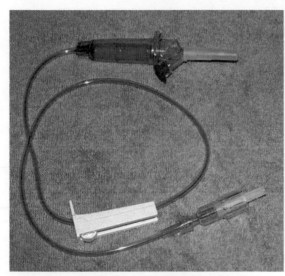

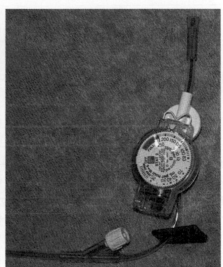

FIGURE 6-14
A, Primary set with a roller clamp to regulate the IV set. **B,** Primary set with a port for adding piggyback medications.

A

B

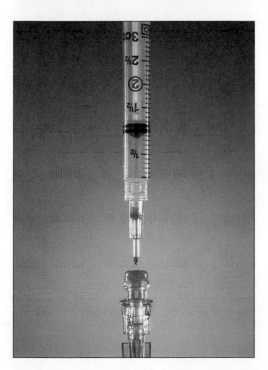

FIGURE 6-15 InterLink® IV Access System, an example of a needleless system. *(From Becton, Dickinson, and Company, Franklin Lakes, NJ.)*

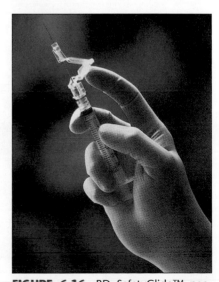

FIGURE 6-16 BD SafetyGlide™ needle. *(From Becton, Dickinson, and Company, Franklin Lakes, NJ.)*

GRAVITY PIGGYBACK INFUSIONS

The acronym for intravenous piggyback is IVPB (Figure 6-17). When special medications are ordered intermittently, the primary IV can be bypassed by introducing the medication through a special entry or portal. Piggyback (PB) medications are infused intermittently via the existing IV line. A secondary IV tube with a needle attachment is inserted into the portal or entry site. The PB infusion amount is usually 50 to 250 mL of medicated solution.

Elevating the IVPB 12 inches above the existing IV allows the PB to infuse by gravity (Figure 6-18). When all of the medication has been infused, the existing IV will resume to the rate set for the PB infusion. The nurse must remember to regulate the primary IV to the previous rate. If an infusion device is used, the IV can be programmed to resume to the primary infusion rate at the completion of the PB.

Piggyback medications are premixed by the pharmacy, drug manufacturer, or nurse. The manufacturer's insert provides recommended times for IVPBs to infuse if the physician does not state the rate in the order.

> **REMEMBER** Gravity-flow sets are delivered in drops per minute.

PIGGYBACK PREMIXED IVs

Piggyback IV additions are premixed by the pharmacy or the manufacturer. The medication is diluted in 50 to 250 mL of an iso-osmotic sterile solution. The amount of solution used depends on the type of medication, the presence of fluid restrictions, and the weight of the patient.

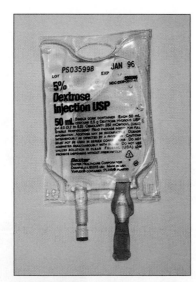

FIGURE 6-17 50 mL of solution for IV piggyback infusion.

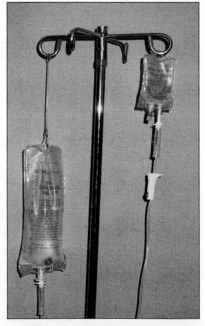

FIGURE 6-18 Gravity flow IV piggyback. The IV piggyback is elevated above the existing IV, allowing it to infuse by gravity.

IVPB admixtures (Figure 6-19) are usually prepared in bulk by the pharmacist for more efficient use of time. If more than one day's supply is prepared, the IVPB can be frozen without altering its stability.

Premixed frozen IVPBs should be thawed in the refrigerator or at room temperature. Never thaw in a microwave oven or in hot or warm water.

All IVPB admixtures must be visually inspected before starting. Check the order, label, medication, strength, and quantity. Make sure that the admixture is clear and free from particles and the expiration date has not passed.

NURSE-ACTIVATED PIGGYBACK SYSTEMS

The Abbott ADD-Vantage and the Baxter Mini-Bag Plus (Figure 6-20) are used in home care as well as in hospitals and long-term care centers. The IVPB mini-bag has a vial of medication attached to a special port. The pharmacy dispenses the IVPB with the unreconstituted drug vial attached to the mini-bag. At the time of delivery, the nurse breaks the seal between the vial and the mini-bag. This allows the medication to flow into the mini-bag. The medication vial remains attached to the mini-bag, which is a safety feature created to decrease potential medication errors. Figure 6-21 shows the steps for assembling and using the ADD-Vantage system.

ELECTRONIC INFUSION DEVICES

Electronic infusion devices are used in hospitals, extended care facilities, home care, and ambulatory care settings. They deliver a set amount of intravenous fluids per hour. Some examples of electronic infusion devices are shown in Fig-

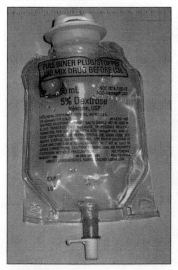

FIGURE 6-19 50 mL of dextrose. Medication can be added for infusion as an IV piggyback.

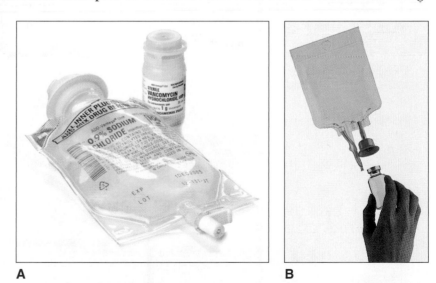

A   B

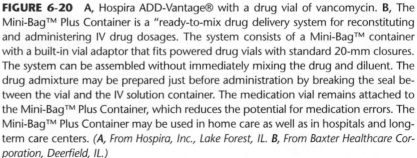

FIGURE 6-20 **A,** Hospira ADD-Vantage® with a drug vial of vancomycin. **B,** The Mini-Bag™ Plus Container is a "ready-to-mix drug delivery system for reconstituting and administering IV drug dosages. The system consists of a Mini-Bag™ container with a built-in vial adaptor that fits powered drug vials with standard 20-mm closures. The system can be assembled without immediately mixing the drug and diluent. The drug admixture may be prepared just before administration by breaking the seal between the vial and the IV solution container. The medication vial remains attached to the Mini-Bag™ Plus Container, which reduces the potential for medication errors. The Mini-Bag™ Plus Container may be used in home care as well as in hospitals and long-term care centers. *(A, From Hospira, Inc., Lake Forest, IL. B, From Baxter Healthcare Corporation, Deerfield, IL.)*

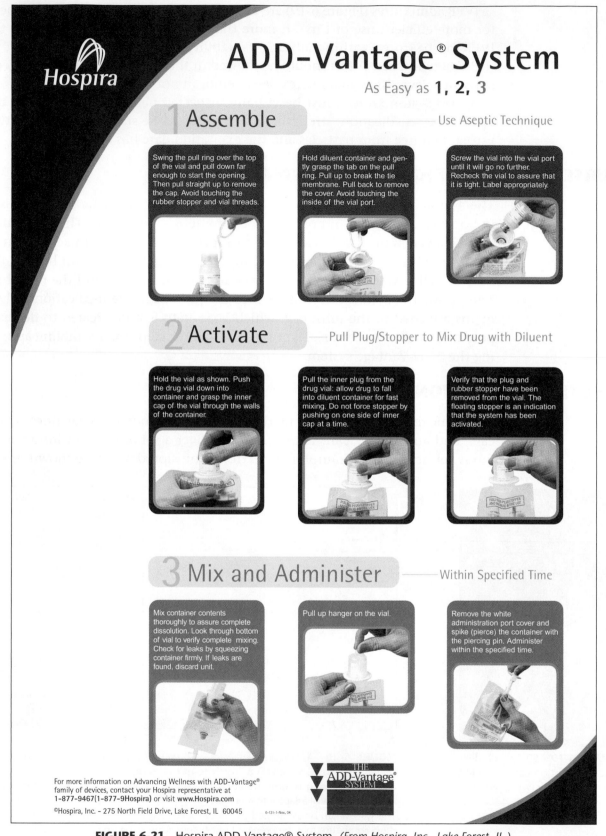

ADD–Vantage® System
As Easy as 1, 2, 3

1 Assemble — Use Aseptic Technique

Swing the pull ring over the top of the vial and pull down far enough to start the opening. Then pull straight up to remove the cap. Avoid touching the rubber stopper and vial threads.

Hold diluent container and gently grasp the tab on the pull ring. Pull up to break the tie membrane. Pull back to remove the cover. Avoid touching the inside of the vial port.

Screw the vial into the vial port until it will go no further. Recheck the vial to assure that it is tight. Label appropriately.

2 Activate — Pull Plug/Stopper to Mix Drug with Diluent

Hold the vial as shown. Push the drug vial down into container and grasp the inner cap of the vial through the walls of the container.

Pull the inner plug from the drug vial: allow drug to fall into diluent container for fast mixing. Do not force stopper by pushing on one side of inner cap at a time.

Verify that the plug and rubber stopper have been removed from the vial. The floating stopper is an indication that the system has been activated.

3 Mix and Administer — Within Specified Time

Mix container contents thoroughly to assure complete dissolution. Look through bottom of vial to verify complete mixing. Check for leaks by squeezing container firmly. If leaks are found, discard unit.

Pull up hanger on the vial.

Remove the white administration port cover and spike (pierce) the container with the piercing pin. Administer within the specified time.

For more information on Advancing Wellness with ADD-Vantage® family of devices, contact your Hospira representative at 1-877-9467(1-877-9Hospira) or visit www.Hospira.com

©Hospira, Inc. - 275 North Field Drive, Lake Forest, IL 60045

THE ADD-Vantage® SYSTEM

FIGURE 6-21 Hospira ADD-Vantage® System. *(From Hospira, Inc., Lake Forest, IL.)*

ure 6-22. They are individually programmed to deliver a set amount of IV solution per hour.

CADD-Prizm (see Figure 6-22, *A*) is a battery-operated pump that provides IV medications to confined or ambulatory patients. There are four delivery modes:

- Patient-controlled analgesia (PCA)
- Continuous infusion
- Intermittent infusion
- Total parenteral nutrition

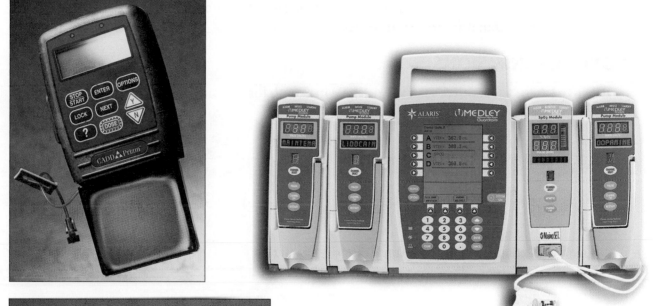

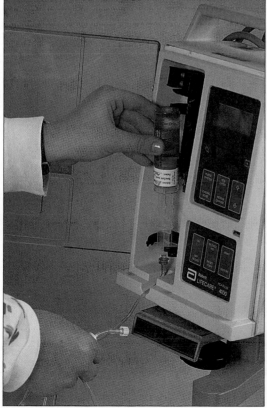

FIGURE 6-22   Electronic infusion devices. **A**, CADD-Prizm VIP ambulatory battery-operated infusion device used for IV parenteral nutrition. **B**, Medley™ Medication Safety System. **C**, Nurse using a PCA electronic infusion device. *(A, From SIMS Deltec, Inc., St Paul, MN. B, From ALARIS Medical Systems, Inc., San Diego, CA. C, From Potter PA, Perry AG:* Fundamentals of nursing, *ed 6, St Louis, 2005, Mosby.)*

Total Parenteral Nutrition Device

The total parenteral nutrition (TPN) delivery mode allows the infusion of nutritional elements slowly at the beginning of the administration. This keeps the glucose level from rising too rapidly. The system slowly tapers up and then tapers down toward the end of the infusion.

Pressure-Flow Infusion Device

The ambulatory infusion device system was developed for ambulatory use. It can be put in a pocket, inside a shirt, or in any other convenient place where it can be concealed. The flow rate is pre-set. Figure 6-23 shows an example of an ambulatory infusion device.

PIGGYBACK INFUSIONS

Examples ■ Ordered: Cefazolin 1 g IV in 50 mL for 30 min. At how many mL/hr should the infusion pump be set?

KNOW   WANT TO KNOW

$50 \text{ mL} : 30 \text{ min} : : x \text{ mL} : 60 \text{ min}$ **OR** $\frac{50}{30} = \frac{x}{60} = \frac{300}{3} = 100 \text{ mL/hr}$

$3\cancel{0} \, x = 300\cancel{0}$

$x = 100 \text{ mL/hr}$

PROOF

$3\cancel{0} \times 10\cancel{0} = 30$

$5\cancel{0} \times 6\cancel{0} = 30$

Set the infusion pump for 100 mL/hr.

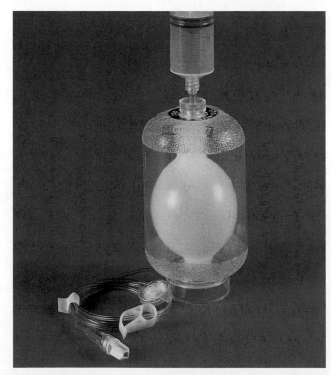

FIGURE 6-23 MedFlo® Postoperative pain management system, ambulatory infusion device. *(From Smith & Nephew Endoscopy, Andover, MA.)*

■ Ordered: Ampicillin 500 mg IV in 100 mL NS for 45 min. At how many mL/hr should the infusion pump be set?

KNOW   WANT TO KNOW
100 mL : 45 min :: x mL : 60 min   Convert minutes into a decimal

$45 x = 100 \times 60 = 6000$ **OR** 45 min $\div 60 = 0.75$

$45 x = 6000$

$x = 133.3 = 133$ mL/hr 100 mL $\div 0.75 = 133$ mL/hr

PROOF
$45 \times 133.3 = 5998.5$
$60 \times 100 = 6000$

Set the infusion pump at 133 mL/hr.

CLINICAL ALERT

Electronic infusion devices are set to infuse mL/hr. When administering a small amount of medication for less than 1 hour, the device must be set at mL/hr even though the medication will infuse in less than 1 hour.

ANSWERS ON PAGE 419

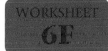

Infusion Device and Solute g/mL and gtt/min Calculations

Use the two-step formula to answer the following questions.

1. Ordered: 100 mL with 1 g cephalothin to be infused for 30 min by microdrip (microdrip = 60 gtt/min).
   a. How many gtt/min will be infused on a gravity flow if the drop factor is used?
   b. At how many mL/hr will you set the infusion device?

2. Ordered: Aqueous penicillin 600,000 units in 100 mL IVPB to be infused for 1 hr. At how many mL/hr will you set the infusion device?

3. Ordered: 250 mL NS to be infused at 150 mL/hr. The drop factor is 15 gtt/mL. How long will it take to infuse?

4. Ordered: Ampicillin 1 g in 50 mL IVPB ADD-Vantage® System to be infused for 20 min.
   a. At how many mL/hr would you set the infusion device?
   b. How many gtt/min will be administered on a gravity flow if the drop factor is 15?

5. Ordered: Keflin 2 g in 100 mL IVPB to be infused for 1 hr. The drop factor is 15. How many gtt/min is this? At how many mL/hr will you set the infusion device?

Continued

190 Drug Calculations

ANSWERS ON PAGE 419

WORKSHEET 6F

Infusion Device and Solute g/mL and gtt/min Calculations (Continued)

6. Ordered: Gentamicin 80 mg in 50 mL IVPB to be infused for 30 min.
   a. At how many mL/hr will you set an infusion device?
   b. How many gtt/min will infuse for a gravity flow if the drop factor is 60?

7. Ordered: 200 mL Foscavir to infuse for 90 min. The drop factor is microdrip.
   a. How many gtt/min will infuse?
   b. At how many mL/hr will you set the infusion pump?

8. Ordered: 1000 mL 0.9% saline to infuse for 12 hr. The drop factor is 15 gtt/mL.
   a. How many gtt/min will infuse?
   b. At how many mL/hr will you set the infusion pump?
   c. How many milliliters of sodium chloride will the patient receive?

9. Ordered: 2000 mL D5W to be infused for 8 hr. The drop factor is 15 gtt/mL.
   a. How many mL/hr will infuse?
   b. How many gtt/min will infuse?
   c. How many milliliters of dextrose will the patient receive in 8 hours?

10. Ordered: Kantrex 300 mg in 150 mL IVPB. Label reads to infuse for 40 to 60 min. The drop factor is microdrip.
    a. What is the fastest rate for the IVPB to infuse? At what rate will you set the infusion device?
    b. What is the slowest rate for the IVPB to infuse? At what rate will you set the device?

ANSWERS ON PAGE 421

WORKSHEET 6G

Multiple-Choice Practice

Circle the letter of the correct answer in the following problems.
Remember: To convert tenths of an hour into minutes, multiply by 60.
Example: 0.65 hr × 60 = 39 min

1. Ordered: 2500 mL to be infused for 24 hr. Available: An IV tubing with 15 gtt/mL. At what rate will you set the IV device?
   a. 52 gtt/min   b. 35 gtt/min   c. 26 gtt/min   d. 104 gtt/min

2. Administer 50 mL of an IV antibiotic for 15 min. The IV set is calibrated at 15 gtt/mL. At how many gtt/min will you set the rate?
   a. 100 gtt/min   b. 60 gtt/min   c. 25 gtt/min   d. 50 gtt/min

3. Ordered: 50 mL piggyback to be infused for 30 min. The drop factor is 20. At how many gtt/min will you set the rate?
   a. 17 gtt/min   b. 100 gtt/min   c. 20 gtt/min   d. 33 gtt/min

ANSWERS ON PAGE 421

WORKSHEET
6G

Multiple-Choice Practice (Continued)

4. Ordered: 300 mL of 0.9% NS for 6 hr. The IV set is microdrip. At how many gtt/min will you set the rate?
   a. 60 gtt/min   b. 50 gtt/min   c. 30 gtt/min   d. 45 gtt/min

5. Ordered: Dobutrex 150 mg in 150 mL Ringer's lactate (RL). The infusion device is set at 12 mL/hr. How long will it take to infuse?
   a. 6 hr, 15 min   b. 12 hr, 50 min   c. 8 hr, 15 min   d. 12 hr, 30 min

6. The IV is infusing at 30 gtt/min. The drop factor is 20 gtt/mL. The IV bag label reads 500 mL of 0.45% NS. How many hours will it take to infuse?
   a. 5 hr, 50 min   b. 3 hr, 36 min   c. 4 hr, 40 min   d. 5 hr, 30 min

7. Calculate the infusion time for an IV of 1000 mL of D5W infusing at 25 gtt/min with a drop factor of 10 gtt/mL.
   a. 6 hr, 40 min   b. 6 hr, 10 min   c. 5 hr, 57 min   d. 4 hr, 17 min

8. A pint of blood (500 mL) is hung at 1100 hours. The flow rate is 42 gtt/min. The drop factor on the administration set is 10 gtt/mL. When will the infusion be complete?
   a. 1733 hours   b. 1920 hours   c. 1300 hours   d. 1654 hours

9. Tridil is infusing at 30 mL/hr. The IV label reads: *500 mL D5W with Tridil 5 mcg/3 mL*. How many hours will it take to infuse?
   a. 15 hr, 10 min   b. 18 hr, 45 min   c. 16 hr, 40 min   d. 12 hr, 48 min

10. Ordered: Amicar 5 g in 250 mL for 2 hr. At how many mL/hr should the infusion device be set?
    a. 150 mL/hr   b. 100 mL/hr   c. 175 mL/hr   d. 125 mL/hr

CRITICAL THINKING EXERCISES

It is the change of shift. The patient with congestive heart failure (CHF) is being infused by an IV of 1000 mL D5W. The patient complains of being very short of breath. After checking the IV rate, you find that it is infusing at 175 mL/hr. Taking into consideration the patient's diagnosis, you check the IV order and it reads 500 mL D5W in 24 hr.

Ordered:

Given:

Error(s):

Potential injuries:

Preventive measures:

Discussion

- What would your first action be?
- What other factors relate to this incident?
- At what rate shoud the IV be infusing?

1. Ordered: 3000 mL for 24 hr. The drop factor is 15. How many drops/min will infuse via a gravity device?

2. Ordered: 75 mL to be infused for 45 min. The drop factor is 10. At how many mL/hr will you set the infusion device? How many drops/min will infuse via a gravity device if the drop factor is 10?

3. Ordered: 1000 mL to be infused for 12 hr IV. At how many mL/hr will you set the infusion device? How many drops/min will be administered via a gravity device if the drop factor is 20?

4. Ordered: 1200 mL to be infused for 8 hr. The drop factor is microdrip. How many drops/min will infuse using a gravity device?

5. Ordered: Infuse 2000 mL D5W for 24 hr. The drop factor is 10. At how many mL/hr will you set the infusion device? How many drops/min will be administered using a gravity device?

6. Ordered: 1500 mL NS to infuse for 12 hr. The drop factor is 15. How many mL/hr will be administered? How many drops/min will infuse?

7. Ordered: 3000 mL D5W to infuse for 24 hr with 0.5 g of penicillin in each 1000 mL. The drop factor is 60, by microdrip. How many mL/hr will infuse? How many drops/min will be administered?

8. Ordered: 200 mL cefazolin to infuse for 45 min via the infusion device. At how many mL/hr will you set the infusion device?

9. Ordered: 1000 mL to run for 12 hr on microdrip. At how many drops/min will you regulate the flow?

10. Ordered: 250 mL to infuse for 90 min. How many mL/hr will infuse if the electronic infusion device is used? How many drops/min will infuse with microdrip?

Refer to the Intravenous Calculations section of the enclosed student CD-ROM for additional practice problems.

Advanced Intravenous Calculations

Objectives

- Calculate milligrams per kilogram and micrograms per kilogram per minute and per hour.
- Calculate hourly drug dose and hourly flow rate for IV solutions.
- Estimate and calculate infusion rates and drug doses using ratio and proportion.
- Calculate time/dose intervals for direct IV push (bolus) medications administered by a syringe.
- Evaluate existing infusions for correct flow rate and/or drug dose, and obtain order to change if incorrect.
- Analyze IV medication errors using critical thinking.

INTRODUCTION

This chapter builds on the mastery of the basic IV calculations learned in Chapter 6. Taking the time to work through each set of problems will facilitate the acquisition of the logic needed to solve complex IV solution calculations. When each step has been mastered, you will be able to identify and use basic safe calculation shortcuts.

Advanced IV Calculations

Advanced IV calculations are used to determine the amount of IV drug and flow rate per minute and/or per hour for potent medications based on the patient's weight, condition, and response to treatment. If an infusion device is not available, microdrip tubing should be used with a volume-control device. (See Figure 11-4 on page 310 for an illustration of equipment.) Some medications are delivered directly into a vein with a syringe.

The choice of administration and equipment depends not only on the orders and the patient's condition but also on hospital policy, state board policy, the literature and pharmacy recommendations, and the equipment available.

The nurse must be able to evaluate orders and existing solutions for safe and correct dose/flow rates, preferred routes, and compatibilities with existing solutions.

Titrated Infusions

Dose/flow rate adjustments may be made, particularly with powerful solutions of medications, based on the patient's condition, weight, and physiologic response to the medication. For example, an order may call for an IV to be **titrated** (adjusted) to maintain a certain blood pressure range. The most potent IV medications are administered and adjusted in micrograms per kilogram per minute or milligrams per kilogram per minute. For purposes of reducing errors and simplifying mathematics in flow rate calculations, many of these infusions now have a standardized **total drug/total volume ratio** of 1:1, 1:2, and 1:4 (e.g., 250 mg/250 mL [1:1]; 250 mg/500 mL [1:2], 250 mg/1000 mL [1:4]). If the patient requires fluid restriction, the physician may order a stronger concentration of drug to solution (4:1 or 2:1 drug in solution, such as 1 g:250 mL [4:1] or 500 mg:250 mL [2:1]).

> ### CLINICAL ALERT
>
> If you consult flow rate and compatibility charts, examine the source and the date published. If the publisher is a reputable source, such as the laboratory that furnishes the IV solutions in use, and if the chart is current, then take further care to examine the layout and content of the tables to ensure that the information needed is selected.

IV solutions that contain powerful medications are preferably diluted and administered by a volumetric infusion pump. There are several sophisticated devices on the market (Figure 7-1). The data to be entered can range from the traditional mL/hr to drug doses ordered per minute in mg/min or mcg/min, along with the patient's weight, if necessary (mg/kg/min) (Figure 7-2).

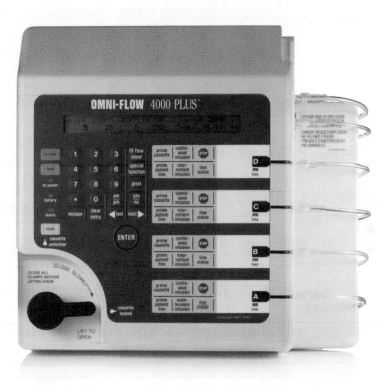

FIGURE 7-1   Omni-Flow® 4000 Plus Medication Management System 4-Channel IV Pump. *(From Hospira, Inc., Lake Forest, IL.)*

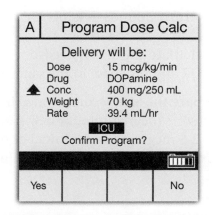

FIGURE 7-2   Plum A+® Drug Confirmation Screen. (Note that this machine shows a delivery rate in tenths of a mL/hr.) *(From Hospira, Inc., Lake Forest, IL.)*

SOLVING TITRATED INFUSION PROBLEMS

STEPS
1. Calculate the safe dose range (SDR) per kilogram per minute (mcg/kg/min or mg/kg/min) from the literature.

2. Compare the SDR in the literature with the physician's order, using the same terms (micrograms or milligrams) and evaluate for the SDR as shown below.

3. If the order is safe, calculate the hourly drug and flow rate using the formula below.

HOURLY DRUG AND FLOW RATE FORMULA FOR TITRATED INFUSIONS

HAVE　　　　　　　　　　　　　WANT TO HAVE

TD　:　TV　::　HD　:　HV

Total drug : Total volume :: Hourly drug : Hourly volume

in　　　　　　　　　　One of these will be x.

Lowest reduced ratio　　　One of these will be known.

REMEMBER IV orders may necessitate converting mcg or mg/min to mg/hr.

Example Ordered: 3 mcg/kg/min of Intropin (dopamine HCl) for a new patient with heart failure. Available: 400 mg dissolved in 500 mL D5W. The literature recommends an initial dose of 2 to 5 mcg/kg/min, (not to exceed a total of 50 mcg/kg/min). The dose is to be titrated to the patient's systolic blood pressure at the level ordered by the physician. This patient weighs 242 lb. What flow rate should be set?

Step 1
a. **Convert** pounds to kilograms using a calculator (2.2 lb = 1 kg).
242 lb ÷ 2.2 = 110 kg
b. **Calculate** the SDR if needed.
(SDR and order are in the same terms. Calculation is not needed.)

Step 2 **Compare** the SDR recommended in the literature with the order:
Ordered: 3 mcg/kg/min for new patient
SDR: 2-5 mcg/kg/min for initial dosing
Decision: Safe to give. Order is within the SDR.

◢ CLINICAL ALERT

Titrated infusions seldom require a high flow rate. It is essential that the flow rates be correct. Speeding up or slowing down an IV without a physician's order, so as to compensate for incorrect flow rate, is hazardous. Be aware that abrupt changes in the flow rates of IV fluids and therefore in medication levels can cause serious side effects.

Step 3   **a.** **Calculate** the ordered hourly drug dose in milligrams (same terms as drug [400 mg] on hand) using a calculator (recalling that 1000 mcg = 1 mg).
3 mcg × 110 kg × 60 min ÷ 1000 = 19.8 mg/hr, rounded to 20 mg/hr.

b. Calculate the hourly flow rate (HV) after reducing the total drug/total volume ratio to lowest terms.

HAVE		WANT TO HAVE
TD : TV	::	HD : HV
400 mg : 500 mL	::	20 mg : x mL
4 : 5	::	20 : x
		x = 25 mL/hr

Set the flow rate on the IV infusion device to 25 mL/hr.

Alternative   If the hourly volume is known but the hourly drug dose is not, just place the
Step 3   unknown (x) under the hourly drug dose and fill in the hourly volume ordered in this equation. Check the answer with the literature for the SDR (e.g., the order was for 25 mL/hr or is infusing at 25 mL/hr when you arrive; how much drug is the patient receiving per hour and per minute so that the SDR can be checked?).

Use the same formula. Read the total drug, total volume, and hourly volume on the IV devices in the patient's room:

HAVE   WANT TO HAVE
TD : TV :: HD : HV
400 mg : 500 mL :: x mg : 25 mL
(reduce ratio) 4 : 5 :: x : 25
5x = 100 x = 20 mg/hr of drug being infused

20 mg/hr ÷ 110 kg ÷ 60 min × 1000 = 3 mg/kg/min

The SDR states 2 to 5 mcg/kg/min. Now you know that the order was followed properly, and that the flow rate is correct and within the SDR. The next few worksheets provide the necessary basic skills practice to understand and perform these calculations rapidly.

ANSWERS ON PAGE 423

WORKSHEET
7A

Advanced IV Calculation Practice

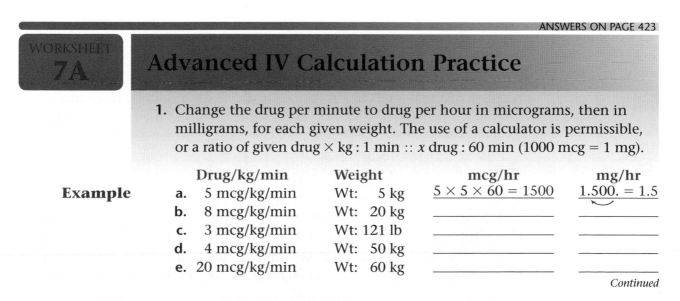

1. Change the drug per minute to drug per hour in micrograms, then in milligrams, for each given weight. The use of a calculator is permissible, or a ratio of given drug × kg : 1 min :: x drug : 60 min (1000 mcg = 1 mg).

		Drug/kg/min	Weight	mcg/hr	mg/hr
Example	**a.**	5 mcg/kg/min	Wt: 5 kg	5 × 5 × 60 = 1500	1.500. = 1.5
	b.	8 mcg/kg/min	Wt: 20 kg	_____	_____
	c.	3 mcg/kg/min	Wt: 121 lb	_____	_____
	d.	4 mcg/kg/min	Wt: 50 kg	_____	_____
	e.	20 mcg/kg/min	Wt: 60 kg	_____	_____

Continued

ANSWERS ON PAGE 423

Advanced IV Calculation Practice (Continued)

2. Reduce the total drug/total volume ratio to lowest terms (e.g., 1000 : 250 = 4 : 1)

	TD : TV	Lowest Ratio
Example	**a.** 250 mg : 1000 mL	1 : 4
	b. 500 mg : 500 mL	_____
	c. 100 mg : 1000 mL	_____
	d. 250 mg : 500 mL	_____
	e. 500 mg : 1000 mL	_____

3. Estimate the value of *x* (hourly volume) after reducing the ratio of total drug to total volume. The ratio of hourly drug to hourly volume will be the same as total drug to total volume.

	TD : TV :: HD : HV	ANSWER
Example	**a.** 250 mg : 1000 mL :: 10 mg : *x* mL	1 : 4 :: 10 : 40 mL/hr
	b. 500 mg : 500 mL :: 30 mg : *x* mL	_____ mL/hr
	c. 100 mg : 1000 mL :: 5 mg : *x* mL	_____ mL/hr
	d. 250 mg : 500 mL :: 3 mg : *x* mL	_____ mL/hr
	e. 500 mg : 250 mL :: 10 mg : *x* mL	_____ mL/hr

4. If you came on duty and evaluated these IV solutions and rates in a patient-care setting, you would estimate the hourly drug after first reducing the total drug/total volume ratio and then examining the rate set on the infusion device.

Estimate the hourly drug *(x)*.

	TD : TV :: HD : HV	ANSWER
Example	**a.** 250 mg : 250 mL :: *x* mg : 20 mL	1 : 1 :: 20 : 20 20 mg/hr
	b. 1000 mg : 500 mL :: *x* mg : 6 mL	_____ mg/hr
	c. 250 mg : 500 mL :: *x* mg : 18 mL	_____ mg/hr
	d. 400 mg : 1000 mL :: *x* mg : 10 mL	_____ mg/hr
	e. 500 mg : 250 mL :: *x* mg : 18 mL	_____ mg/hr

5. Change micrograms to milligrams by moving the decimal three places to the left. Reduce the total drug/total volume ratio to the lowest terms. Finally, estimate the hourly volume. (The hourly drug must always be calculated in the same terms as the total drug.)

	TD : TV :: HD : HV	ANSWER
Example	**a.** 250 mg : 1000 mL :: (4000 mcg) 4 mg : *x* mL	1 : 4 :: 4 : 16 mL/hr
	b. 500 mg : 500 mL :: (9000 mcg) __ mg : *x* mL	_____ mL/hr
	c. 1000 mg : 500 mL :: (20,000 mcg) __ mg : *x* mL	_____ mL/hr
	d. 250 mg : 500 mL :: (15,000 mcg) __ mg : *x* mL	_____ mL/hr
	e. 400 mg : 250 mL :: (8000 mcg) __ mg : *x* mL	_____ mL/hr

ANSWERS ON PAGE 423

WORKSHEET
7B

IV Drug/Flow Rates

Tip: Being able to convert drug, weight, time, and volume parameters within the metric system with ease facilitates advanced IV calculations.

1. Fill in the table by using a calculator and/or by moving decimals.

	mg/hr	mcg/hr	mg/min	mcg/min
a.	0.050.	50	0.050 ÷ 60 = 0.0008	0.8
b.			0.4	
c.	30			
d.				20
e.	7.5			

2. Fill in the table using a calculator.

	kg	mg/hr	mg/kg/min	mcg/kg/min
a.	85	25	25 ÷ 85 ÷ 60 = 0.005	5
b.	70		10	
c.	62			0.1
d.	55	75		
e.	48			50

3. Fill in the table for these IV drug/flow rate calculations using the TD : TV :: HD : HV formula.

	IV Contents	TD : TV Reduced Ratio	HD (mg/hr)	HV (mL/hr)	mg/mL
a.	500 mg/1000 mL	1 : 2	5	1 : 2 :: 5 : 10	500 ÷ 1000 = 0.5
b.	250 mg/500 mL			30	
c.	400 mg/250 mL		24		
d.	500 mg/500 mL			75	
e.	500 mg/250 mL		16		

CLINICAL ALERT

Remember that the difference between a microgram (mcg) and a milligram (mg) is "× 1000." The difference between drug per minute and hourly drug is "× 60."

The difference between mcg/kg/min and mcg/min is equal to "× the weight in kilograms." Manipulating these differences is critical for safe medication administration.

ANSWERS ON PAGE 424.

WORKSHEET
7C

Medication Doses Infusing in Existing Solutions

It is often necessary to verify the amount of drug being delivered in an existing solution. The amount of drug in the IV solution is frequently a milligram dose, whereas the amount of drug the patient is receiving is a microgram dose or a microgram/kilogram dose.

Note the example in Problem 1 and do the following in the remaining problems:

- Set up your TD : TV :: HD : HV ratio and determine mg/hr. Prove your answer.

- Move decimals to change milligrams to micrograms (×1000).

- Use a calculator to change hourly drug (HD) to drug/minute (divide by 60).

- Use a calculator to determine kilograms, and divide micrograms by kilogram weight to obtain mcg/kg/min.

Example

1. An IV of Drug X 100 mg in 1000 mL is infusing at 20 mL/hr. The physician asks, How many *mg/hr* is the patient receiving? How many *mcg/min*? How many *mcg/kg/min*? The patient weighs 143 lb today.
   a. TD : TV reduced ratio: 100 : 1000 = 1 : 10
   b. TD : TV :: HD : HV   1 mg : 10 mL :: 2 mg : 20 mL
   c. mg/hr: 2   **PROOF** 1 × 20 = 20
   d. mcg/hr: 2 × 1000 = 2000   10 × 2 = 20
   e. mcg/min: 2000 ÷ 60 = 33.3
   f. mcg/kg/min: 33.3 ÷ 65 kg = 0.5

2. An IV of Drug X 250 mg in 500 mL is infusing at 15 mL/hr. The patient weighs 110 lb today.
   a. TD : TV :: HD : HV reduced ratio: **PROOF**
   b. mcg/hr:
   c. mcg/min:
   d. mcg/kg/min:

3. An IV of Drug X 400 mg in 1000 mL is infusing at 5 mL/hr. The patient weighs 121 lb today.
   a. TD : TV :: HD : HV reduced ratio: **PROOF**
   b. mcg/hr:
   c. mcg/min:
   d. mcg/kg/min:

WORKSHEET
7C

Medication Doses Infusing
in Existing Solutions (Continued)

4. An IV of Drug X 1000 mg in 250 mL is infusing at 10 mL/hr. The patient weighs 132 lb today.
   a. TD : TV :: HD : HV reduced ratio: PROOF
   b. mcg/hr:
   c. mcg/min:
   d. mcg/kg/min:

5. An IV of Drug X 500 mg in 250 mL is infusing at 8 mL/hr. The patient weighs 175 lb today. (Calculate kilograms to nearest tenth.)
   a. TD : TV :: HD : HV reduced ratio: PROOF
   b. mcg/hr:
   c. mcg/min:
   d. mcg/kg/min:

WORKSHEET
7D

Critical Care IV Practice

Evaluate the following orders and infusions for safety. Use a calculator to determine kilogram weights to the nearest tenth. Change micrograms to milligrams, when applicable, by moving decimals. Use a calculator to determine the SDR when needed. Double check and label all calculations. Prove the hourly flow rate calculation. If requested, decide whether the order/infusion is:

1. Safe/Correct

2. Unsafe/Incorrect. Consult with physician.

Example   1. Ordered: Dopamine HCl (Intropin) 4 mcg/kg/min IV for a 110-lb patient. The literature states that the usual dose is 2 to 5 mcg/kg/min. Available: Dopamine 200 mg in 250 mL D5W.

a. Patient's weight in kg:	$110 \div 2.2 = 50$
b. SDR/min:	100 – 250 mcg/min
c. Is the order safe?	Yes. 4 mcg × 50 = 200 mcg/min.
	200 mcg/min is within the SDR
d. Hourly drug order in mcg:	12,000 (200 mcg × 60 min)
e. Hourly drug order in mg*:	12 (decimal moved 3 places to left)
f. TD : TV reduced ratio:	4 : 5 (200 mg : 250 mL)
g. Hourly flow rate to be set on infusion device:	12 mL/hr (4 : 5 : 12 : x)
	$4x = 60$
	$x = 15$ mL/hr

*Because the available drug (250 mg) is in mg, the hourly drug order must also be entered in mg.

Continued

ANSWERS ON PAGE 424

Critical Care IV Practice (Continued)

2. Ordered: Dobutamine HCl (Dobutrex) 5 mcg/kg/min IV for a 132-lb patient. Available: Dobutamine 250 mg in 250 mL D5W. The flow rate is currently infusing at 36 mL/hr.
   a. Patient's weight in kg:
   b. Hourly drug order in mcg:
   c. Hourly drug order in mg*:
   d. TD : TV reduced ratio:
   e. Hourly flow rate to be set on infusion device:
   f. Is current infusion correct?
   g. Evaluation and decision:

3. Ordered: Lidocaine 4 mg/min. Available: 1 g of lidocaine in 500 mL of D5W.
   a. TD : TV reduced ratio (mg : mL):
   b. Hourly drug ordered:
   c. Hourly flow rate to be set on infusion device:

4. Ordered: Isuprel (isoproterenol hydrochloride) 5 mcg/min. Available: Isoproterenol hydrochloride 1 mg in 250 mL D5W.
   a. TD : TV reduced ratio:
   b. Hourly drug ordered in mcg and in mg: PROOF
   c. TD : TV :: HD : HV ratio:
   d. Hourly flow rate to be set on infusion device:

5. Ordered: Initial infusion of norepinephrine at 50 mL/hr. Available: Norepinephrine 1 mg in 250 mL normal saline (NS). The SDR is 8 to 12 mcg/min initially.
   a. TD : TV :: HD : HV ratio:
   b. Hourly drug being infused in mg: PROOF
   c. Hourly drug order in mcg/hr:
   d. Hourly drug order in mcg/min:
   e. SDR for this patient:
   f. Evaluation and decision:

*Because the available drug (250 mg) is in mg, the hourly drug order must also be entered in mg.

CLINICAL ALERT
Document IVs carefully according to hospital policies. Consult the prescriber if the flow rate needs adjustment.

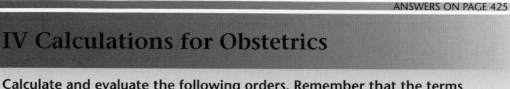

IV Calculations for Obstetrics

Calculate and evaluate the following orders. Remember that the terms must be the same in your TD : TV :: HD : HV ratio and proportion.

Example

1. Ordered: Magnesium sulfate 2 g/hr IV. Available: Magnesium sulfate 40 g/250 mL Ringer's lactate solution on an infusion device infusing at 13 mL/hr.
   a. TD : TV :: HD : HV   40̸ g : 250̸ mL :: 2 g : x mL
   b. mL/hr ordered (HV): $4x = 50$, $x = 12.5$ mL/hr
   c. mL/hr infusing: 13 mL/hr   **PROOF** $4 \times 12.5 = 50$
   d. Evaluation and decision: Rate is correct. $25 \times 2 = 50$

2. Ordered: Pitocin (oxytocin) 20 milliunits/min. Available: 1000 mL D5NS with 10 units of Pitocin (1000 milliunits = 1 unit). The IV is infusing at 100 mL/hr. (Hint: Change units to milliunits to obtain the total drug equivalent for the equation.)
   a. TD : TV reduced ratio:
   b. TD (milliunits) : TV :: HD (milliunits) : HV ordered:
   c. Evaluation and decision: **PROOF**

3. Ordered: Terbutaline 10 mcg/min for 30 min. Available: Terbutaline 5 mg in 500 mL/D5W.
   a. TD : TV reduced ratio:
   b. Hourly drug ordered in mcg:
   c. Hourly drug ordered in mg:
   d. TD : TV :: HD : HV ratio: **PROOF**
   e. Hourly flow rate to be set on infusion device:

4. Ordered: Magnesium sulfate 25 mL/hr. Call the doctor when 2 g have been infused. Available: 500 mL D5W with 20 g of magnesium sulfate on infusion device.
   a. TD (g) : TV reduced ratio in infusion:
   b. TD : TV :: HD : HV (existing infusion):   **PROOF**
   c. g/hr ordered at 25 mL/hr:
   d. Length of time 2 g to be infused:

5. Ordered: Pitocin (oxytocin) 2 milliunits/min. Available: 10 units Pitocin in 1000 mL of D5NS.
   a. milliunits/mL of Pitocin in IV container:
   b. TD : TV reduced ratio:
   c. Hourly drug ordered:
   d. TD : TV :: HD : HV ratio: **PROOF**
   e. Flow rate on infusion device to be set:

ANSWERS ON PAGE 425

More IV Practice Problems

Calculate and evaluate the following infusion problems.

1. Ordered: Esmolol hydrochloride at 39 mL/hr. Available: 5 g in 500 mL 5% D Ringer's lactated solution. The patient weighs 143 lb. The SDR is 50 to 200 mcg/kg/min.
   a. Patient's weight in kg:
   b. SDR for this patient in mcg/min:
   c. SDR in mg/hr:
   d. TD : TV :: HD : HV ratio ordered:
   e. Hourly drug delivered in mg:
   f. mg/min ordered:
   g. mcg/min ordered:
   h. mcg/kg/min ordered:
   i. Evaluation and decision:

2. Ordered: Nitroglycerin IV at 10 mcg/min. Available: Nitroglycerin IV 50 mg in 500 mL D5W. The infusion is flowing at 6 mL/hr.
   a. TD : TV :: HD : HV ratio ordered:
   b. Hourly drug ordered in mg:
   c. TD : TV :: HD : HV infusing
   d. mcg/min being delivered:
   e. Is flow rate correct?
   f. Evaluation and decision:

3. Ordered: Pronestyl (procainamide hydrochloride) at 50 mL/hr. Available: 1 g in 500 mL D5W. The SDR for maintenance is 1 to 6 mg/min.
   a. TD : TV :: HD : HV ratio:
   b. Hourly drug delivered in mg:
   c. mg/min ordered:
   d. Evaluation and decision:

4. Ordered: Nipride (sodium nitroprusside) at 0.3 mcg/kg/min. Available: 50 mg sodium nitroprusside in 250 mL NS. The infusion is flowing at 15 mL/hr. The patient weighs 220 lb.
   a. Weight in kg:
   b. Hourly drug ordered in mg:
   c. TD : TV :: HD : HV ratio ordered:
   d. TD : TV :: HD : HV ratio infusing:
   e. Hourly drug infusing in mg:
   f. Evaluation and decision:

5. Ordered: Cardizem (diltiazem hydrochloride) at 15 mg/hr. Available: Diltiazem hydrochloride 125 mg in 25 mL diluent to be added to 100 mL D5W. Infusion is flowing at 15 mL/hr.
   a. TD : TV :: HD : HV ratio:
   b. Evaluation and decision:

Direct IV (Bolus) Administration with a Syringe

Direct IV administration (IV push) is used to administer small amounts of diluted or undiluted medication over a brief period (seconds or minutes).

Medications such as meperidine, Dilantin, or furosemide may be prepared in a syringe and then delivered directly via a vein, an intermittent heparin lock, or the proximal port of an existing continuous IV.

Many of the medications that are administered in this manner must be diluted. A wide barrel (diameter) syringe such as a 5-mL or 10-mL syringe is preferred in order to reduce pressure during administration. Check agency policies for syringe sizes for flushes and other direct IV push medications.

It is crucial that the literature be consulted for safe-dose limits, rates of flow, dilutions, compatible solutions, and routes and that the patient's response be closely monitored during the administration and afterwards.

To reduce needlestick injuries, the trend is to use infusion systems with safety features (Figure 7-3).

There are two ways to time IV push medications for direct administration of medication through a syringe. Regardless of the method you select, the first step is always to calculate and prepare the correct volume.

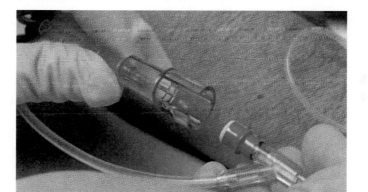

A

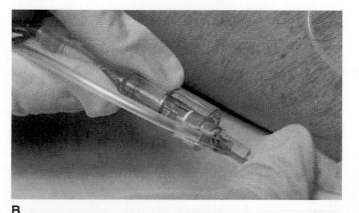

B

FIGURE 7-3   A, Shielded needle infusion system. **B,** Connection into an injection port. *(From Elkin MK, Perry AG, Potter PA: Nursing interventions and clinical skills, ed 4, St Louis, 2007, Mosby.)*

TIMING IV PUSH MEDICATIONS— METHOD 1 (mL PER MINUTE)

This method calculates the amount in milliliters to be slowly and gradually pushed over each minute.

Formula

$$TV \quad : \quad TM \quad :: \quad x \text{ mL} \quad : 1 \text{ min}$$
$$\text{Total volume} : \text{Total minutes} :: x \text{ volume (mL)} : 1 \text{ min}$$

Example Ordered: Digoxin 0.5 mg IV over 5 min. Dilute to 4 mL sterile water for injection.

$$TV : TM :: x \text{ mL} : 1 \text{ min}$$
$$4 \text{ mL} : 5 \text{ min} :: \text{ mL} : 1 \text{ min}$$

$$\frac{\cancel{5}}{\cancel{5}}x = \frac{4}{5}$$

$x = 0.8$ mL to be pushed slowly each minute

> **PROOF** $4 \times 1 = 4$
> $5 \times 0.8 = 4$

Schedule

1600 : 00	4 mL in syringe
1601	3.2 mL remaining
1602	2.4 mL remaining
1603	1.6 mL remaining
1604	0.8 mL remaining
1605	0 remaining

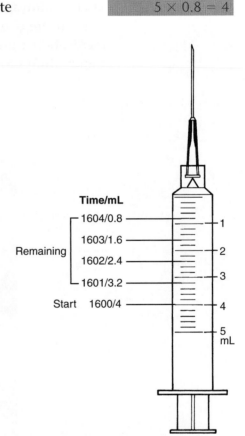

Time/mL
Remaining
1604/0.8 ——— 1
1603/1.6 ———
1602/2.4 ——— 2
1601/3.2 ——— 3
Start   1600/4 ——— 4
5 mL

The schedule above reflects a start time of 1600 hours. It is helpful to write your start time and a schedule of "markers" (increments of time and volume) when you need to push over several minutes. Write this before beginning to inject and have it in front of you to avoid errors caused by distraction.

Safety syringes and needleless syringes are being used to reduce needlestick injuries (Figure 7-4).

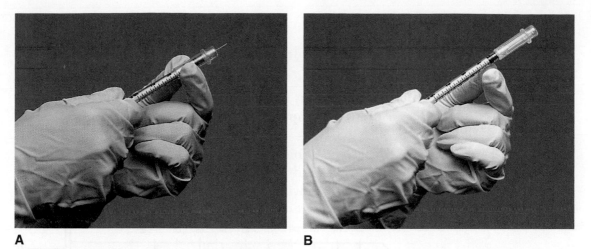

A   **B**

FIGURE 7-4   Needle with plastic guard to prevent needle sticks. **A,** Position of guard before injection. **B,** After injection, the guard locks in place, covering the needle. *(From Elkin MK, Perry AG, Potter PA: Nursing interventions and clinical skills, ed 4, St Louis, 2007, Mosby.)*

TIMING IV PUSH MEDICATIONS—
METHOD 2 (SECONDS PER CALIBRATION)

Many IV push medications have dilutions that permit 1 mL/min so that the timing is easy to maintain. Occasionally, when the timing is to be very slow and is not 1 mL/min, counting seconds per calibration permits more precise timing of the injection.

RULE   Divide the number of seconds of total time of administration by the number of calibrated increments in a syringe prepared with medication (lines on the syringe within each milliliter). This will yield the seconds per increment to be pushed.

Formula $\dfrac{\text{Total seconds}}{\text{Total increments}}$ = Seconds to deliver each increment

Example   Give 0.5 mg digoxin IV over 5 min. Directions say to dilute to 4 mL of sterile water for injection. There are 20 calibrations in 4 mL on this syringe.

$$\frac{300 \text{ seconds}}{20 \text{ calibrations (0.2 mL ea)}} = 1 \text{ calibration (0.2 mL) every 15 seconds}$$

Use the second hand on your watch and/or count each cycle (1 to 15) as you administer the medication, 1 calibration (0.2 mL) every 15 seconds.

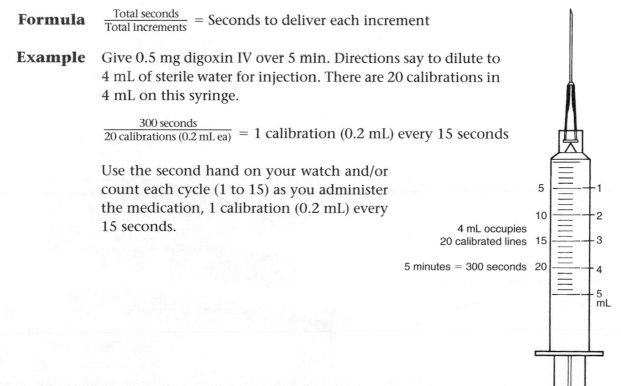

4 mL occupies
20 calibrated lines   15

5 minutes = 300 seconds   20

ANSWERS ON PAGE 426

WORKSHEET
7G

IV Push Calculations

Solve the following problems using the syringes shown to calculate the seconds per calibration, if applicable, and mL/min to be administered.

1. Ordered: 10% calcium chloride (10 mL) over 5 min.
   a. For how many seconds will you administer each calibration?
   b. How many mL/min will be injected?

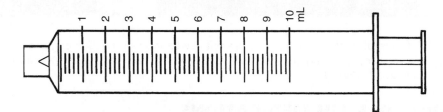

2. Ordered: Digoxin 0.5 mg IV over 10 min. (The literature specifies a minimum of 5 min for administration.) Available: Digoxin 250 mcg/mL.
   a. Total mL you will inject:
   b. Total seconds for injection:
   c. Seconds per calibration:
   d. mL/min to be injected:

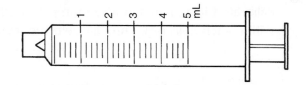

3. Ordered: Phenytoin sodium IV loading dose of 900 mg at 50 mg/min on an infusion device (Figure 7-5). Available: Phenytoin 100 mg/mL.
   a. Total mL to be injected:
   b. Total time for injection:
   c. mL/min to be administered:

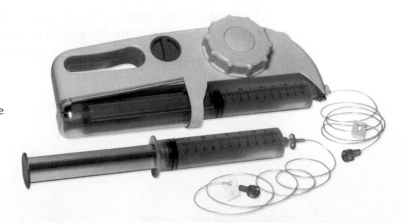

FIGURE 7-5 Freedom 60 syringe infusion device system. *(From Repro-med Systems, Inc., Chester, NY.)*

ANSWERS ON PAGE 426

WORKSHEET
7G

IV Push Calculations (Continued)

4. Ordered: Furosemide 20 mg IV undiluted over 2 min. Available: Furosemide 10 mg/mL.

   a. Total mL to be injected:

   b. Total time in seconds:

   c. Seconds per calibration:

   d. mL/min to be administered:

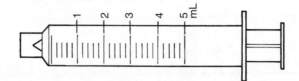

5. Ordered: Meperidine HCl 10 mg IV. The literature states that a single dose should be administered over 5 min and that the dose must be diluted to 5 mL with sterile water or normal saline for injection. Available: Meperidine 50 mg/mL.

   a. Total mL to be injected:

   b. Total time in seconds.

   c. Seconds per calibration:

   d. mL/min to be administered:

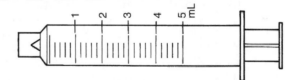

ANSWERS ON PAGE 426

Multiple-Choice Practice

Use a calculator. Estimate your answers for each applicable step in the mathematics. Establish the reduced total drug/total volume ratio for the infusions, move decimals to convert between micrograms and milligrams, and use logical shortcuts such as multiplying by 60 to change minutes to hours where applicable.

1. Ordered: Isoproterenol HCl IV at 5 mcg/min. How many mg/hr would be infused?
   a. 0.5 mg
   b. 50 mg
   c. 0.3 mg
   d. 300 mg

2. Available: Aminophylline 250 mg in 1000 mL of D5W. How many milligrams are in each milliliter of the IV solution (mg/mL)?
   a. 0.25 mg
   b. 0.5 mg
   c. 1 mg
   d. 4 mg

3. Available: 1 g of lidocaine in 500 mL of D5W. What is the total drug ratio to the total volume of IV solution?
   a. 2:1
   b. 4:1
   c. 1:2
   d. 1:4

4. Available: Norepinephrine 1 mg in 250 mL of NS. The SDR is 8 to 12 mcg/min initially. What is the minimum flow rate recommendation in mL/hr? *Hint: Change the SDR to milligrams after you obtain the SDR in mcg/hr so that you can compare milligrams to milligrams.*
   a. 48 mL/hr
   b. 60 mL/hr
   c. 120 mL/hr
   d. 480 mL/hr

5. Ordered: Furosemide 30 mg IV push over 2 min. Available: Furosemide 10 mg/mL. How many mL/min are to be administered?
   a. 0.5 mL/min
   b. 0.7 mL/min
   c. 1 mL/min
   d. 1.5 mL/min

ANSWERS ON PAGE 00

WORKSHEET 7H

Multiple-Choice Practice (Continued)

6. Ordered: Lanoxin IV push 0.5 mg over 5 min. Available: Lanoxin 250 mcg/mL. How many mL/min will be injected?
   a. 0.25 mL/min
   b. 0.4 mL/min
   c. 1 mL/min
   d. 1.5 mL/min

7. Procainamide hydrochloride is infusing at 40 mL/hr (per the prescriber order) for maintenance in an adult with an arrhythmia. Available: 1 g in 500 mL D5W. The SDR for maintenance is 1 to 6 mg/min. What decision will the nurse make?
   a. The order is within SDR. Proceed with the IV.
   b. The order is above the SDR. Hold the infusion and clarify with the physician.
   c. The order is below SDR. Start the infusion and consult with the physician.
   d. The order is unclear. Consult with a knowledgable colleague.

8. Ordered: Procainamide hydrochloride at 60 mg/hr on an infusion device. Available: 1 g in 1000 mL D5W. What flow rate in mL/hr will the nurse set?
   a. 30 mL/hr
   b. 60 mL/hr
   c. 100 mL/hr
   d. 120 mL/hr

9. Ordered: Magnesium sulfate 30 mL/hr. Call the physician when 3 g have been infused. Available: 500 mL D5W with 20 g of magnesium sulfate on an infusion device. In how much time will you expect to call the physician at this flow rate? *Hint: Determine how much drug per hour is infusing.*
   a. 30 min
   b. 1 hr 50 min
   c. 2 hr 30 min
   d. 3 hr

10. Ordered: Dobutamine HCl 2.5 mcg/kg/min for a 70-kg patient. Available: Dobutamine HCl IV concentration 500 mcg/mL. What flow rate will you set in mL/hr?
    a. 10 mL/hr
    b. 11 mL/hr
    c. 20 mL/hr
    d. 21 mL/hr

CRITICAL THINKING EXERCISES

1. During a bedside emergency for ventricular fibrillation, a physician called for several medications to be given by IV direct push. Also ordered were two IV sites to be maintained (one in each arm), one with D5W. As the orders were called out, one nurse prepared the medications and handed them to the nurse who was assisting, who then administered the medications. At one point, the nurse was handed two syringes of medication. She was told that one was bretylium tosylate and that the other syringe contained KCl 30 mEq. The KCl was administered undiluted to the patient by direct push, and the bretylium was placed in D5W.

   Error(s):

   Causes of error(s):

   Potential injuries:

   Nursing actions:

   Preventive measures:

2. A patient in the ICU weighing 60 kg was to receive an IV infusion of Dobutrex ordered to start at 3 mcg/kg/min. The nurse programmed the IV pump to infuse at 3 mg/kg/min.

   Error(s):

   Causes of error(s):

   Potential injuries:

   Nursing interventions:

   Recommendations for the patient safety committee to prevent this type of error:

CHAPTER 7 **Final**   ANSWERS ON PAGE 429

Solve the following problems using a calculator, moving decimals, reducing ratios, and labeling your answers. Prove your work.

Make a decision:

A. Safe to give

B. Unsafe; consult with physician

1. Ordered: Dobutamine HCl 5 mcg/kg/min. Available: Dobutamine HCl 2000 mcg/mL in an infusion device. Patient's weight is 50 kg.
   a. mcg/hr needed:
   b. Flow rate to be set on IV infusion device: _____ hr

2. Ordered: Potassium chloride 10 mEq to be administered to a 44-lb child with hypokalemia. Administer over 4 hr. Dilute in 100 mL of D5W. The literature states that the rate should not exceed 3 mEq/kg/24 hr for a child.

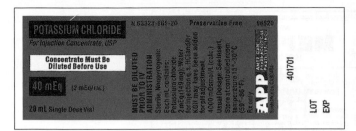

    a. Patient's weight in kg:
    b. SDR for this child per 24 hr:
    c. Total drug ordered:
    d. Decision (Safe/Unsafe):
    e. Amount of drug in mL to be added to IV (refer to label for mEq/mL):
    f. Hourly flow rate on infusion device in mL:

3. Ordered: Dopamine HCl at 2 mcg/kg/min. Infusing when you enter the room: Dopamine HCl at 15 mL/hr. Available: Dopamine HCl 400 mg/ 500 mL. Patient's weight is 80 kg.
    a. mg/hr needed:
    b. Actual mg/hr infusing:
    c. Flow rate ordered:
    d. Actual flow rate in mL/hr:
    e. Decision (correct or needs order for change):

4. Ordered: Dopamine IV at 4 mcg/kg/min for a patient in septic shock who weighs 110 lb today. The SDR is 2 to 10 mcg/kg/min. The IV solution contains 200 mg in 250 mL of solution. The IV is flowing at 15 mL/hr when you enter the room.

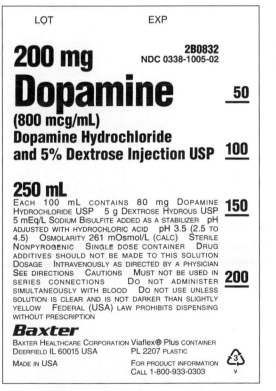

    a. Patient's weight in kg:
    b. SDR for this patient:
    c. Ordered drug rate/min:
    d. Decision (Safe/Unsafe):
    e. TD : TV ratio:
    f. mg/hr of drug ordered:
    g. Hourly flow rate needed:
    h. Decision (correct or needs order for change):

5. Ordered: Meperidine HCl 30 mg IV to be administered for pain at the rate of 10 mg/min. Must be diluted to at least 5 mL with sterile water for injection.

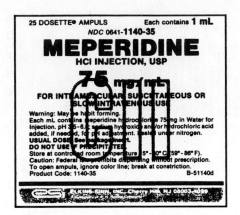

a. Total amount of meperidine to be prepared (in mL, round to nearest tenth):

b. Total amount of diluted volume to be administered in mL:

c. Total number of minutes for injection:

d. Use the syringe provided to calculate the number of seconds per calibration to be administered to nearest whole number of seconds:

e. Amount in mL/min to be administered gradually:

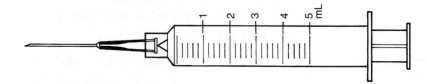

Refer to the Advanced Calculation section of the enclosed student CD-ROM for additional practice problems.

Parenteral Nutrition

Objectives

- Calculate grams of protein, dextrose, and lipids per order.
- Calculate the percentage of protein, dextrose, and lipids per infusion.
- Discuss the reasons that different concentrations of additives are used in peripheral and central lines.
- Calculate the percentage of additives per infusion.
- Calculate the kilocalories for protein, dextrose, and lipids per infusion.
- Calculate the total kilocalories per infusion.
- Compare the ordered amount of parenteral nutrition with the infusion label.

INTRODUCTION

The IV requirements for patients who are unable to ingest food are calculated on a daily basis. Concentrations of nutrients are calculated to show the differing strengths and percentages of additives for peripheral and central lines. The percentage of additives is calculated to ensure that the electrolyte and mineral requirements are being met. Standard orders for peripheral and central lines are compared. Medication administration records are discussed. The importance of parenteral orders and verification of the labels on the bag are stressed.

Total Parenteral Nutrition

Total parenteral nutrition (TPN) permits the venous administration of dextrose, amino acids, lipids, electrolytes, and vitamins to sustain life when the gastrointestinal system must be bypassed or during serious illness or injury (e.g., burns). A TPN bag is shown in Figure 8-1.

A routine maintenance IV solution of 1000 mL with 5% dextrose delivered over an 8-hour period provides approximately 200 calories derived from dextrose. If a patient is restricted from ingesting anything by mouth (npo) and receives 3 liters of D5W a day, the 600 total calories received would not be enough to promote or maintain health for a sustained period. In contrast, TPN may deliver as much as 1 cal/mL, depending on the concentration of nutrients.

TPN is administered via a central vein such as the subclavian or internal jugular. This is known as *central parenteral nutrition (CPN)*. Peripheral administration, known as *peripheral parenteral nutrition (PPN)*, is given via peripheral

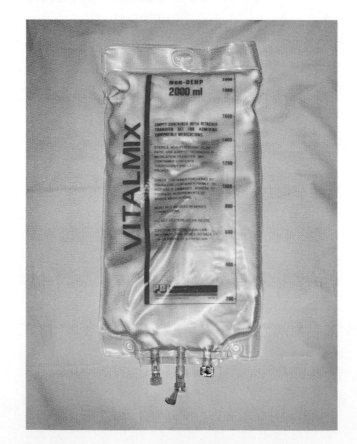

FIGURE 8-1 TPN bag. The content label is put on the bag by the pharmacist.

216

veins. The choice depends on the patient, the vein condition, and how long the patient will need the therapy. The larger central veins are selected for longer term therapy and higher concentrations of nutrients. The contents of TPN are customized according to the patient's condition and need, the venous route, relevant laboratory values, and the patient's weight. Orders for the contents may be changed daily.

PPN is used for nutritional therapy of 2 weeks or less. A PPN solution must be kept at the following concentration levels to prevent vein irritation: amino acids, 5.5%; dextrose, 10%; lipids, 10%. CPN permits high levels of concentration because it is infused into large veins. CPN solutions are hypertonic and have high osmolarity. CPN is used when nutrition therapy is needed for longer than 2 weeks. CPN maximum concentrations are as follows: amino acids, 8.5% to 10%; dextrose, 20% to 70%; lipids, 20%. Dextrose administered with amino acids spares the protein for tissue repair. Parenteral nutrition must always be administered by an infusion pump, **never** by gravity. There are many types of electronic delivery devices. Figure 8-2 shows two of them.

A three-in-one solution, or total nutrition admixture, combines lipids, amino acids, and dextrose. The solution is white because of the lipids, which make precipitation difficult to observe. The three-in-one solution is used for both hospital and home therapy. The lipids can also be administered separately (Figure 8-3). Lipids help control hyperglycemia, which is a complication of paren-

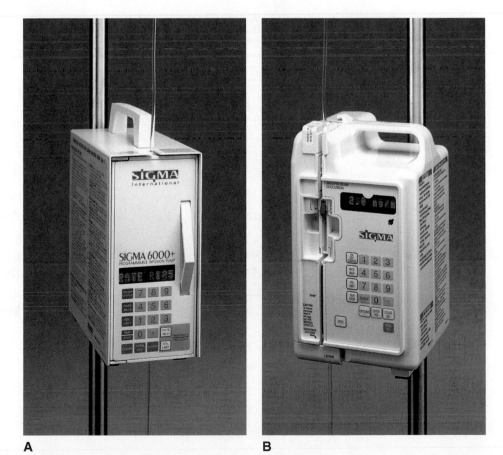

A   **B**

FIGURE 8-2   **A,** Sigma International 6000 programmable infusion device. **B,** Sigma 8000 automatic dose-related calculation device. *(From Sigma International, Inc., Medina, NY.)*

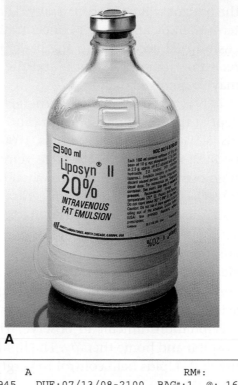

A

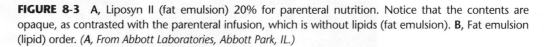

```
             A                    RM#:        (N ED )
RX# NO1922945   DUE:07/13/08-2100  BAG#:1  @: 16. ml/hr
-------------------------------------------------------
FAT EMULSIONS 20%            200ML

* CHANGE TUBING/BOTTLE EVERY 12 HOURS.
* INFUSE AT 17CC/HR X 12 HOURS DAILY.


PREP BY:____.RPH:____.07/13/08 at: ____. RX.MSALAR
  *** RETURN IV TO PHARMACY IF NOT USED IN 24 HOURS***
```

B

FIGURE 8-3 A, Liposyn II (fat emulsion) 20% for parenteral nutrition. Notice that the contents are opaque, as contrasted with the parenteral infusion, which is without lipids (fat emulsion). **B,** Fat emulsion (lipid) order. *(A, From Abbott Laboratories, Abbott Park, IL.)*

teral nutrition. Lipids are isotonic and can therefore be administered either peripherally or centrally. If a fat embolus could be a problem, monitor the patient closely.

The nurse's responsibility is to check the physician's order to determine if the pharmacy has filled the order according to the directions in Figure 8-4. Compare the order with the label (Figure 8-5).

Calculate grams, percentage of concentration, and kilocalories per bag of TPN.

Example   Refer to Figure 8-4, a sample physician's order form.

TPN ORDER SHEET

HOME HEALTH	DATE
PATIENT	ADDRESS

TPN FORMULA:

AMINO ACIDS: ☐ 5.5% ☐ 8.5% ☑ 10% ☐ WITH STANDARD ELECTROLYTES	*425* mL
DEXTROSE: ☐ 10% ☐ 20% ☐ 40% ☐ 50% ☑ 70% (check one)	*357* mL
LIPIDS: ☐ 10% ☑ 20% FOR ALL-IN-ONE FORMULA	*125* mL

FINAL VOLUME qsad STERILE WATER FOR INJECTION *400 mL*	*1307* mL

Calcium Gluconate	0.465 mEq/mL	*5* mEq
Magnesium Sulfate	4 mEq/mL	*5* mEq
Potassium Acetate	2 mEq/mL	mEq
Potassium Chloride	2 mEq/mL	mEq
Potassium Phosphate	3 mM/mL	*22* mM
Sodium Acetate	2 mEq/mL	mEq
Sodium Chloride	4 mEq/mL	*35* mEq
Sodium Phosphate	3 mM/mL	mM
TRACE ELEMENTS CONCENTRATE	☐ 4 ☐ 5 ☐ 6	mL

Patient Additives:

☐ MVC 9 + 3 10 mL Daily

☐ HUMULIN-R *10* units DAILY

☐ FOLIC ACID _____ mg
   _____ times weekly

☐ VITAMIN K _____ mg
   _____ times weekly

☐ OTHER: *MVI 12 10 mL/daily*

☐ OTHER: _____

Directions:

INFUSE: ☑ DAILY

☐ _____ TIMES WEEKLY

OTHER DIRECTIONS:

_____

_____

_____

_____

Rate: ☐ CYCLIC INFUSION: OVER _____ HOURS (TAPER UP AND DOWN)	" " "	☐ CONTINUOUS INFUSION: AT _____ mL PER HOUR	" "	☑ STANDARD RATE: AT *110* mL PER HOUR FOR *12* HOURS

LAB ORDERS:

☐ STANDARD LAB ORDERS
   SMAC-20, CO2, Mg+2 TWICE WEEKLY
   CBC WITH AUTO DIFF WEEKLY
   UNTIL STABLE, THEN:
   SMAC-20, CO2, Mg+2 WEEKLY
   CBC WITH AUTO DIFF MONTHLY

☐ OTHER: _____
_____
_____

VALIDATION:

_____
DOCTOR'S SIGNATURE

Print Name: _____

Office Address: _____

_____

Phone: _____

WHITE: Home Health   CANARY: Physician

FIGURE 8-4 Sample physician's order form for TPN. An example of the calculations is on page 220.

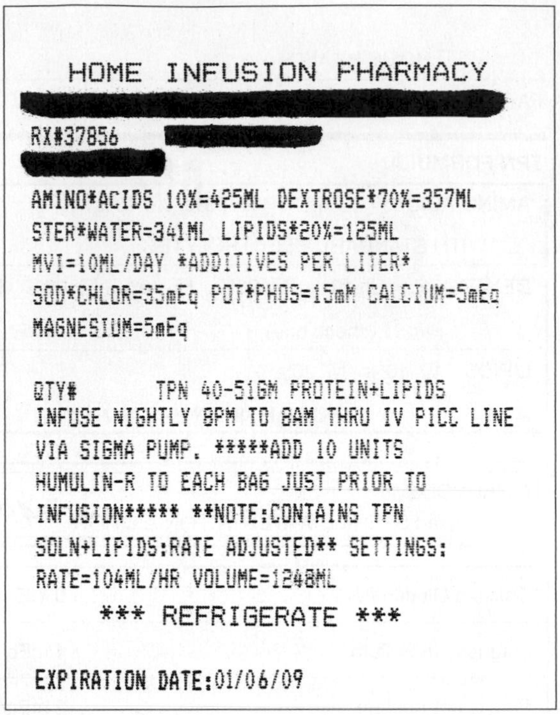

FIGURE 8-5 TPN bag label. It is the nurse's responsibility to check the label on the TPN bag with the physician's order. Quantities of nutrients and additives are calculated based on 1 liter. The total volume (TV) is calculated by adding the amount over 1 liter as a decimal (e.g., 1248 mL = 1.248 L).

```
      HOME  INFUSION  PHARMACY
    ▄▄▄▄▄▄▄▄▄▄▄▄▄▄▄▄▄▄▄▄▄▄▄▄▄▄▄▄
    RX#37856    ▄▄▄▄▄▄▄▄▄▄▄
    ▄▄▄▄▄▄▄▄▄▄▄

    AMINO*ACIDS 10%=425ML DEXTROSE*70%=357ML
    STER*WATER=341ML LIPIDS*20%=125ML
    MVI=10ML/DAY *ADDITIVES PER LITER*
    SOD*CHLOR=35mEq POT*PHOS=15mM CALCIUM=5mEq
    MAGNESIUM=5mEq


    QTY#       TPN 40-51GM PROTEIN+LIPIDS
    INFUSE NIGHTLY 8PM TO 8AM THRU IV PICC LINE
    VIA SIGMA PUMP. *****ADD 10 UNITS
    HUMULIN-R TO EACH BAG JUST PRIOR TO
    INFUSION***** **NOTE:CONTAINS TPN
    SOLN+LIPIDS:RATE ADJUSTED** SETTINGS:
    RATE=104ML/HR VOLUME=1248ML
          *** REFRIGERATE ***


    EXPIRATION DATE:01/06/09
```

TOTAL GRAMS PER BAG

Formula: % × mL = g/L

Step 1
Amino acids (AA) 10% in 425 mL

0.10 × 425 = 42.5 g/L

Formula: g/L × TV*/L = g/bag

Step 2
42.5 g/L × 1.307 TV/L = 55.5 g/bag

There are 55.5 g of AA in 1307 mL of TPN.

Shortcut method: % × mL = g/L × TV/L = g/bag

AA 10% in 425 mL

0.10 × 425 = 42.5 g/L × 1.307 TV/L = 55.5 g

To calculate the answer for g/L, multiply by the TV to determine the total g/bag.

There are 55.5 g of AA in 1307 mL of TPN.

Shortcut method: % × mL = g/L × TV/L = g/bag

Dextrose 70% in 357 mL

0.70 × 357 = 249.9 g/L × 1.307 TV/L = 326.6 g/bag

To calculate the answer for g/L, multiply by the TV to determine the total g/bag.

There are 326.6 g of dextrose in 1307 mL of TPN.

---

*TV, total volume.

Shortcut method: $\% \times mL = g/L \times TV/L = g/bag$

Lipids 20% in 125 mL

Step 1	Step 2

$0.20 \times 125 = 25 \text{ g/L} \times TV/L \; 1.307 = 32.68 \text{ g/bag}$

There are 32.68 g of lipids in 1307 mL.

PERCENTAGE OF CONCENTRATION PER BAG

Formula: $\frac{g/bag}{TV} = \%/bag$

AA $\frac{55.5}{1307} = 0.04246 = 4.25\%$ of bag is AA (PRO)

Dextrose $\frac{326.6}{1307} = 0.2498 = 25\%$ dextrose (CHO)

Lipids $\frac{32.8}{1307} = 0.02509 = 2.5\%$ lipids (FAT)

PERCENTAGE OF ADDITIVES

Formula:	Step 1	$mEq/L \times TV/L = mEq/bag$
	Step 2	$mEq/bag \div TV = \%$ in bag

Shortcut method:	$mEq/L \times TV/L \div TV = \%$ in bag
Calcium gluconate	$5 \text{ mEq} \times 1.307 \text{ TV} = 6.53 \text{ mEq/bag}$
	$6.53 \div 1307 = 0.00499 = 0.5\%$ in bag
Magnesium sulfate	$5 \text{ mEq} \times 1.307 = 6.53 \div 1307 = 0.5\%$ in bag
Potassium phosphate	$22 \text{ mEq} \times 1.307 = 28.75 \div 1307 = 2.2\%$ in bag
Sodium chloride	$35 \text{ mEq} \times 1.307 = 45.75 \div 1307 = 3.5\%$ in bag

A milliequivalent (mEq) is a measurement of weight that represents 1000th of a gram.

mL/hr TO SET THE PUMP

$$\frac{TV}{Total \; Time \; (hr)} = mL/hr \quad \frac{1307}{12} = 109 \; mL/hr$$

KILOCALORIES (kcal) PER BAG

Formula: $kcal/g \times g/bag = kcal/bag$

1 g CHO = 4 kcal	$326.6 \text{ g} \times 4 \text{ kcal} = 1306 \text{ kcal of CHO}$
1 g PRO = 4 kcal	$55.5 \text{ g} \times 4 \text{ kcal} = 222 \text{ kcal of PRO}$
1 g FAT = 9 kcal	$32.68 \text{ g} \times 9 \text{ kcal} = 294 \text{ kcal of FAT}$

Total kcal = 1822/bag of TPN

> ### ⬡ CLINICAL ALERT
>
> Begin TPN at a slow rate of 40 to 50 mL/hr and gradually increase by 25 mL/hr q6h to the ordered rate, according to hospital protocol. Maintain a steady rate of infusion (within 10% of the ordered dose) to reduce the chance of a sudden onset of hyperglycemia.

VALIDATION OF TPN LABEL WITH THE PHYSICIAN'S ORDER

Validate the contents listed on the TPN bag label (see Figure 8-5), with the physician's order (Figure 8-6).

The 341 mL of qsad (quantity sufficient additive) sterile water includes the volume for the additives of calcium gluconate, magnesium sulfate, potassium phosphate, sodium chloride, and multivitamins. In this order, the pharmacist included all of the additives (except for the 10 units of insulin, which the nurse will add immediately before administration).

Example Refer to Figure 8-6, a sample physician's order form.

1. $\dfrac{\% \text{ of AA} \times mL = g/L}{0.10 \times 425 = 42.50 \text{ g/L}} \rightarrow \dfrac{g/L \times TV/L = g/bag}{42.50 \times 1.248 = 53 \text{ g/bag}}$

$\dfrac{g/bag \div TV = \% \text{ of concentration}/bag}{53 \div 1248 = 4.25\% \text{ of concentration of AA/bag}}$

2. $\dfrac{\% \text{ of dextrose} \times mL = g/L}{0.70 \times 357 = 250 \text{ g/L}} \rightarrow \dfrac{g/L \times TV/L = g/bag}{250 \times 1.248 = 312 \text{ g/bag}}$

$\dfrac{g/bag \div TV = \% \text{ of concentration}/bag}{312 \div 1248 = 25\% \text{ of concentration of dextrose (CHO)/bag}}$

3. $\dfrac{\% \text{ of lipids} \times mL = g/L}{0.20 \times 125 = 25 \text{ g/L}} \rightarrow \dfrac{g/L \times TV/L = g/bag}{25 \times 1.248 = 31.2 \text{ g/bag}}$

$\dfrac{g/bag \div TV = \% \text{ of concentration}/bag}{31.2 \div 1248 = 2.5\% \text{ of concentration of lipids/bag}}$

Additives

$mEq/L \times TV/L = mEq/bag$ | $mEq/bag \div TV = \%/bag$

Calcium gluconate 5 mEq × 1.248 = 6.24 mEq/bag | 6.24 ÷ 1248 = 0.5%/bag

Magnesium sulfate 5 mEq × 1.248 = 6.24 mEq/bag | 6.24 ÷ 1248 = 0.5%/bag

Potassium phosphate 15 mEq × 1.248 = 18.72 mEq/bag | 18.72 ÷ 1248 = 1.5%/bag

Sodium chloride 35 mEq × 1.248 = 43.68 mEq/bag | 43.68 ÷ 1248 = 3.5%/bag

Remember to add the 10 units of regular insulin.

Kilocalories

Formula: **kcal/g × g/bag 5 kcal/bag**

1 kcal of PRO = 4 g	53 g of PRO × 4 = 212 kcal
1 kcal of CHO = 4 g	312 g of CHO × 4 = 1248 kcal
1 kcal of FAT = 9 g	31.2 g of FAT × 9 = 281 kcal

Total kcal = 1739/bag of TPN

TPN ORDER SHEET

HOME HEALTH

DATE

PATIENT

ADDRESS

TPN FORMULA:

AMIMO ACIDS: ☐ 5.5% ☐ 8.5% ☑ 10% ☐ WITH STANDARD ELECTROLYTES	mL *425*	
DEXTROSE: ☐ 10% ☐ 20% ☐ 40% ☐ 50% ☑ 70% (check one)	mL *357*	
LIPIDS: ☐ 10% ☑ 20% FOR ALL-IN-ONE FORMULA	mL *125*	

FINAL VOLUME qsad STERILE WATER FOR INJECTION *400 mL*	*1248* mL

Calcium Gluconate	0.465 mEq/mL	*5* mEq
Magnesium Sulfate	4 mEq/mL	*5* mEq
Potassium Acetate	2 mEq/mL	mEq
Potassium Chloride	2 mEq/mL	mEq
Potassium Phosphate	3 mM/mL	*15* mM
Sodium Acetate	2 mEq/mL	mEq
Sodium Chloride	4 mEq/mL	*35* mEq
Sodium Phosphate	3 mM/mL	mM
TRACE ELEMENTS CONCENTRATE	☐ 4 ☐ 5 ☐ 6	mL

Patient Additives:

☐ MVC 9 + 3 10 mL Daily

☐ HUMULIN-R _*10*_ units DAILY

☐ FOLIC ACID _____ mg
 _____ times weekly

☐ VITAMIN K _____ mg
 _____ times weekly

☐ OTHER: _*MVI 10 mL/daily*_

☐ OTHER: _____

Directions:

INFUSE: ☐ DAILY

☐ _____ TIMES WEEKLY

OTHER DIRECTIONS:

_____
_____
_____
_____

Rate: ☐ CYCLIC INFUSION:
 OVER _____ HOURS
 (TAPER UP AND DOWN) | ☐ CONTINUOUS INFUSION:
 AT _____ mL PER HOUR | ☑ STANDARD RATE:
 AT _*104*_ mL PER HOUR
 FOR _*12*_ HOURS

LAB ORDERS:

☐ STANDARD LAB ORDERS
 SMAC-20, CO2, Mg+2 TWICE WEEKLY
 CBC WITH AUTO DIFF WEEKLY
 UNTIL STABLE, THEN:
 SMAC-20, CO2, Mg+2 WEEKLY
 CBC WITH AUTO DIFF MONTHLY

☐ OTHER: _____
_____
_____

VALIDATION:

_____
DOCTOR'S SIGNATURE

Print Name: _____

Office Address: _____
_____

Phone: _____

WHITE: Home Health   CANARY: Physician

FIGURE 8-6 Sample physician's order form for TPN example calculation on page 222.

NURSING CONSIDERATIONS FOR TPN

- Patients receiving TPN must be monitored for hyperglycemia and serum potassium levels as well as for all electrolytes.
- The TPN and lipid administration set should be changed every 24 hours. When administering lipids only, change tubing every 12 hours.
- The TPN and lipid solutions should be refrigerated at 39° F or 4° C until time of administration.
- The fat emulsions filter should be a 1.2-micron size.
- TPN solutions should be filtered with a 0.22-micron filter.

RULE Always compare the order with the label to ensure correct percentage of nutritional elements.

CLINICAL ALERT

The admixture of fat emulsions with the dextrose and amino acids may produce bacterial growth. Discard the solution after 24 hours.

ANSWERS ON PAGE 430

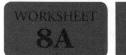

WORKSHEET 8A

Central Parenteral Nutrition Calculations

Use Figure 8-7 to answer the following questions.

1. What are the total grams per bag of:
   a. Amino acids (AA)
   b. Dextrose
   c. Lipids

2. What are the percentages of concentration per bag of:
   a. AA
   b. Dextrose
   c. Lipids

3. What are the percentages of concentration per bag of:
   a. Calcium gluconate
   b. Magnesium sulfate
   c. Potassium acetate
   d. Sodium chloride

4. How many kilocalories are there per bag of:
   a. CHO
   b. PRO
   c. FAT
   d. What is the total number of kilocalories per bag?

5. For how many mL/hr will you set the infusion device?

A sample MAR for parenteral nutrition is shown in Figure 8-8.

TPN ORDER SHEET

HOME HEALTH	DATE
PATIENT	ADDRESS

TPN FORMULA:

		mL
AMINO ACIDS: ☑ 5.5% ☐ 8.5% ☐ 10%		**400**
☐ WITH STANDARD ELECTROLYTES		
DEXTROSE: ☑ 10% ☐ 20% ☐ 40% ☐ 50% ☐ 70%		mL
(check one)		**350**
LIPIDS: ☑ 10% ☐ 20%		mL
FOR ALL-IN-ONE FORMULA		**200**

FINAL VOLUME qsad STERILE WATER FOR INJECTION *400 mL*	**1350** mL

Calcium Gluconate	0.465 mEq/mL	**5** mEq
Magnesium Sulfate	4 mEq/mL	**10** mEq
Potassium Acetate	2 mEq/mL	mEq
Potassium Chloride	2 mEq/mL	**20** mEq
Potassium Phosphate	3 mM/mL	mM
Sodium Acetate	2 mEq/mL	mEq
Sodium Chloride	4 mEq/mL	**30** mEq
Sodium Phosphate	3 mM/mL	mM
TRACE ELEMENTS CONCENTRATE	☐ 4 ☐ 5 ☐ 6	mL

Patient Additives:

☐ MVC 9 + 3 10 mL Daily

☐ HUMULIN-R _____ units DAILY

☐ FOLIC ACID _____ mg
 _____ times weekly

☐ VITAMIN K _____ mg
 _____ times weekly

☐ OTHER: _____

☐ OTHER: _____

Directions:

INFUSE: ☐ DAILY

 ☐ _____ TIMES WEEKLY

OTHER DIRECTIONS:

_____

_____

_____

_____

Rate: ☐ CYCLIC INFUSION: "   ☐ CONTINUOUS INFUSION: "   ☑ STANDARD RATE:
 OVER _____ HOURS   "   AT _____ mL PER HOUR   "   AT _____ mL PER HOUR
 (TAPER UP AND DOWN)   "   "   FOR **12** HOURS

LAB ORDERS:

☐ STANDARD LAB ORDERS
 SMAC-20, CO2, Mg+2 TWICE WEEKLY
 CBC WITH AUTO DIFF WEEKLY
 UNTIL STABLE, THEN:
 SMAC-20, CO2, Mg+2 WEEKLY
 CBC WITH AUTO DIFF MONTHLY

☐ OTHER: _____
_____
_____

VALIDATION:

_____
DOCTOR'S SIGNATURE

Print Name: _____

Office Address: _____

_____

Phone: _____

WHITE: Home Health   CANARY: Physician

FIGURE 8-7   Sample physician's order for Worksheet 8A.

			M	MEDICATION
Acct: Admitted: Att Phys: Diagnosis: Allergies:		MR#: Age: HT: WT:	A R	AMINISTRATION RECORD

Page: 3
From: 10/10/08 0730
Thru: 10/11/08 0730

Start Date/Time	Stop Date/Time	RN/ LPN	Medication	0731-1530	1531-2330	2331-0730
10/05/08 1800	11/04/08 1759		**PICC Line Flush** **(1 Inject)** **FLush** **Q12H** **IV** **#022** **Flush PICC Q 12 HRS with NS 10 ML** **when PICC line used for TPN**		1800	0600
10/09/08 1800	11/08/08 1759		**Amino Acid 8.5% 600 ML** **(600 ML)** **Dextrose 50% 600 ML** **(600 ML)** **Sodium Chloride CO 58 MEQ** **(14.5 ML)** **Potassium Acetate 12 MEQ** **(6 ML)** **Magnesium Sulfate 6 MEQ** **(1.5 ML)**		1800	
			Calcium Gluconate 6 MEQ **(12.84 ML)** **Infuvite Multivitamin 10 ML** **(10 ML)** **Trace Elements 1 ML** **(1 ML)** **Sodium Phosphate 26 MEQ** **(6.5 ML)** **Insulin Humulin Regu 21 units** **(0.21 ML)**			
			50 ML/HR **Q24H** **#047** **IV** **Central**			
			Store in Refrigerator			

The preprinted MAR from the pharmacy shows the contents of the TPN, the time it is to
be started and the times and amount of NS to be used to flush the Central and PICC Lines.
The nurse will initial next to the pre-printed time as well as initial and sign the bottom of
the MAR. The MAR is for 24 hours only.

Order Date	RN INIT.	Date/Time To Be Given	One Time Orders and Pre-Operatives Medication-Dose-Route	Actual Time Given	Site Codes			Dose Omission Code
					Arm	LA	RA	A = pt absent
					Deltoid	LD	RD	H = hold
					Ventrogluteal	LVG	RVG	M = med absent
					Gluteal	LG	RG	N = NPO
					Abdomen	LUQ	RUQ	O = other
					Abdomen	LLQ	RLQ	R = refused
								U = unable to tolerate

INIT	Signature	INIT	Signature

60321 (8/98)A   CHART

FIGURE 8-8   Sample medication administration record (MAR).

ANSWERS ON PAGE 430

WORKSHEET
8B

Peripheral Parenteral Nutrition Calculations

Use Figure 8-9 to answer the following questions.

1. What are the total grams per bag of:
   a. Amino acids (AA)
   b. Dextrose
   c. Lipids

2. What are the percentages of concentration per bag of:
   a. AA
   b. Dextrose
   c. Lipids

3. What are the percentages of concentration per bag of:
   a. Calcium gluconate
   b. Magnesium sulfate
   c. Potassium phosphate
   d. Sodium chloride

4. How many kilocalories are there per bag of:
   a. PRO
   b. CHO
   c. FAT
   d. What is the total number of kilocalories per bag?

5. For how many mL/hr will you set the infusion device?

TPN ORDER SHEET

HOME HEALTH

DATE

PATIENT

ADDRESS

TPN FORMULA:

AMINO ACIDS: □ 5.5% ☑ 8.5% □ 10% □ WITH STANDARD ELECTROLYTES	mL *500*
DEXTROSE: □ 10% □ 20% □ 40% ☑ 50% □ 70% (check one)	mL *500*
LIPIDS: ☑ 10% □ 20% FOR ALL-IN-ONE FORMULA	mL *250*

FINAL VOLUME qsad STERILE WATER FOR INJECTION	*1500* mL

Calcium Gluconate	0.465 mEq/mL	*5* mEq
Magnesium Sulfate	4 mEq/mL	*15* mEq
Potassium Acetate	2 mEq/mL	*8.3* mEq
Potassium Chloride	2 mEq/mL	mEq
Potassium Phosphate	3 mM/mL	*35* mM
Sodium Acetate	2 mEq/mL	mEq
Sodium Chloride	4 mEq/mL	*35* mEq
Sodium Phosphate	3 mM/mL	mM
TRACE ELEMENTS CONCENTRATE	□ 4 □ 5 □ 6	mL

Patient Additives:

□ MVC 9 + 3 10 ml Daily

□ HUMULIN-R *10* units DAILY

□ FOLIC ACID _____ mg
_____ times weekly

□ VITAMIN K _____ mg
_____ times weekly

☑ OTHER: *MVI 12 1.5mL/daily*

□ OTHER: _____

Directions:

INFUSE: ☑ DAILY

□ _____ TIMES WEEKLY

OTHER DIRECTIONS:

_____
_____
_____
_____

Rate: □ CYCLIC INFUSION:
OVER *12* HOURS
(TAPER UP AND DOWN)

□ CONTINUOUS INFUSION:
AT _____ mL PER HOUR

☑ STANDARD RATE:
AT _____ mL PER HOUR
FOR *12* HOURS

LAB ORDERS:

☑ STANDARD LAB ORDERS
SMAC-20, CO2, Mg+2 TWICE WEEKLY
CBC WITH AUTO DIFF WEEKLY
UNTIL STABLE, THEN:
SMAC-20, CO2, Mg+2 WEEKLY
CBC WITH AUTO DIFF MONTHLY

□ OTHER: _____
_____
_____

VALIDATION:

_____
DOCTOR'S SIGNATURE

Print Name: _____

Office Address: _____

_____

Phone: _____

WHITE: Home Health   CANARY: Physician

FIGURE 8-9 Sample physician's order form for Worksheet 8B.

ANSWERS ON PAGE 431

WORKSHEET
8C

Central Parenteral Nutrition Calculations

Refer to Figure 8-10 to answer the following questions. Use the formulas on pages 220 and 221.

1. Total grams per bag:
   a. How many total grams of amino acids (AA) are there per bag?
   b. How many total grams of dextrose are there per bag?

2. Percentage of concentrations per bag:
   a. What is the percentage of amino acids per bag?
   b. What is the percentage of dextrose per bag?

3. Percentage of additives per bag:
   a. Sodium chloride
   b. Potassium phosphate
   c. Potassium chloride
   d. Magnesium sulfate
   e. Calcium gluconate

4. Kilocalories per bag:
   a. AA
   b. CHO
   c. Total kcal

5. How many hours will it take for the contents of the parenteral nutrition bag to be infused?

Amino Acid 10%	(900 ML)
Dextrose 70%	(430 ML)
Sterile Water For Injection	(70 ML)
Sodium Chloride Conc 140 MEQ	(35 ML)
Potassium Phosphate 41 MEQ	(9.318 ML)
Potassium Chloride 43 MEQ	(21.5 ML)
Magnesium Sulfate 7 MEQ	(1.75 ML)
Calcium Gluconate 7 MEQ	(14.98 ML)
Insulin Humulin Regular 20 units	(0.2 ML)
Infuvite Multivitamin A 10 ML	(10 ML)

Total: 1492.748

** Continued **

DO NOT START AFTER 24 HOURS

Rate: 55 ml/hr   Freq: Q24H
Modified Central TPN
Hang Date/Time: 1800 11/19/08
Expir:
Init: DF
Refrigerate
Prep. By: /

DO NOT START AFTER 24 HOURS

FIGURE 8-10   Sample CPN label for Worksheet 8C. Notice that the three-in-one formula with lipids is not used. The time to hang the CPN is 1800 hours.

ANSWERS ON PAGE 432

WORKSHEET
8D

Peripheral Parenteral Nutrition Calculations

Refer to Figure 8-11 to answer the following questions. Use the formulas on pages 220 and 221.

1. Total grams per bag:
   a. Amino acids
   b. Dextrose

2. Percentage of concentrations per bag:
   a. Amino acids
   b. Dextrose

3. Percentage of additives per bag:
   a. Sodium chloride
   b. Potassium phosphate
   c. Potassium acetate
   d. Calcium gluconate
   e. Magnesium sulfate

4. Kilocalories per bag:
   a. AA
   b. CHO
   c. Total kcal

Amino Acid 8% (Hepatic)	(600 ML)
Dextrose 20%	(600 ML)
Sodium Chloride Conc 42 MEQ	(10.5 ML)
Potassium Phosphate 26 MEQ	(5.909 ML)
Potassium Acetate 10 MEQ	(5 ML)
Calcium Gluconate 6 MEQ	(12.84 ML)
Magnesium Sulfate 6 MEQ	(1.5 ML)
Infuvite Multivitamin A 10 ML	(10 ML)
Insulin Humulin Regular 24 units	(0.24 ML)

Total: 1245.989

** Continued **

DO NOT START AFTER 24 HOURS

Rate: 50 ml/hr   Freq: Q24H
Peripheral
Hang Date/Time: 1800 11/19/08
Expir:
Init: MM

Prep. By: /_____

DO NOT START AFTER 24 HOURS

FIGURE 8-11 Sample PCN label for Worksheet 8D. Peripheral central line is to be infused at 1800 hours.

5. How many hours will it take for the contents to be infused?

ANSWERS ON PAGE 433

WORKSHEET
8E

Multiple-Choice Practice

1. Have: CPN solution with 8.5% AA in 375 mL. The total volume (TV) is 1500 mL. How many grams of protein are in the solution?
   a. 50 g/bag   b. 77.7 g/bag   c. 62 g/bag   d. 47.8 g/bag

2. What is the percentage of concentration of grams per bag of the AA in question 1?
   a. 4.6%   b. 3%   c. 8.2%   d. 4.7%

3. Have: CPN solution with 40% dextrose in 400 mL. The TV is 1450. How many grams of dextrose are in the solution?
   a. 232 g/bag   b. 130 g/bag   c. 160 g/bag   d. 260 g/bag

ANSWERS ON PAGE 433

WORKSHEET
8E

Multiple-Choice Practice (Continued)

4. What is the percentage of concentration per bag for dextrose in question 3?
   a. 18%   b. 16%   c. 160%   d. 180%

5. Have: A three-in-one TPN solution with 20% lipids in 175 mL. The TV is 1200 mL. How many grams of lipids are in the solution?
   a. 42 g/bag   b. 48 g/bag   c. 52 g/bag   d. 36 g/bag

6. What is the percentage of concentration of grams per bag for lipids in question 5?
   a. 2.7%   b. 3.5%   c. 5.6%   d. 7%

7. Have: Calcium gluconate additive of 6 mEq/L. The TV of the TPN is 1350 mL. What is the percentage of calcium gluconate in the bag?
   a. 0.3%   b. 1%   c. 0.4%   d. 0.6%

8. Have: Magnesium sulfate additive 10 mEq/L. The TV is 1258 mL. What is the percentage of magnesium sulfate in the bag?
   a. 1%   b. 10.2%   c. 1.8%   d. 11%

9. Have: Potassium acetate 12 mEq/L. The TV is 1385 mL. What is the percentage of potassium acetate in the bag?
   a. 2.2%   b. 3.6%   c. 1.2%   d. 2.6%

10. The TV of the parenteral nutrition (PN) solution is 1275 mL. The infusion rate is 110 mL/hr. The infusion is started at 1800 hr. What time will it be completed?
    a. 0659 hr   b. 0459 hr   c. 0535 hr   d. 0345 hr

CRITICAL THINKING EXERCISES

Your patient, Mary Braun, is receiving peripheral parenteral nutrition (PPN). On assessment, she complains that the IV site burns. When the site is checked, the solution is infusing well and is infusing at the correct rate. The label on the solution is 8.5% amino acids and 70% dextrose.

Error(s):

Causes of error(s):

Nursing interventions:

Preventive measures:

Discussion
What will your first action be?
Why are the percentages of amino acids and dextrose important?
What is the percentage difference?

CHAPTER 8 **Final**

ANSWERS ON PAGE 433

Calculate and solve the following problems using a calculator, moving decimals, reducing ratios, and labeling your answers. Prove your work.*

1. A TPN order reads amino acids 8.5% in 550 mL. The total volume of the TPN infusion is 1430 mL.
   a. How many grams of AA will the patient receive through the central line?
   b. How many kilocalories of protein will the patient receive?

2. A TPN order reads dextrose 10% in 475 mL.
   a. How many grams of dextrose will be infused?
   The total volume is 1550 mL in the peripheral line.
   b. How many kilocalories of dextrose will the patient receive?

3. A PPN order reads: Amino acids 5% in 350 mL. The TV is 1280 mL.
   a. How many grams of AA will the patient receive?
   b. How many kilocalories of protein will the patient receive?

4. The TPN order reads: Dextrose 40% in 400 mL. The TV is 1325 mL.
   a. How many grams of dextrose will the patient receive?
   b. How many kilocalories of carbohydrate will the patient receive?

5. The TPN formula has potassium chloride 4 mEq. The TV is 1250 mL.
   What is the percentage of potassium chloride in the bag?

6. The parenteral nutrition formula has 25 mEq of sodium chloride (NaCl).
   The TV of the bag is 1425 mL.
   What is the percentage of NaCl in the bag?

7. A TPN solution has 48 g of protein, 255 g of carbohydrate, and 38.6 g of fat.
   How many total kilocalories will the patient receive?

8. A three-in-one TPN solution has lipids 20% in 110 mL. The TV is 1145 mL.
   a. How many grams of lipids will the patient receive?
   b. How many kilocalories of fat will the patient receive?

9. The TPN of 1420 mL is to start at 1800 hr. The rate is 108 mL/hr.
   What time will the infusion be completed?

10. A TPN of 1320 mL is infusing at 120 mL/hr.
    How many hours will it take to infuse?

---

*It may be acceptable to withdraw small amounts of large-volume IV solutions equal to the number of milliliters of drug to be added so as to simplify calculations and flow rates. Follow your hospital's policy.

Insulin

Objectives

- Identify sites for insulin injections.
- Identify the different types of insulin.
- Compare the actions of fast-, intermediate-, and long-acting insulins.
- Read calibrations on 30-, 50-, and 100-unit insulin syringes.
- Prepare single- and mixed-dose insulin injections.
- Calculate units of insulin based on CHO grams.
- Interpret the sliding scale using the BMBG method.
- Calculate IV insulin for units/hr and mL/hr and duration.
- Use electronic intravenous devices to administer insulin dosages.
- Analyze medication errors using critical thinking.

Insulin

Insulin is an aqueous solution of the principal hormone of the pancreas. Insulin affects metabolism by allowing glucose to leave the blood and enter the body cells, preventing hyperglycemia.

Diabetes Mellitus

Diabetes mellitus is a deficiency of insulin and is classified according to cause. In type 1, which usually affects people before the age of 30, the pancreatic beta cells do not produce insulin. Insulin injections must be taken every day to control blood glucose levels.

The onset of type 2 diabetes usually occurs after 30 years of age; however, obesity has contributed to a rise in the diagnosis of type 2 diabetes in children and young adults. The pancreas produces *some* insulin but not enough to metabolize the glucose. In some cases, the insulin that is produced is not effective; this is known as *insulin resistance.* Of people with diabetes, 95% have type 2, and 40% of people with type 2 diabetes take insulin injections in conjunction with oral diabetes medications.

The most common complication of insulin therapy is hypoglycemia. This may be caused by injecting too much insulin (a risk in home care), by missing or delaying meals, or by being involved in more physical activity than usual. To treat hypoglycemia, a patient should always carry sugar in some form. The treatment of choice, if the patient can swallow, is glucose tablets (4 to 5 g carbohydrate [CHO] per tablet). A glucose gel of 15 g is also available for the treatment of hypoglycemia. If the blood glucose level gets very low, unconsciousness may occur. At that point, the patient will need a glucagon injection. Emergency kits are available for home use (Figure 9-1).

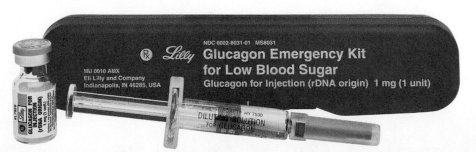

FIGURE 9-1 Glucagon emergency kit for home use. *(Copyright Eli Lilly and Company. All rights reserved. Used with permission.)*

Injection Sites

The abdomen is the preferred site for insulin injections. When insulin injections are required on a daily basis, it is important to rotate within that site (Figure 9-2). The abdomen absorbs insulin more rapidly and is safer as an injection site than the upper arm, back, or thigh. If use of the abdomen is medically contraindicated, alternative sites may be used.

Types of Insulin

The source of insulin is either human or animal. This is known as the *species* of the insulin. Human insulin is manufactured to be the same as insulin produced by the body. Human insulin is made in one of two ways:

- By recombinant DNA technology, a chemical process used to produce unlimited amounts of human insulin; or
- By a process that chemically changes animal insulin into human insulin.

Humalog insulin (lispro) is recombinant DNA insulin with a rapid action of 5 to 15 minutes, allowing patients to dose and eat.

Recombinant DNA insulins cause fewer allergies than those from animal sources.

All insulin is supplied in units denoting strength. Insulin is given via special insulin syringes (Figure 9-3) and pens (Figure 9-4). Figure 9-5 shows examples of the different types of cartridges used with insulin pens. Attached needles are usually 24- to 26-gauge with a $\frac{5}{16}$- or $\frac{1}{2}$-inch needle. There is also an inhaled form of insulin (Exubera), as shown in Figure 9-6.

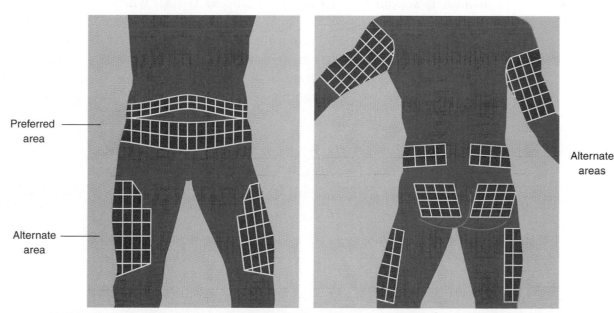

Preferred area

Alternate area

Alternate areas

FIGURE 9-2   Insulin injection areas. *(Copyright Eli Lilly and Company. All rights reserved. Used with permission.)*

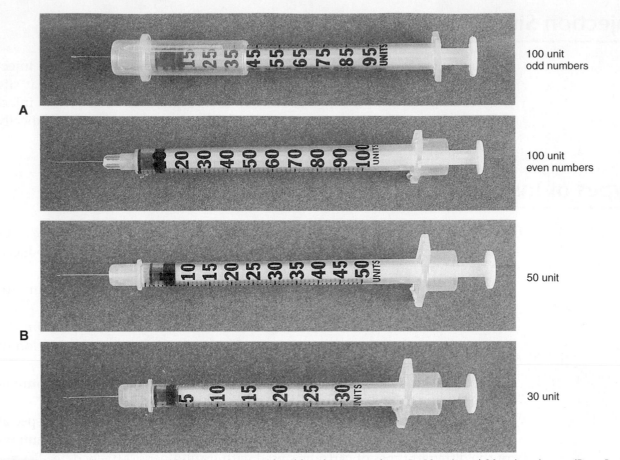

FIGURE 9-3 Insulin syringes. **A**, 100-unit syringes with odd and even numbers. **B**, 50-unit and 30-unit syringes. *(From Becton, Dickinson, and Company, Franklin Lakes, NJ.)*

Insulin is supplied in 10 mL vials labeled U-100, which means there are 100 units/mL (Figure 9-5). Insulin is also supplied in 10 mL vials of U-500, which means there are 500 units/mL. This strength is used for those whose blood glucose levels fluctuate to very high levels. This type of insulin is rarely used. Table 9-1 lists the duration of activity of various types of insulins and other injectables. See examples of various U-100 insulins on pages 241 and 242.

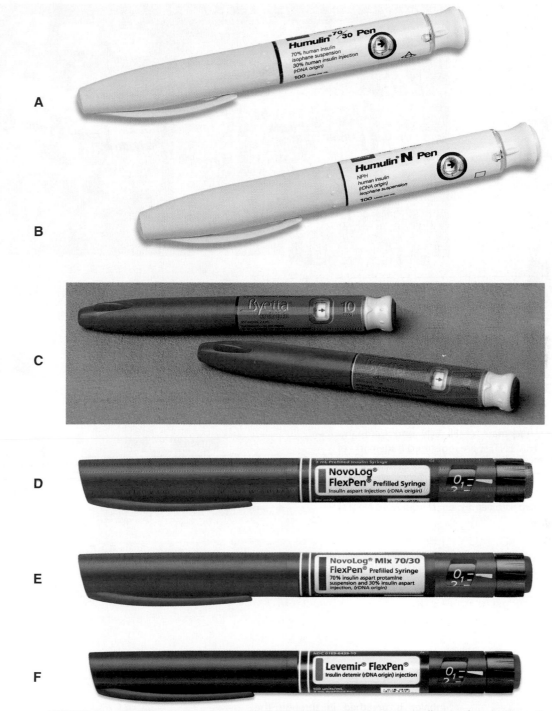

FIGURE 9-4 Prefilled insulin pens. **A,** Humulin 70/30 short- and intermediate-acting. **B,** Humulin N intermediate-acting. **C,** Incretin mimetic. **D,** Novolog® rapid-acting. **E,** Novolog® 70/30 short- and intermediate-acting. **F,** Levemir® long-acting. *(A and B, Copyright Eli Lilly and Company. All rights reserved. Used with permission. **C,** From Amylin Pharmaceuticals, Inc., San Diego, CA. **D-F,** From Novo Nordisk Inc., Princeton, NJ.)*

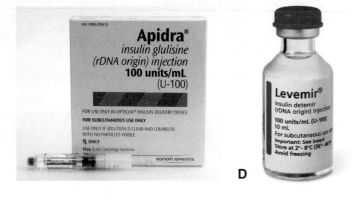

FIGURE 9-5 **A,** Lantus (insulin glargine). The Lantus vial is taller and narrower than the NPH, Regular, and Humalog vials. Lantus is written in purple letters. **B,** Insulin vials and cartridges used in insulin pens. HUMULIN® L LENTE® and HUMULIN® U ULTRALENTE® have been discontinued and are not longer available. Please see www.lillydiabetes.com for more information. HUMULIN® is a registered trademark of Eli Lilly and Company. LENTE® and ULTRALENTE® are registered trademarks of Novo Nordisk Pharmaceuticals. **C,** Rapid-acting Apidra. **D,** Long-acting Levemir. *(A and C from Sanofi Aventis U.S. Inc., Bridgewater, NJ. B, Copyright Eli Lilly and Company. All rights reserved. Used with permission. D from Novo Nordisk Inc., Princeton, NJ.)*

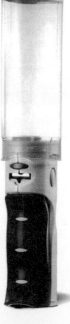

FIGURE 9-6 Insulin from an Exubera inhaler is breathed in through the mouth. Exubera is a short-acting insulin that is taken at mealtimes to replace injected insulin. Blood sugar must still be monitored when taking Exubera. *(Permission granted by Pfizer Inc.)*

TABLE 9-1   Insulins and Other Injectables for Diabetes Management

Type	Onset	Peak	Duration	Appearance	When to Take	Mixed with
Insulins						
Rapid-acting						
Aspart or Novolog	5-15 min	1-3 hr	3-5 hr	Clear	15 min	NPH
Lispro or Humalog	15 min	1-2 hr	3-4 hr		before	
Glulisine or Apidra	15 min	1-2 hr	3-4 hr		a meal	
Short-acting						
Regular	30-60 min	2-4 hr	6-8 hr	Clear	30 min before a meal	NPH
Intermediate-acting						
NPH	1-4 hr	4-10 hr	10-16 hr	Cloudy	30 min before a meal	Regular, rapids
Long-acting						
Glargine or Lantus	1-2 hr	Peakless	Up to 24 hr 5-23 hr	Clear	At bedtime	**Do not mix**
Detemir or Levemir	$1\frac{1}{2}$ hr	6-8 hr	(dose dependent)	Clear	At supper or bedtime	**Do not mix**
Short- and intermediate-acting						
70/30	1-4 hr	2-4 hr and again 6-10 hr	3-4 hr and 10-16 hr	Cloudy	30 min before a meal	Already mixed
50/50						
Rapid- and intermediate-acting						
75/25	15 min- 4 hr	1-2 hr and 6-10 hr	3-4 hr and 10-16 hr	Cloudy	15 min before a meal	Already mixed
70/30 Novolog Mix	15 min- 4 hr	30-90 min and 6-10 hr	4-5 hr and 10-16 hr	Cloudy	15 min before a meal	Already mixed
Inhaled						
Exubera Inhaler 1 and 3 mg blister packs (1 mg dose is approximately equal to 3 units of rapid-acting insulin)	15 min	1-2 hr	5-6 hr	Tablet	15 min before a meal	Use with mouthpiece

Continued

TABLE 9-1   Insulins and Other Injectables for Diabetes Management—cont'd

Brand Name	Generic Name	Dosing	Action	When to Take
Other				
Symlin	Pramlintide acetate	Given subcutaneously. Prefilled pen. Titrate starting at 15 mcg to 60 mcg. (Reduce the rapid- or short-acting insulin by 50%.)	This is a synthetic version of human Amylin, a hormone co-secreted with insulin by the beta cells in the pancreas. Works with insulin to help maintain normal glucose concentrations. It has three actions: (1) helps control blood glucose levels by reducing the postmeal release of glucose from the liver; (2) slows the absorption of carbohydrate by slowing the rate of stomach emptying; (3) reduces appetite.	Is taken with meals or snacks when more than 30 g of carbohydrates are eaten.
Byetta	Exenatide	Given subcutaneously. Prefilled pen. 5 mcg × 1 month, then 10 mcg	This is a new class of drugs called incretin mimetics. These drugs mimic the action of gut hormones that stimulate the release of insulin in response to increased blood glucose levels. These drugs work by slowing the emptying of the stomach, suppressing the release of glucose from the liver after eating, and stimulating the beta cells of the pancreas to produce more insulin when blood glucose levels rise. They also reduce food intake, thus decreasing body weight.	Within 60 min before breakfast and the evening meal

NPH, Neutral protamine Hagedorn. (From Lee Wiysel, RN, CDE, Diabetes Education Specialist, The John C. Lincoln North Mountain Campus.)

Types of U-100 Insulins

RAPID-ACTING

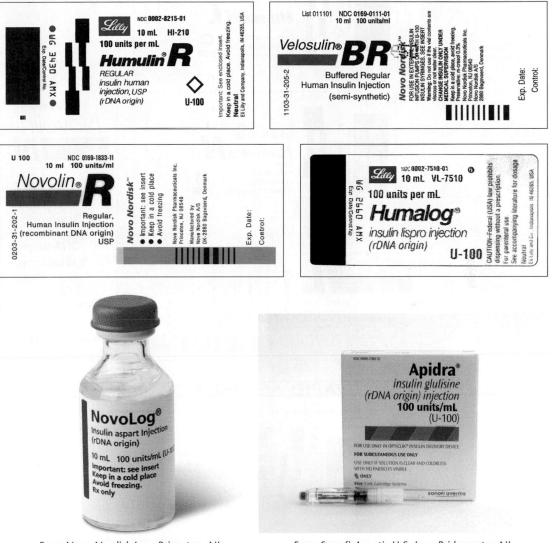

From Novo Nordisk Inc., Princeton, NJ.   *From Sanofi-Aventis U.S. Inc., Bridgewater, NJ.*

> ### ⬢ CLINICAL ALERT
>
> Regular insulin should always be clear. Discard if unclear.
>
> Mix insulins only with those of the same name because they may have differ-ing amounts of preservatives. For example, Humulin R should be combined only with Humulin L or N. Humulin is a brand name.

INTERMEDIATE-ACTING

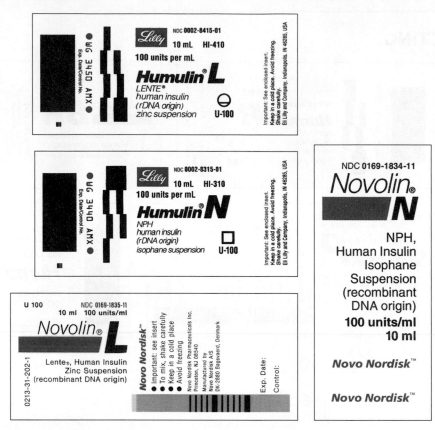

INTERMEDIATE- AND RAPID-ACTING MIXTURES

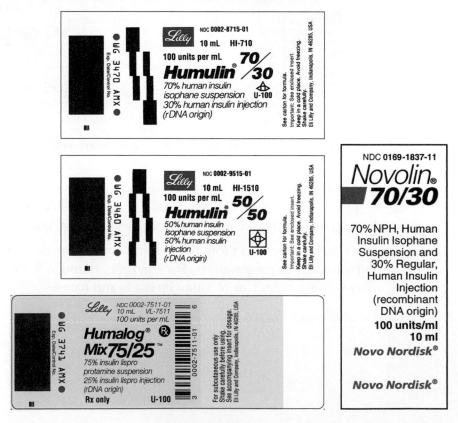

The insulin combination of NPH and Regular is used to give a 24-hour effect.

In 1 mL of Humulin 70/30, there are 70 units of intermediate-acting insulin and 30 units of rapid-acting insulin. In 1 mL of Humulin 50/50, there are 50 units of intermediate-acting insulin and 50 units of rapid-acting insulin.

Note: Mix before administration by rolling *gently* between the palms. Never shake because this creates bubbles.

CLINICAL ALERT

Insulin comes in various strengths (e.g., U-100 and U-500). Read labels carefully to avoid giving the wrong strength.

LONG-ACTING

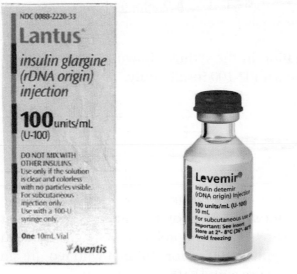

From Novo Nordisk Inc., Princeton, NJ.

CLINICAL ALERT

Lantus must NOT be mixed in the same syringe with any other insulin or be diluted. It is NOT intended for IV administration. Caution: Lantus is clear like Regular Humalog. Lantus is given anytime for 24-hour coverage without a peak. Consistency in administration is necessary.

Insulin Syringes

Insulin is usually given in a 1 mL or 0.5 mL insulin syringe calibrated to U-100 insulin. The 0.5 mL insulin syringe is used for smaller doses because the calibrations are larger and easier to read. The most commonly used insulin syringes are 50- and 100-unit syringes, as shown in Figure 9-3.

TYPES OF U-100 INSULIN SYRINGES

Each calibration in the syringe shown in Figure 9-7 represents 1 unit. This syringe is used for small doses of 50 units or less and is used with U-100 insulin only. Needles are usually 24 to 26 gauge for subcutaneous injections. Clip-on magnifiers for syringes are available to enlarge the calibrations and numbers.

FIGURE 9-7 50-unit syringe.

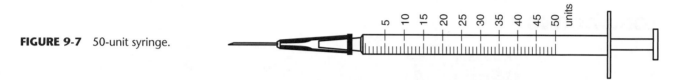

Each calibration in the syringe shown in Figure 9-8 equals 2 units. This syringe is for use with U-100 insulin only.

FIGURE 9-8 100-unit syringe.

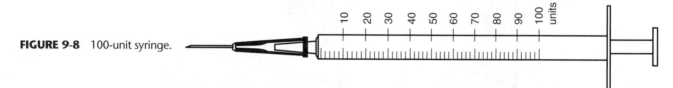

Each calibration in the syringe shown in Figure 9-9 represents 1 unit. This syringe is used for small doses of 30 units or less as a safety feature for people with diabetes who have vision problems (a Magni-Guide may also be useful for those people [Figure 9-10]) or for children who require small doses of insulin. This syringe is for use with U-100 insulin only.

FIGURE 9-9 30-unit syringe.

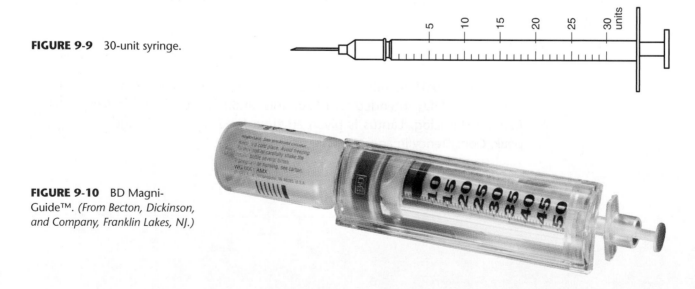

FIGURE 9-10 BD Magni-Guide™. *(From Becton, Dickinson, and Company, Franklin Lakes, NJ.)*

Insulin Orders

A typical order for insulin must include the following:

A. The *name* of the insulin: Humulin, Novolin, Lantus.

B. The *type* of the insulin: regular, lispro, aspart, N, detemir, or glargine.

C. The *number* of units or amount the patient will receive: 10 units.

D. The *time* to be given: AM, $\frac{1}{2}$ hr before a meal.

E. The *route* is subcutaneous unless IV is specified.

Example   Prepare 30 units of Humulin R insulin subcutaneously $\frac{1}{2}$ hr before a meal. Using a 100 unit syringe, 50 unit syringe, or 30 unit syringe fill the syringe to the 30 units calibration (Figure 9-11). (All insulins come in U-100 so orders no longer specify U-100.)

> ## ⬡ CLINICAL ALERT
>
> Units must be spelled out (not abbreviated by a U) because this can be a source of medication errors (e.g., mistaking the U for a zero).

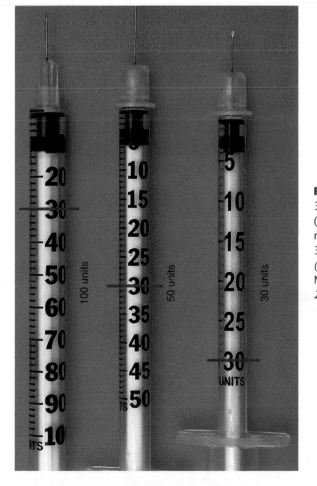

FIGURE 9-11   From left to right: 30 units measured on a 100 unit syringe (each calibration is 2 units), a 50 unit syringe (each calibration is 1 unit), and a 30 unit syringe (each calibration is 1 unit). *(From Macklin D, Chernecky C, Infortuna H. Math for clinical practice, ed 1, St Louis, 2005, Mosby.)*

ANSWERS ON PAGE 434

WORKSHEET
9A

Single-Dose Measures

Read the syringes and write your answers in the spaces provided.

1. Units measured: _____

2. Units measured: _____

3. Units measured: _____

4. Units measured: _____

5. Units measured: _____

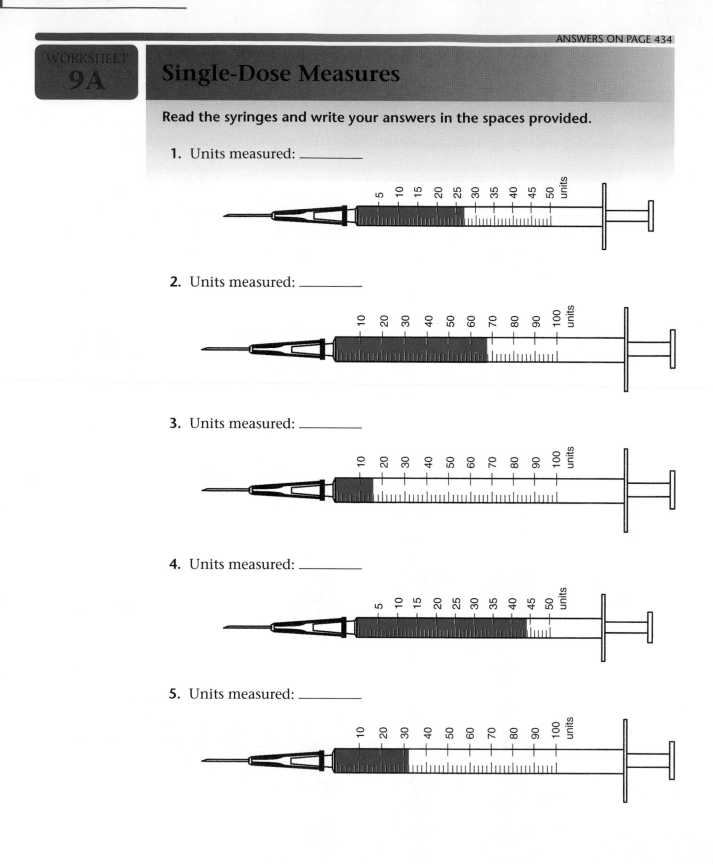

ANSWERS ON PAGE 434

WORKSHEET
9A

Single-Dose Measures (Continued)

6. Units measured: _____

7. Units measured: _____

8. Units measured: _____

9. Units measured: _____

10. Units measured: _____

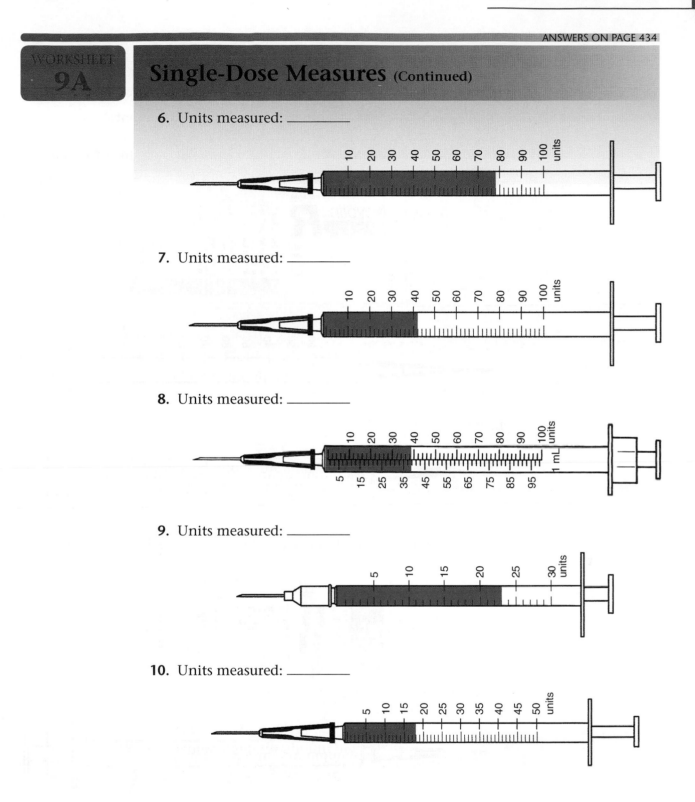

ANSWERS ON PAGE 434

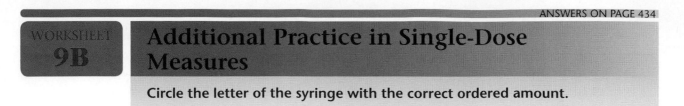

WORKSHEET 9B

Additional Practice in Single-Dose Measures

Circle the letter of the syringe with the correct ordered amount.

1. Ordered: 12 units of Novolin Regular subcutaneous 30 min before a meal.

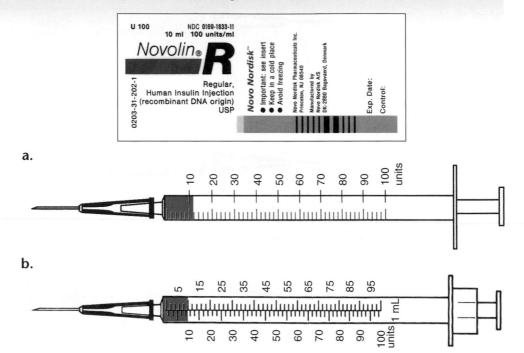

a.

b.

2. Ordered: 6 units of Humulin Regular subcutaneous $\frac{1}{2}$ hr before a meal.

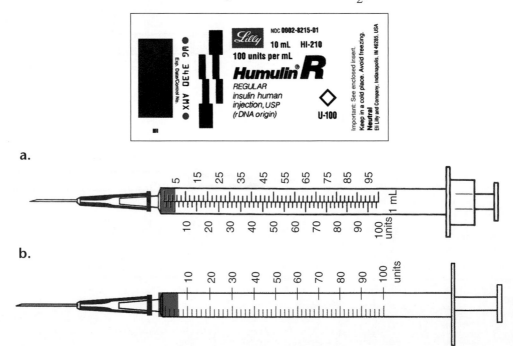

a.

b.

ANSWERS ON PAGE 434

WORKSHEET 9B

Additional Practice in Single-Dose Measures (Continued)

3. Ordered: 13 units of Humulin NPH subcutaneous at 1100 hr.

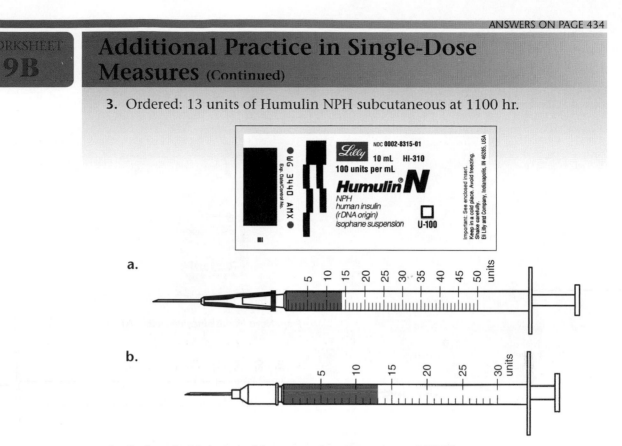

4. Ordered: 12 units of Lantus subcutaneous at 2200 hr.

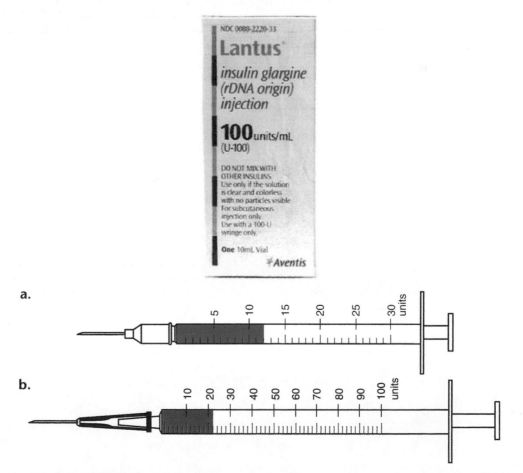

Continued

ANSWERS ON PAGE 434

WORKSHEET 9B

Additional Practice in Single-Dose Measures (Continued)

5. Ordered: 40 units of detemir subcutaneous at 0930.

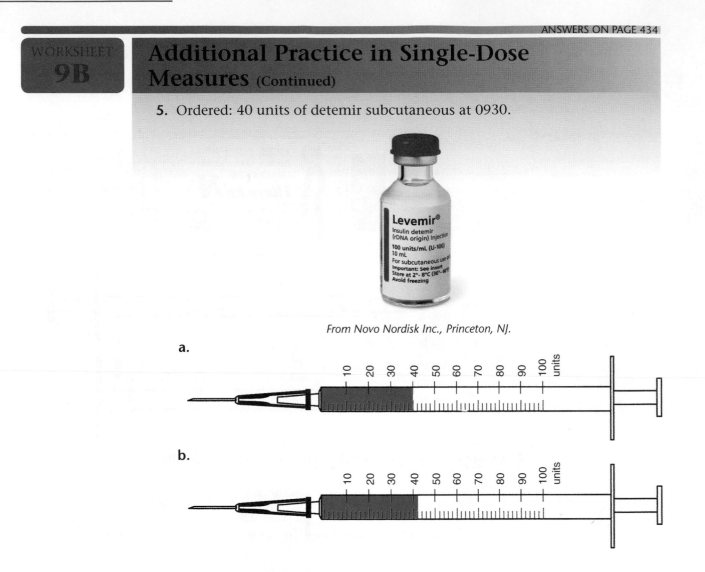

From Novo Nordisk Inc., Princeton, NJ.

a.

b.

Mixing Insulin

Insulin dosages are drawn up *exactly* as ordered. An incorrect dosage could be devastating to the patient. Frequently, regular or rapid-acting insulin is combined with an intermediate-acting insulin. This gives insulin coverage (glucose control) within 15 to 60 minutes and lasts 10 to 16 hours. This technique of combining the two types of insulin is important for the nurse, patient, and family to master. The regular insulin vial should *not* be contaminated with the longer-acting insulin; therefore, the regular insulin should be drawn up first. The mixing procedure is illustrated in Figures 9-12 and 9-13.

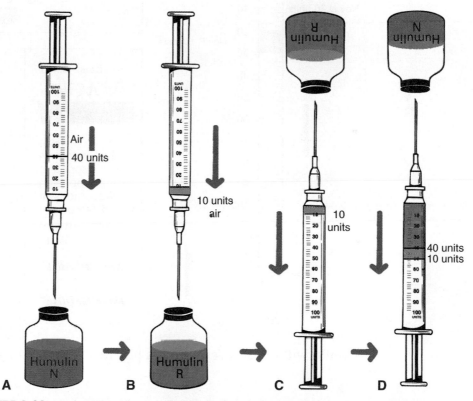

FIGURE 9-12   Order: Give 10 units of Humulin R and 40 units of Humulin N via subcutaneous injection. **A,** Inject 40 units of air into Humulin N first. Do **not** allow needle to touch insulin. Withdraw needle. **B,** Inject 10 units of air into Humulin R. **C,** With needle still in place, invert vial and withdraw 10 units of R. Withdraw needle. **D,** Insert needle into vial of Humulin N, invert vial and withdraw 40 units. Total amount in syringe equals 50 units.

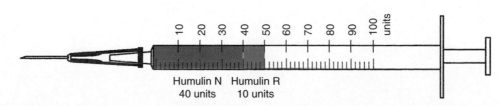

FIGURE 9-13   100-unit syringe showing the mixing of two insulins. Remember: clear to cloudy when drawing up insulins.

Example Ordered: 10 units of Novolin Regular and 20 units of Novolin N.
Total units: 30 units
Source: DNA and DNA
Which insulin will you draw up first? *Regular* (see Figure 9-12)

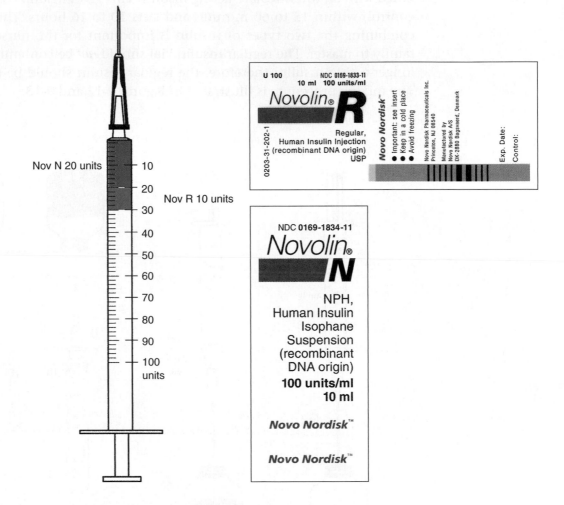

Nov N 20 units

Nov R 10 units

U 100   NDC 0169-1833-11
10 ml   100 units/ml

Novolin® **R**

Novo Nordisk™

Regular,
Human Insulin Injection
(recombinant DNA origin)
USP

● Important: see insert
● Keep in a cold place
● Avoid freezing

Novo Nordisk Pharmaceuticals Inc.
Princeton, NJ 08540

Manufactured by
Novo Nordisk A/S
DK-2880 Bagsvaerd, Denmark

Exp. Date:

Control:

0203-31-202-1

NDC 0169-1834-11

Novolin®
N

NPH,
Human Insulin
Isophane
Suspension
(recombinant
DNA origin)

**100 units/ml
10 ml**

Novo Nordisk™

Novo Nordisk™

Insulin will not stay separated as pictured in the syringe.

CLINICAL ALERT

Draw up regular insulin first before N is added (see Figure 9-12).

Regular insulin should not be contaminated with Humulin N or any N insulin. A multiple-dose vial of regular insulin can be used for IV infusion, and contamination with intermediate-acting insulin could be fatal.

ANSWERS ON PAGE 434

WORKSHEET
9C

Mixing Insulin

Calculate the total number of units in the following problems. Circle the letter of the syringe with the correct amount.

1. Ordered: 10 units of Humalog and 38 units Humulin N $\frac{1}{2}$ hr before breakfast. Total units: _____

   a.

   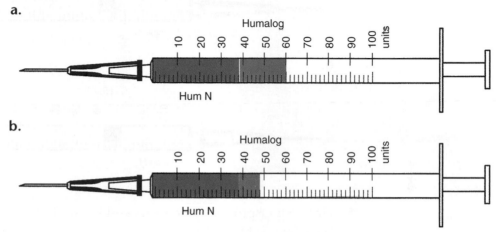

   b.

2. Ordered: Humalog R 14 units and Humulin N 25 units.
   Total units: _____

   a.

   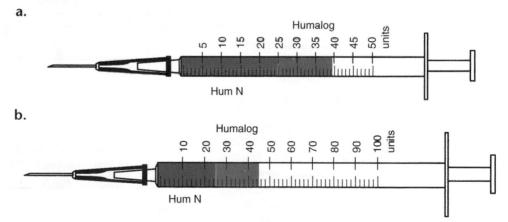

   b.

3. Ordered: Novolin R 8 units and Novolin N 15 units. Total units: _____

   a.

   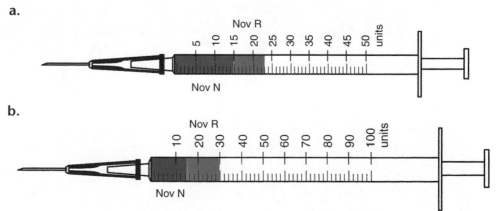

   b.

Continued

ANSWERS ON PAGE 434

WORKSHEET
9C

Mixing Insulin (Continued)

4. Ordered: Novolin 8 units and Novolin N 30 units. Total units: _____

a.

b.

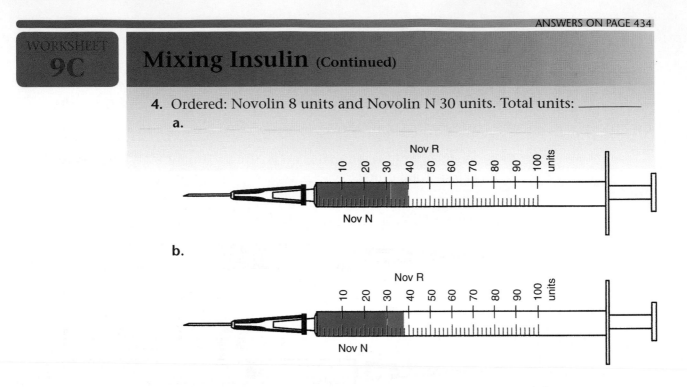

5. Ordered: Lispro insulin 8 units and Humulin N 60 units $\frac{1}{2}$ hr before breakfast. Total units: _____

a.

b.

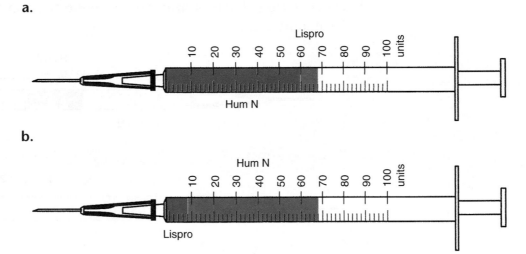

ANSWERS ON PAGE 434

WORKSHEET 9C

Mixing Insulin (Continued)

Shade in insulin dose on syringe. All orders are for U-100 insulin.

6. Ordered: 15 units of Novolog at 0830 before breakfast. Available: Novolog (aspart). How many units will you administer? When will it peak?

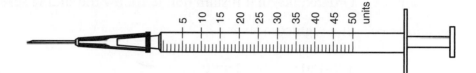

7. Ordered: 10 units of Apidra before meals. Available: Aprida U-100. How many units will you give? When will the action begin (onset)?

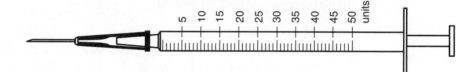

8. Ordered: Fixed combination of 70/30, 44 units daily. Available: Fixed 70/30. How many units will you give? When will it peak? What is the duration?

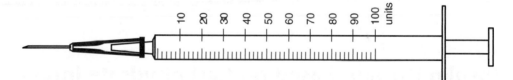

9. Ordered: Novolin R 10 units and Novolin N 40 units subcutaneous every AM $\frac{1}{2}$ before meals. How many total units will you give? What is the duration?

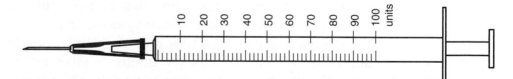

10. Ordered: Humulin R insulin 12 units and Humulin N 30 units every AM before breakfast. How many total units will you give? When will this peak? What is the duration?

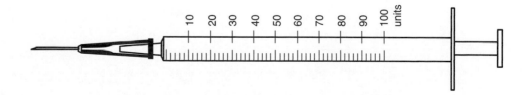

Sliding-Scale Calculations

Insulin administered according to a sliding scale is predicated on the type of diabetes, insulin resistance, weight, age, renal status, and activity level. Blood glucose levels determine how much insulin to give. Blood glucose readings may be taken several times a day to determine daily insulin requirements. Sliding scales can vary greatly because they are individualized.

Example   Ordered: Regular insulin q6h to follow the sliding scale.

Sliding Scale   Blood glucose level

0-100	No coverage
100-150	2 units
151-200	4 units
201-250	6 units
251-300	8 units
301-above	Call physician

For a blood glucose level above 425, give 15 units regular insulin stat and call physician. Repeat blood glucose measurement 4 hr after it peaks.

At 1700 hr, the patient's blood glucose level was 280 mg/dL. How much insulin should be given? Shade the amount in the syringe.

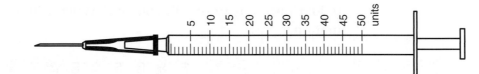

Insulin Dosage Based on Carbohydrate Intake

Because blood glucose levels fluctuate during the day, insulin doses should also fluctuate rather than being a constant dose every day. In order to keep the blood glucose level as close to the desired range as possible, carbohydrate intake must be calculated for each meal based on current blood glucose levels. This technique produces a more constant glucose level, which will help to minimize the detrimental effects of wide variations in blood glucose levels during the day. However, blood glucose levels must be taken before each meal and at bedtime. Usually, an insulin pump is used. If the carbohydrate ratio is high, the insulin pump can provide a bolus dose.

The health care provider will set the parameters because they are individualized for each patient, depending on metabolic needs.

Example   Based on blood glucose level (BGL) and carbohydrate (CHO) intake.
- Desired blood glucose level is 130 mg/dL
- Order: Give 1 unit of insulin for every 20 mg/dL above 130 mg.
   Give 1 unit of insulin for every 10 g of CHO consumed.

Lunch
- $\frac{3}{4}$ cup of potato salad   21 g
- 2 slices of whole wheat bread   42 g
- 2 slices of Swiss cheese   2 g
- 2 slices of ham   2 g
- Mustard   1 g
- 1 12 oz can of Pepsi   42 g
- Total   109 g CHO

Step 1

Desired BGL is 130 mg/dL. The BSL before lunch was 145 mg/dL. The difference between 130 and 145 is 15. The order states to give 1 unit of insulin for each 15 mg/dL above the desired 130 mg/dL. Therefore, 1 unit of insulin is required to treat the blood glucose level.

R & P Formula	**Easy Method**
15 mg : 1 unit :: 15 mg: x units	Divide the BGL difference by the order.
$15x = 15$	15 divided by 15 = 1 unit
$x = 1$ unit	

Step 2

Total CHO for lunch is 109 g
Order: give 1 unit of insulin for each 10 g of CHO consumed.

R & P Formula	**Easy Method**
10 g : 1 unit :: 109 g : x units	Divide the total grams of CHO by the order.
$10x = 109$	109 divided by 10 = 10.9 = 11 units
$x = 10.9 = 11$ units	
Round to nearest whole number	

Give: 1 unit because the blood glucose level is above 15 g and give 11 units for the amount of CHO consumed. Give a total of 12 units of insulin.

ANSWERS ON PAGE 435

WORKSHEET
9D

Insulin Dosage Based on CHO Intake

Use the following order to answer questions 1, 2, and 3. Round answers to the nearest whole number. Calculate the total number of insulin units required on the basis of the BGL and the CHO intake.

Ordered: BGL of 130 mg/dL is desired.

Give 1 unit of insulin for each 10 mg above 130 mg.

Give 1 unit of insulin for every 8 g of CHO consumed.

1. Breakfast   BGL is 150 mg/dL
   $\frac{3}{4}$ cup Total cereal   CHO = 23 g
   8 oz low-carb milk   3 g
   $\frac{1}{2}$ cup blueberries   1 g
   1 slice wheat toast   21 g
   1 pat butter   0 g
   1 cup black coffee   0 g
   Total units _____

2. Lunch   BGL is 135 mg/dL
   8 oz yogurt   CHO = 25 g
   $\frac{1}{3}$ cup dried cranberries   33 g
   2 apple slices   1 g
   5 grapes   1 g
   5 saltines   11 g
   Plain ice tea   0 g
   Total units_____

3. Dinner   BGL is 145 mg/dL
   1 pork chop   CHO = 0 g
   $\frac{3}{4}$ cup mashed potatoes   34 g
   $\frac{3}{4}$ cup broccoli   0 g
   8 oz plain ice tea   0 g
   Total units_____

   Bedtime snack   BGL is 145 mg/dL
   $\frac{3}{4}$ cup lowfat ice cream   CHO = 15 g
   Total units_____

ANSWERS ON PAGE 435

WORKSHEET 9D

Insulin Dosage Based on CHO Intake (Continued)

Use the following order to calculate the total insulin units in questions 4 and 5.

Ordered: The desired BGL is 140 mg/dL

Give 1 unit of insulin for every 10 mg above 140 mg/dL.

Give 1 unit of insulin for every 10 g of CHO consumed.

4. Breakfast   BGL is 135 mg/dL
   2 eggs   CHO = 1 g
   2 slices wheat toast   42 g
   2 slices bacon   0 g
   2 cups black coffee   0 g
   Total units _____

5. Lunch   BGL is 160 mg/dL
   4 oz hamburger patty   CHO = 0 g
   1 hamburger bun   28 g
   $\frac{1}{2}$ cup cole slaw   20 g
   1 small serving fries   45 g
   Total units _____

ANSWERS ON PAGE 435

WORKSHEET 9E

Insulin Dosage Based on Blood Glucose and CHO Intake

Calculate the insulin requirements in questions 1, 2, and 3. The BGL readings and CHO requirements are based on the following orders. Mark each syringe with the total dose required.

Ordered: Give 1 unit of insulin for every 20 mg BGL above 160 mg/dL.
Give 1 unit of insulin for every 15 g of CHO consumed.

1. BGL is 190 mg/dL; 98 g of CHO were consumed.
   How many total units of insulin are required?

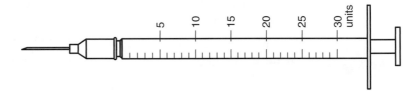

2. BGL is 210 mg/dL; 118 g of CHO were consumed.
   How many total units of insulin are required?

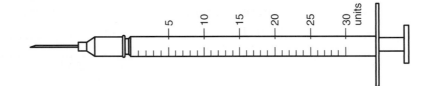

3. BGL is 180 mg/dL; 40 g of CHO were consumed. How many total units of insulin are required?

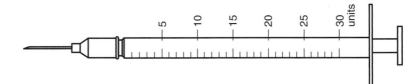

ANSWERS ON PAGE 435

WORKSHEET 9E

Insulin Dosage Based on Blood Glucose and CHO Intake (Continued)

Calculate the total insulin requirements in questions 4 through 7. The BGL reading and CHO requirements are based on the following orders. Mark each syringe with the total dose required.

Ordered: Give 1 unit of insulin for every 30 mg BGL above 150 mg/dL.
Give 1 unit of insulin for every 10 g of CHO consumed.

4. BGL is 240 mg/dL; 58 g of CHO were consumed. How many total units of insulin are required?

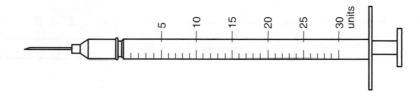

5. BGL is 180 mg/dL; 120 g of CHO were consumed. How many total units of insulin are required?

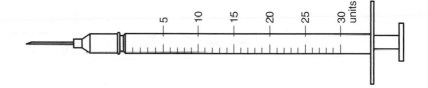

6. BGL is 260 mg/dL; 58 g of CHO were consumed. How many total units of insulin are required?

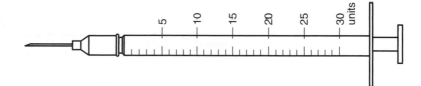

7. BGL is 160 mg/dL; 28 g of CHO were consumed. How many total units of insulin are required?

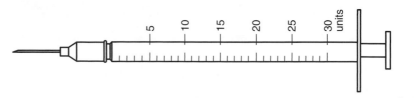

Continued

ANSWERS ON PAGE 435

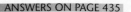

WORKSHEET
9E

Insulin Dosage Based on Blood Glucose and CHO Intake (Continued)

Calculate the total insulin requirements for questions 8, 9, and 10. The BGL and CHO requirements are based on the following orders. Mark each syringe with the total dose required.

Ordered: Give 1 unit of insulin for every 20 mg BGL above 130 mg/dL.
Give 1 unit of insulin for every 8 g of CHO consumed.

8. BGL is 140 mg/dL; 45 g of CHO were consumed. How many total units of insulin are required?

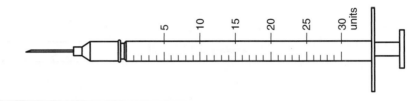

9. BGL is 160 mg/dL; 80 g of CHO were consumed. How many total units of insulin are required?

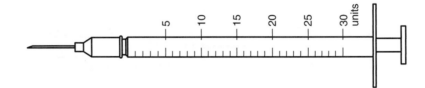

10. BGL is 120 mg/dL; 85 g of CHO were consumed. How many total units of insulin are required?

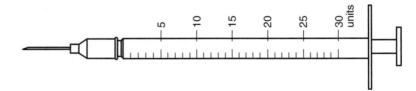

Estimating Insulin-to-Carbohydrate Ratio

This formula is based on estimates of insulin needs according to CHO intake and weight. It is a simple formula that gives estimates for categories of weight based on Table 9-2. Also given is the kilogram ratio for the same number of pounds. Table 9-2 is used to compute all of the problems on Worksheet 9F.

Example Breakfast = 44 CHO. The patient's weight is 165 lb. Refer to Table 9-2. The ratio is 1 unit of insulin to 11 g of CHO consumed.

R & P Method

Total grams of CHO (Divided by) unit-to-CHO Ratio = Insulin Needs

1 unit : 11 CHO :: x units : 44 CHO   or   44 (divided by) 11 = 4 units

$11x = 44$

$x = 4$ units of R insulin

TABLE 9-2 Insulin Units Required Based on CHO Intake and Weight

Weight in Pounds	Weight in Kg	Unit: grams of CHO
100-109	45.5-49.5	1:16
110-129	50-58.6	1:15
130-139	59-63.2	1:14
140-149	63.6-67.7	1:13
150-159	68.2-72.3	1:12
160-169	72.7-76.8	1:11
170-179	77.3-81.4	1:10
180-189	81.8-85.9	1:9
190-198	86.4-90	1:8
200-239	90.9-108.6	1:7
240+	109.1+	1:6

ANSWERS ON PAGE 436

Insulin Dosage Based on CHO Intake and Weight

Calculate the insulin requirements for the following CHO intake related to the patient's weight. Refer to Table 9-2 on the previous page. Use either method shown in the example.

1. The patient ate 26 g CHO for breakfast. She weighs 142 lb. How many units of R are required?

2. The patient weighs 83 kg and ate 80 g CHO for lunch. How many units of R are required?

3. The patient ate 18 g CHO for lunch. She weighs 108 lb. How many units of R are required?

4. The patient consumed 90 g CHO for dinner and weighs 240 lb. How many units of R are required?

5. The patient weighs 162 lb. The total CHO intake during a 24-hour period was 160 g. How many units of R has the patient received in 24 hours?

6. The patient's total CHO intake during 24 hours was 145 g. How many units of R did she receive? The patient weighs 100 kg.

7. The physician calls at 1500 hours and wants to know how many total units of R his patient has received for the day. You calculate the following: breakfast included 45 g CHO, and he ate half of the CHO plus three quarters of his lunch, which had 72 g CHO. The patient weighs 190 lb. How many total units of R has the patient received?

8. You estimate that the patient ate half of his carbohydrates for lunch. The total CHO on his lunch menu was 50 g. His weight is 81 kg. How many units of R should he receive?

9. The patient weighs 70 kg. He has consumed 44 g CHO for breakfast, 72 g CHO for lunch, and 48 g CHO for dinner. His bedtime snack had 15 g CHO. What is the total amount of CHO the patient has consumed? What is the total amount of R he requires for the day?

10. Breakfast included 38 g CHO. The patient ate half of the CHO on the tray. Lunch included 50 g of CHO, and she ate one quarter of the CHO on the tray. Dinner included 48 g CHO, and she ate one third of the CHO. She weighs 112 lb. What is the total amount of CHO the patient has consumed? What is the total amount of R she requires for the three meals?

IV Insulin

During acute phases of illness, regular insulin is given by the IV route to ensure a controlled supply of medication that will vary depending on laboratory monitoring. A piggyback infusion is always administered with an IV-controlled infusion device. Discard the first 2 to 3 mL of combined infusion through IV tubing to prevent the insulin from binding to the tubing.

RULE   Begin the problem with the known amount of medication in the total solution.

The pharmacy standard insulin drip: 100 units Human Regular in 100 mL of NS.

Example   Ordered: Regular human insulin 5 units/hr IV drip. Pharmacy has delivered 100 mL 0.9% NS with 100 units of regular human insulin.
* How many mL/hr will infuse 5 units/hr?
* For how many hours will the IV infuse?

KNOW	WANT TO KNOW		PROOF

Step 1:   100 units : 100 mL :: 5 units : x mL

$100x = 100 \times 5 = 500$

$100x = 500$

$x = 5$ mL/hr = 5 units of insulin

PROOF
$100 \times 5 = 500$
$100 \times 5 = 500$

Step 2:   HAVE   WANT TO HAVE

5 mL : 1 hr :: 100 mL : x hr

$5x = 100$

$x = 20$ hr

PROOF
$20 \times 5 = 100$
$1 \times 100 = 100$

CLINICAL ALERT

Only clear regular insulin can be used intravenously. Discard if cloudy (Figure 9-14).

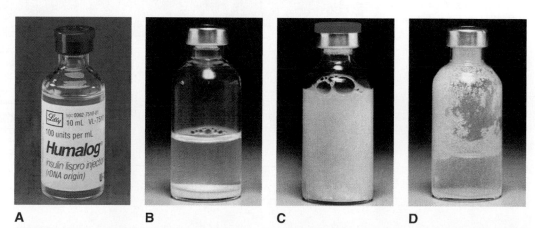

A   **B**   **C**   **D**

FIGURE 9-14   **A,** Regular and Humalog (lispro), Novolog (aspart), and Aprida (glulisine) should always look clear. **B,** Insulin at the bottom of the bottle; do not use if insulin stays on the bottom of the bottle after gentle rolling. **C,** Clumps of insulin; do not use if there are clumps of insulin in the liquid or on the bottom of the vial. **D,** Bottle appears frosted; do not use if particles of insulin are on the bottom or sides of the bottle and give it a frosty appearance. *(Copyright Eli Lilly and Company. All rights reserved. Used with permission.)*

ANSWERS ON PAGE 437

WORKSHEET
9G

IV Insulin Calculations

Answer questions 1 through 3 using Figure 9-15.

1. The patient's BMBG level is 310 mg/dL at 0820 hr.
   a. At what rate will you set the IV infusion device?
   b. At 0920 hr the BMBG is 270 mg/dL. What will be the rate for the IV infusion device?

2. The patient's blood glucose level is 235 mg/dL at 0400 hr.
   a. At what rate will you set the infusion rate?
   b. In 1 hour, the BMBG level is 270 mg/dL. What will be the new IV rate?
   c. At 0600 hr the physician called and inquired about the BMBG level. He asked how many units of insulin the patient had received since the IV was started. What will you tell the physician?

3. Your patient is receiving insulin IV. The standard rate of 100 units in 100 mL of NS is sent from the pharmacy. The BMBG q1h is as follows: 350 mg/dL, 330, 270, 210, 190, 165, 145, 120, 120 mg/dL. How many total units has the patient received?

Obtain initial Bedside Monitoring Blood Glucose (BMBG) IMMEDIATELY prior to starting insulin infusion. (Call physician if <70 or >340 mg/dL). Check serum K+ every day or _____.

Maintenance IV fluid (addition of dextrose and K+ is recommended).

☐ D5 0.45 NS +___ mEq KC/L@ 50 mL/hr or _____ mL/hr.
☐ Other _____ mL/hr.

Insulin Infusion—Use pharmacy standard Insulin Drip: 100 units Human Regular in 100 mL NS (1 unit = 1 mL). Begin infusion per algorithm below. Use standard column unless the "stress" or "customized" ☐ is checked below.

FIGURE 9-15 Standard Insulin Infusion Chart. *(Modified from Scottsdale Healthcare, Scottsdale, AZ.)*

BG (mg/dL)	Std. Infusion Rate (units/hour)	☐ Stress Infusion Rate (units/hour)	☐ Customized (units/hour)
<80	0.2	0.2	_____
80-100	0.5	1.0	_____
101-140	1.0	2.0	_____
141-180	1.5	3.0	_____
181-220	2.0	4.0	_____
221-260	2.5	5.0	_____
261-300	3.0	6.0	_____
301-340	4.0	8.0	_____
>340	5.0	10.0	_____

WORKSHEET
9G

IV Insulin Calculations (Continued)

4. The pharmacy has sent 50 mL of NS with 100 units of insulin. The order is for 5 units/hr until the BMBG level is stable at 130 mg/dL.
   a. At how many mL/hr will you set the IV infusion device?
   b. It took 16 hours for the BMBG level to stabilize at 130 mg/dL. How many total units of insulin did the patient receive during the 16 hours?

5. Ordered: 100 units Human Regular insulin in 50 mL of NS to be infused at 3 mL/hr until the blood glucose level is stable at 120 mg/dL.
   a. How many units/hr will be delivered?
   b. If it took 8 hours for the blood glucose level to stabilize at 120 mg/dL, how many total units of insulin did the patient receive?

For Problems 6 through 10, calculate the following:

• mL/hr necessary to infuse the ordered amount via an infusion device

• length of time the IV is to infuse

6. Ordered: Humulin R IV at 10 units/hr. Available: 150 mL of 0.9% NS with 100 units Humulin (lispro) R insulin.

7. Ordered: Humulin R in 50 mL to infuse at 8 units/hr. Available: 50 mL 0.9% NS with 50 units Humulin R insulin.

8. Ordered: Humulin R in 50 mL to infuse at 15 units/hr. Available: 50 mL 0.9% NS with 75 units Humulin R insulin.

9. Ordered: 120 units Humulin R insulin IV at 10 units/hr. Available: 100 mL of NS 0.9% with 120 units Humulin R insulin.

10. Ordered: 150 units Humulin R insulin IV at 12 units/hr. Available: 150 mL of NS 0.9% with 150 units Humulin R insulin.

ANSWERS ON PAGE 438

WORKSHEET
9H

Additional IV Insulin Calculations

Calculate mL/hr, units/hr, and hours to infuse.

1. Ordered: Regular insulin to infuse at 8 units/hr. Available: 500 mL of 0.9% NS with 100 units. How many mL/hr will deliver 8 units/hr?

2. Refer to question 1. The physician has increased the order to 10 units/hr. How many mL/hr will deliver 10 units/hr?

3. Ordered: 2 units of Regular insulin/hr. Available: 50 units of insulin in 250 mL of 0.9% NS. How many mL/hr will deliver 2 units/hr? How many hours will it take to infuse 250 mL?

4. Ordered: Regular insulin 40 units in 500 mL of 0.9% NS to infuse for 15 hr. At how many mL/hr will you set the infusion rate?

5. Ordered: Regular insulin to infuse at 3 units/hr. Available: 500 mL 0.45% NS with 50 units of insulin. The IV was started at 0700 hr. What time will the infusion be completed?

6. Ordered: 1 unit of Regular insulin/hr intravenous piggybank (IVPB). Available: 20 units in 250 mL of 0.45% NS. At what rate should the IV infuse?

7. Ordered: 50 units of Regular insulin to infuse at 2 units/hr. Available: IVPB with 150 mL 0.9% NS. How many mL/hr will infuse? How long will it take to infuse?

8. Ordered: 4 units of Regular insulin/hr. Available: 500 mL 0.45% NS with 30 units of insulin. If the IV was started at 0600 hr, when will it be completed?

9. A 250 mL IVPB of 0.9% NS with 30 units of insulin is to infuse at 20 mL/hr. How many units of insulin will infuse per hour? How long will it take to infuse?

10. Order: IVPB to infuse at 2 units/hr. Available: 250 mL 0.9% NS with 50 units of Regular insulin. At how many mL/hr will you set the infusion device? How long will it take to infuse?

Oral Diabetes Medications

Oral diabetes medications (ODMs) are used to treat persons with type 2 diabetes. They are taken alone or in combination with insulin. Blood glucose levels determine the strength of oral medication needed. ODMs are *not* insulin. Some ODMs stimulate the pancreas to produce insulin and other ODMs make more effective use of the insulin that is produced.

Insulin Infusion Devices

Insulin infusion devices (pumps) allow insulin to be delivered at a constant (basal) rate throughout the day, with additional insulin boluses given before meals. The patient determines the appropriate bolus based on the premeal blood glucose level as well as the carbohydrate content of the meal. The device contains a disposable syringe connected to plastic tubing. The tubing is secured to a subcutaneous cannula, which must be changed every two to three days. Only Velosulin (Buffered Regular), Novolog, or Humalog insulin can be used in the device; therefore ketoacidosis can develop quickly if the insulin infusion is interrupted. Because of this significant risk, **the device must not be stopped or disconnected without supplemental insulin coverage.**

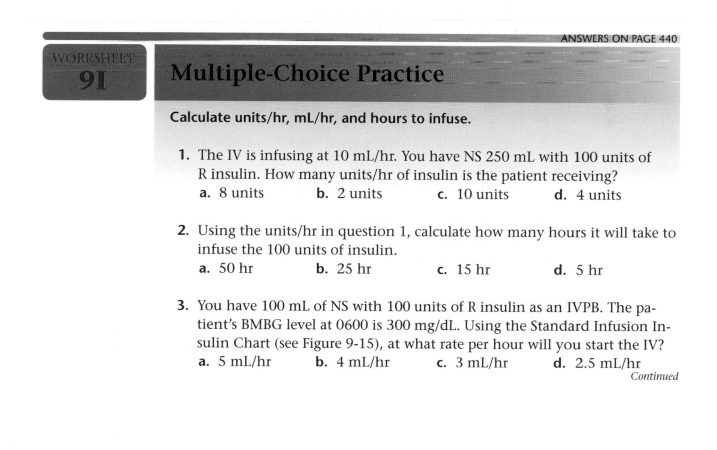

ANSWERS ON PAGE 440

WORKSHEET 91

Multiple-Choice Practice

Calculate units/hr, mL/hr, and hours to infuse.

1. The IV is infusing at 10 mL/hr. You have NS 250 mL with 100 units of R insulin. How many units/hr of insulin is the patient receiving?
   a. 8 units   **b.** 2 units   **c.** 10 units   **d.** 4 units

2. Using the units/hr in question 1, calculate how many hours it will take to infuse the 100 units of insulin.
   a. 50 hr   **b.** 25 hr   **c.** 15 hr   **d.** 5 hr

3. You have 100 mL of NS with 100 units of R insulin as an IVPB. The patient's BMBG level at 0600 is 300 mg/dL. Using the Standard Infusion Insulin Chart (see Figure 9-15), at what rate per hour will you start the IV?
   a. 5 mL/hr   **b.** 4 mL/hr   **c.** 3 mL/hr   **d.** 2.5 mL/hr

Continued

ANSWERS ON PAGE 440

WORKSHEET
91

Multiple-Choice Practice (Continued)

4. Ordered: 30 units of R insulin to be infused over 12 hr.
   Available: 50 mL NS with 30 units of insulin. How many units/hr will be infused?
   a. 1.5 units   **b.** 2.5 units   **c.** 5 units   **d.** 4 units

   At how many mL/hr will you set the infusion device?
   a. 4 mL/hr   **b.** 12 mL/hr   **c.** 41 mL/hr   **d.** 8 mL/hr

5. Ordered: 10 units of R insulin/hr IVPB.
   Available: 500 mL NS with 100 units of R insulin.
   At what rate will you set the IV infusion device?
   a. 50 mL/hr   **b.** 25 mL/hr   **c.** 100 mL/hr   **d.** 5 mL/hr

6. The type of insulin that is used for infusions is
   a. Humulin N   **b.** Levemir
   c. Humulin R   **d.** Lantus

7. Ordered: 15 units of Lantus (glargine) subcutaneous.
   What is the length of effectiveness of the insulin?
   a. 12 hr   **b.** 4 hr   **c.** 36 hr   **d.** 24 hr

8. Ordered: Humulin N 20 units subcutaneous at 0730.
   When will it peak?
   a. 4-5 hr   **b.** 4-10 hr   **c.** 1-3 hr   **d.** 3-4 hr

9. Lantus (glargine) is the preferred insulin because it:
   a. peaks in 15 minutes   **b.** has a duration of 16 hr
   c. is absorbed quickly   **d.** is peakless

10. Lantus (glargine) is usually given subcutaneously:
    a. at breakfast   **b.** at bed time   **c.** at midday   **d.** at anytime

Frequent Blood Glucose Monitoring/Insulin Drip Record

Normal Blood Glucose
M 75-110 mg/dL F 65-105 mg/dL

DATE 12/5/08

Time	Glucose (mg/dL)	Intervention Insulin (units/h) or other	Ketones S/M/L/Neg	Initial
00				
01				
02				
03		IV Insulin Drip Started		
04 15	350	5.0		JB
05 15	303	4.0		JB
06 15	310	4.0		JB
07 15	270	3.0		JB
08 15	180	1.5		JB
09 15	165	1.5		JB
10 15	150	1.5		JB
11				
12 15	140	1.0		JB
13 15	130	1.0		JB
14				
15 15	135	1.0		JB
16				
17 15	140	1.0		JB
18		Converted to Subcutaneous Insulin		
19				
20				
21				
22				
23				
Insulin Total Daily Dose (TDD)				

DATE

Time	Glucose (mg/dL)	Intervention Insulin (units/h) or other	Ketones S/M/L/Neg	Initial
00				
01				
02				
03				
04				
05				
06				
07				
08				
09				
10				
11				
12				
13				
14				
15				
16				
17				
18				
19				
20				
21				
22				
23				
Insulin Total Daily Dose (TDD)				

DATE

Time	Glucose (mg/dL)	Intervention Insulin (units/h) or other	Ketones S/M/L/Neg	Initial
00				
01				
02				
03				
04				
05				
06				
07				
08				
09				
10				
11				
12				
13				
14				
15				
16				
17				
18				
19				
20				
21				
22				
23				
Insulin Total Daily Dose (TDD)				

Initial	Signature	Initial	Signature	Initial	Signature
JB	J Booth				

Original in Medical Chart   Copy to Pharmacy

NOTE: IV insulin should always be used with an infusion device, never via gravity feed.

FIGURE 9-16 Diabetes Flow Sheet. (*Modified from Scottsdale Healthcare, Scottsdale, AZ.*)

CRITICAL THINKING EXERCISES

Analyze the following scenario.

Mr. Johnson's blood glucose level was 350 mg/dL. The orders on his chart read: Give 10 units of Humalog stat and check the BMBG in 1 hour. The nurse gave the insulin at 1400 hr. After the change of shift, at 1430 hr, Mr. Johnson was incoherent. On checking the Diabetes Flow Sheet (Figure 9-16) the nurse found that Mr. Johnson had been given 1 mL of Humalog.

Ordered:

Given:

Error(s):

Discussion
What would be your immediate action?
How did this error occur?
How could this error have been prevented?
Do you think the nurse should have known the safe dosage range?
What were the potential injuries to the patient?

NDC 0002-7510-01
Lilly
10 mL   VL-7510

100 units per mL

Humalog®
insulin lispro injection
(rDNA origin)
U-100

CAUTION—Federal (USA) law prohibits dispensing without a prescription.
For parenteral use
See accompanying literature for dosage
Neutral
Eli Lilly and Co. Indianapolis, IN 46285, USA

CHAPTER 9 Final

ANSWERS ON PAGE 441

1. Ordered: Humalog insulin 15 units stat. Available: Humalog insulin.
   - How many units will you give?
   - Which syringe will give a precise measurement?

   a.

   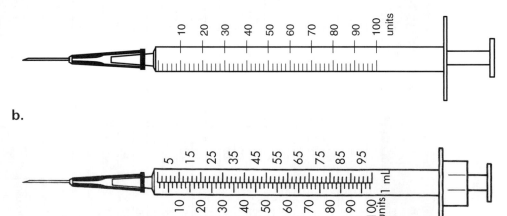

   b.

2. The blood glucose level is 280. How many units of Regular insulin will you give subcutaneously? Use the sliding scale on page 256.

3. Ordered: Novolin R 16 units with Novolin N insulin 30 units at 0700. Shade in the amount of regular insulin. Shade in the amount of N insulin.

4. Ordered: Humalog 18 units before breakfast at 0930.
   • How many units will you give?
   • Which syringe is easier to read?

   a.

   b.

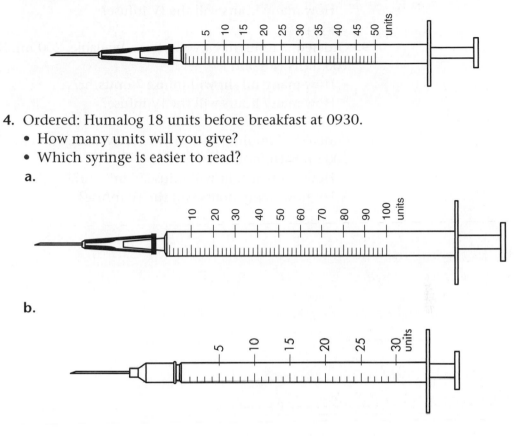

5. Ordered: Glucophage 850 mg tab and Novolin N 15 units before breakfast. How many total units will you give? Shade in the correct amount.

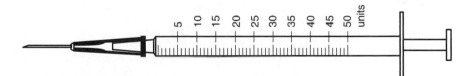

6. Ordered: 10 units/hr Novolin R insulin IV. Available: 500 mL 0.9% saline with 250 units Novolin R regular insulin.
   • How many mL/hr will deliver 10 units/hr?
   • How many hours will the IV infuse?

7. Ordered: 6 units/hr Novolin R IV. Available: 100 units Humulin R insulin in 250 mL of 0.9% saline.
   • How many mL/hr will infuse 6 units of insulin?
   • How many hours will the IV infuse?

8. Ordered: 8 units/hr Novolin R IV. Available: 250 mL NS with 100 units insulin.
   - How many mL/hr will infuse 8 units of insulin?
   - How many hours will the IV infuse?

9. Ordered: 7 units/hr Novolin R IV. Available: 200 mL NS with 100 units Novolin R.
   - How many mL/hr will infuse 7 units/hr?
   - How many hours will the IV infuse?

10. Ordered: Humulin R 9 units/hr IV. Available: 500 mL NS IV solution with 100 units Humulin R.
    - How many mL/hr will infuse 9 units/hr?
    - For how many hours will the IV infuse?

Refer to the Advanced Calculations section of the enclosed student CD-ROM for additional practice problems.

Anticoagulants

Objectives

- Compare the actions of oral, subcutaneous, and intravenous anticoagulants.
- Measure a dose in a tuberculin syringe.
- Measure subcutaneous heparin using various concentrations.
- Titrate intravenous heparin for bolus dose, units/kg, units/hr, and mL/hr.
- Calculate the length of time to infuse.
- Analyze medication errors using critical thinking.

INTRODUCTION

Various concentrations of subcutaneous heparin sodium, Fragmin, and Lovenox are measured with a tuberculin syringe. Titrated heparin sodium for intravenous drip and titrated Fragmin are calculated for bolus and prophylactic regimens. An example of a flow chart, or medical administration record (MAR), is shown.

Injectable Anticoagulants

Heparin sodium injection, USP, is a drug used to interrupt the clotting process. It affects the ability of the blood to coagulate, thereby preventing clots from forming. It is used to treat deep vein thrombosis (DVT) and pulmonary embolism (PE), for cardiac surgery, during hemodialysis, myocardial infarction (MI), and disseminated intravascular coagulation (DIC), and prophylactically for immobilized patients. It may be given in therapeutic doses or in small, diluted doses to maintain the patency of IV or intraarterial (IA) lines.

Because it is inactive orally, heparin sodium is administered intravenously or subcutaneously. If administered intramuscularly, the drug produces a high level of pain and may cause hematomas. The orders for heparin are highly individualized and are based on the weight of the patient and coagulation values. Heparin comes in various strengths, including 1000, 5000, 10,000, 20,000, and 50,000 units/mL. Heparin also comes in 10 and 100 units/mL for IV patency flushes. The vial must be checked carefully before administration. Heparin is fast-acting.

Figure 10-1 shows heparin injection sites. Figure 10-2 demonstrates how subcutaneous heparin injections are documented.

Check laboratory values for clotting times before administering heparin. Heparin therapy must not be interrupted and is incompatible with other medications.

Heparin has a half-life of 1 to 6 hours. To maintain a therapeutic level in the blood, heparin is usually given as a continuous IV drip during hospitalization. The heparin level is titrated on the basis of partial thromboplastin time (PTT) levels, which are taken every 6 hours to correlate with the half-life of heparin. Heparin can be counteracted with protamine sulfate.

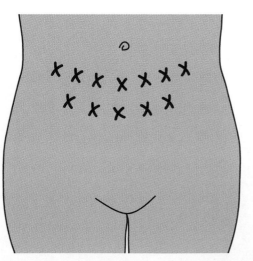

FIGURE 10-1 Subcutaneous injection sites. The abdominal sites are better for absorption of heparin.

			MEDICATION ADMINISTRATION RECORD			

HT :
WT :
ALLERGIES:

ADM. DX :
DIET :

Start Date/Time	Stop Date/Time	RN/ LPN	Medication	0731-1530	1531-2330	2331-0730
12/13/08		NB	Heparin sodium 5,000 units subcut	0800 RLQ		
		NB	Heparin sodium 5,000 units subcut	1400 LLQ		
		KR	Heparin sodium 5,000 units subcut	2000 RLQ		

Order Date	RN INIT.	Date/Time To Be Given	One Time Orders and Pre-Operatives Medication-Dose-Route	Actual Time Given	Site Codes		Dose Omission Code
					Arm	LA RA	A = pt absent
					Deltoid	LD RD	H = hold
					Ventrogluteal	LVG RVG	M = med absent
					Gluteal	LG RG	N = NPO
					Abdomen	LUQ RUQ	O = other
					Abdomen	LLQ RLQ	R = refused
							U = unable to tolerate

INIT	Signature	INIT	Signature
NB	Nancy Berg RN		
KR	Kay Rae RN		

FIGURE 10-2   Sample MAR. *(Modified from Scottsdale Healthcare, Scottsdale, AZ.)*

Lovenox (enoxaparin) and Fragmin (dalteparin) (Figure 10-3) are low-molecular-weight anticoagulants. They are prescribed for the prevention and treatment of DVT and PE and also after knee and hip surgery. Lovenox and Fragmin have a longer half-life than heparin, and because of their low level of activity in the blood, there is a reduced need for PTT tests because the two drugs have more predictable peaks and durations of action. The preferred site for low-molecular-weight anticoagulants is the "love handles," or anterolateral abdominal wall.

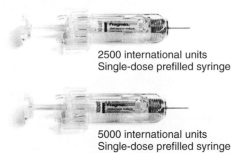

2500 international units
Single-dose prefilled syringe

5000 international units
Single-dose prefilled syringe

FIGURE 10-3   Fragmin single-dose prefilled syringes. *(Used with permission from Pfizer, Inc.)*

CLINICAL ALERT

Lovenox and Fragmin should never be given in the deltoid because they may cause large hematomas.

Example   Ordered: Lovenox 30 mg subcutaneous q12h after hip replacement. The pharmacy has sent 40 mg/0.4 mL in a prefilled syringe. How many milliliters will be administered? How many milliliters will be discarded?

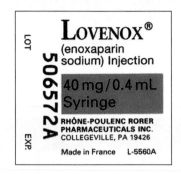

HAVE   WANT TO HAVE
40 mg : 0.4 mL :: 30 mg : x mL

40x = 0.4 × 30 = 12

40x = 12

   x = 0.3 mL

PROOF
40 × 0.9 = 12
0.4 × 30 = 12

0.1 mL will be discarded.

SUBCUTANEOUS HEPARIN INJECTIONS

Example   Ordered: Heparin 3500 units subcutaneous q6h. Available: Vial containing 5000 units/mL. How many milliliters will the patient receive? Shade in the dose on the tuberculin syringe.

KNOW   WANT TO KNOW
5000 units : 1 mL :: 3500 units : x mL

5000x = 3500

   x = 0.7 mL

PROOF
5000 × 0.7 = 3500
1 × 3500 = 3500

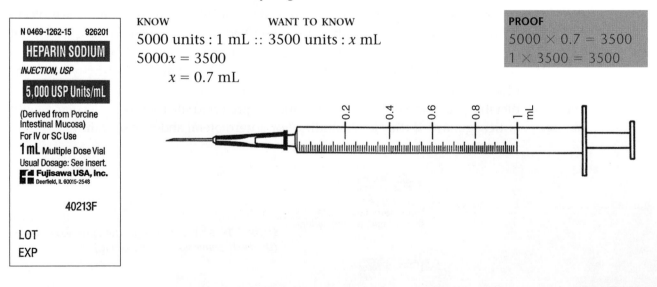

Example   Ordered: Fragmin 8000 international units subcutaneous q6h. How many milliliters will you give? Shade in the dose on the syringe.

KNOW   WANT TO KNOW

10,000 international units : 1 mL :: 8000 international units : x mL

$10x = 1 \times 8 = 8$

$x = 0.8$ mL

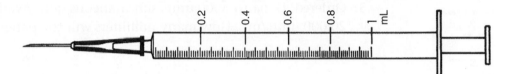

10,000 international units/mL
9.5 mL multidose vial
NDC 0013-2436-06

PROOF
$1 \times 8000 = 8000$
$10,000 \times 0.8 = 8000$

Used with permission from Pfizer, Inc.

⬡ **CLINICAL ALERT**

Do not massage the injection site because this increases the incidence of bleeding and hematoma development.

ANSWERS ON PAGE 443

WORKSHEET
10A

Subcutaneous Injections

Multidose vials are available in 10, 100, 1000, 5000, 10,000, 20,000, and 50,000 units/mL. Read the labels carefully. Answer the following questions and show your proofs (carry out to nearest hundredth). Shade in doses on syringes.

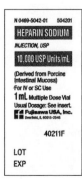

1. Ordered: Heparin 7000 units subcutaneous. Available: Heparin 10,000 units/mL. How many milliliters will the patient receive?

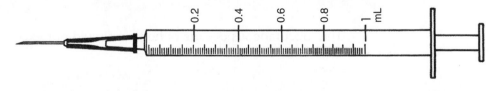

Continued

ANSWERS ON PAGE 443

Subcutaneous Injections (Continued)

2. Ordered: Heparin 15,000 units subcutaneous q8h. Available: Heparin 20,000 units/mL. How many milliliters will the patient receive?

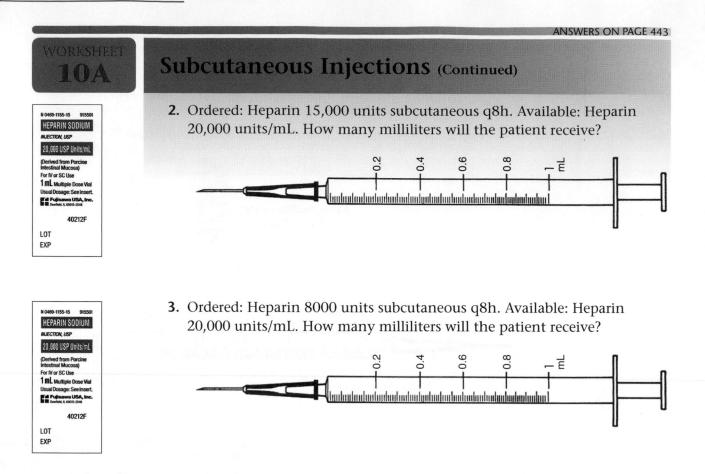

3. Ordered: Heparin 8000 units subcutaneous q8h. Available: Heparin 20,000 units/mL. How many milliliters will the patient receive?

4. Ordered: Heparin 17,000 units subcutaneous stat dose. Available: Heparin 10,000 units/mL and 20,000 units/mL. Which strength will you choose? How many milliliters will the patient receive?

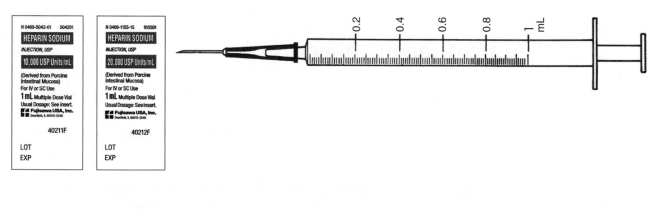

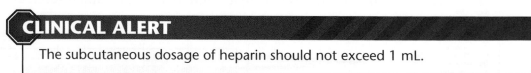

CLINICAL ALERT

The subcutaneous dosage of heparin should not exceed 1 mL.

ANSWERS ON PAGE 443

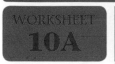

Subcutaneous Injections (Continued)

5. Ordered: Fragmin 7500 units subcutaneous q6hr. Available: Fragmin 10,000 international units/mL. How many milliliters will the patient receive?

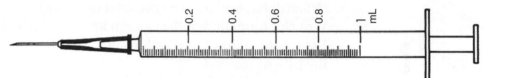

10,000 international units/mL
9.5 mL multidose vial
NDC 0013-2436-06

Used with permission from Pfizer, Inc.

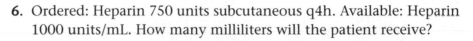

6. Ordered: Heparin 750 units subcutaneous q4h. Available: Heparin 1000 units/mL. How many milliliters will the patient receive?

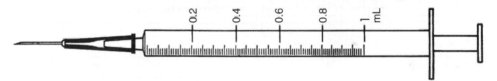

7. Ordered: Heparin 800 units subcutaneous q8hr. Available: Heparin 1000 units/mL in a multidose vial. How many milliliters will the patient receive?

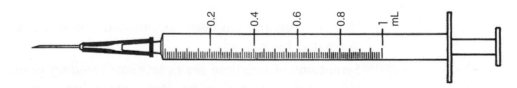

CLINICAL ALERT

Check your patient's chart for allergies. Heparin is made from pork and beef.

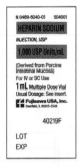

Continued

ANSWERS ON PAGE 443

WORKSHEET
10A

Subcutaneous Injections (Continued)

8. Ordered: Heparin 3000 units subcutaneous q8h. Available: Heparin 5000 units/mL in a multidose vial. How many milliliters will the patient receive?

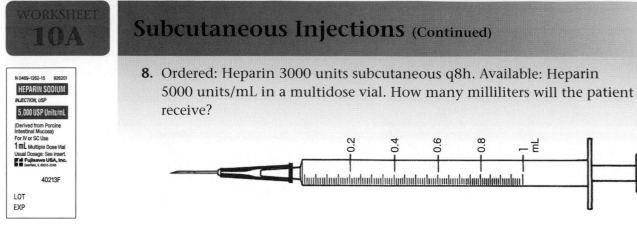

IV Flushes

9. Ordered: Heparin flush 5 units after each medication administration to prevent clot formation in the heparin lock. Available: Heparin 10 units/mL. How many units of medication are in the vial? How many milliliters will the patient receive?

Follow hospital protocol for saline and heparin flushes after medication administration.

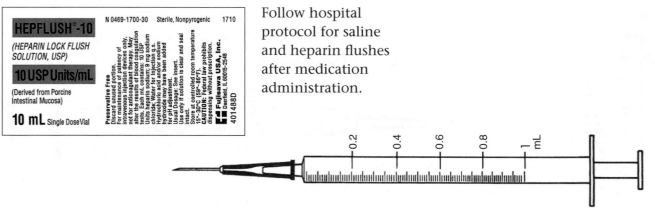

CLINICAL ALERT

Heparin resistance has been documented in elderly patients; therefore, large doses may be ordered.

Symptoms of overdose are nosebleed, bleeding gums, tarry stools, petechiae, and easy bruising. An electric razor should be used for shaving.

ANSWERS ON PAGE 443

WORKSHEET
10A

Subcutaneous Injections (Continued)

IV Flushes

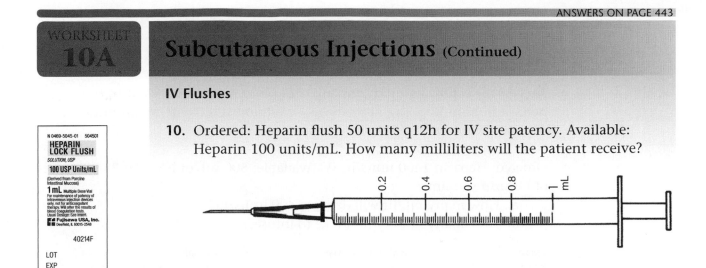

10. Ordered: Heparin flush 50 units q12h for IV site patency. Available: Heparin 100 units/mL. How many milliliters will the patient receive?

IV FLUSHES

Heparin flushes are used to prevent clot formation in central lines and intermittent infusion lines. Inject heparin flush (10 to 100 units) or saline for injection according to hospital protocol after each medication administration or every 8 to 12 hours. Peripheral IV lines are usually flushed with isotonic saline. Heparin locks provide patient mobility.

CLINICAL ALERT

Heparin IV flushes are available in 10 units/mL and 100 units/mL in prepared syringes and multiple-dose vials. Read labels carefully. Hospital protocol will determine the amount to administer.

IV Heparin

When intermittent or continuous IV therapy is used, blood should be drawn for a PTT and a hematocrit level to determine the course of therapy. Therapeutic anticoagulant dosage is regulated according to the results of the PTT and the patient's weight.

Pharmacies are standardizing IV heparin preparations in concentrations of 25,000 units/500 mL and 25,000 units/250 mL. Dispensing charts indicating mL/hr and units/hr are available for each concentration. This will reduce overdosing and underdosing. Protamine sulfate is the antagonist for heparin. It is the nurse's responsibility to have protamine sulfate available.

ANSWERS ON PAGE 445

WORKSHEET
10B

IV Heparin Calculations: mL/hr and Hours to Infuse

Answer the following questions and show your proofs (carry out to the nearest hundredth). The heparin will be administered with an infusion device.

Example   Ordered: Heparin 1400 units/hr IV. Available: 500 mL of NS with 25,000 units of heparin sodium.

      a. How many mL/hr will deliver 1400 units/hr?

      b. How many hours will it take to infuse?

KNOW	WANT TO KNOW
500 mL : 250 units :: x mL : 14 units	
$250x = 500 \times 14 = 7000$	
$250x = 7000$	

PROOF
$500 \times 1400 = 7000$
$250 \times 28 = 7000$

    $x = 28/\text{mL/hr}$. Set infusion pump to deliver 28 mL/hr.

KNOW	WANT TO KNOW
28 mL : 1 hr :: 500 mL : x hr	
$28x = 1 \times 500 = 500$	
$28x = 500$	

PROOF
$500 \times 1 = 500$
$28 \times 17.85 = 499.8 = 500$

    $x = 17.85$ hr $60 \times 0.85 = 51$ The IV will take 17 hr 51 minutes to infuse.

1. Ordered: Heparin sodium 1000 units/hr IV. Available: 1 L of 0.9% saline with 20,000 units of heparin.
   a. How many mL/hr will deliver 1000 units?
   b. How many hours will it take to infuse the bag?

2. Ordered: Heparin sodium 20,000 units IV in 12 hr. Pharmacy has sent 1000 mL of 0.9% normal saline with 20,000 units heparin sodium.
   a. At how many mL/hr should the IV infuse?
   b. How many units/hr will infuse?
   c. The shift reports that 250 mL have been infused. How many hours remain for the infusion?

3. Ordered: Heparin 1500 units/hr IV. Pharmacy has sent 1 L 0.9% saline with 20,000 units of heparin.
   a. How many mL/hr will deliver 1500 units?
   b. How many hours will it take to infuse this bag?

ANSWERS ON PAGE 445

WORKSHEET 10B

IV Heparin Calculations:
mL/hr and Hours to Infuse (Continued)

4. Ordered: Heparin 10,000 units in 15 hr. Pharmacy has sent 1000 mL NS with 10,000 units of heparin. The infusion was started at 0830.
   a. How many units/hr will the patient receive?
   b. How many mL/hr will be infused?
   c. The 0700 hr shift reports that 300 mL have been infused. When will the infusion finish? How many hours remain for the infusion?

5. Ordered: Heparin 1200 units/hr. Available: 500 mL NS with 10,000 units of heparin.
   a. How many mL/hr will infuse 1200 units/hr?
   b. How many hours will it take to infuse this bag?

6. Ordered: Heparin 2500 units/hr IV. Available: 50,000 units per 1000 mL 0.9% NS.
   a. How many mL/hr will deliver 2500 units/hr?
   b. How many hours will it take to infuse?

7. Ordered: Heparin 1000 units/hr IV. Available: 25,000 units/500 mL.
   a. How many mL/hr will deliver 1000 units/hr?
   b. How many hours will it take to infuse?

8. Ordered: Heparin 1300 units/hr IV. Available: 500 mL with 25,000 units of heparin sodium.
   a. How many mL/hr will deliver 1300 units/hr?
   b. How long will it take to infuse?

9. Ordered: Heparin 1800 units/hr IV. Your patient is on fluid restrictions; therefore the pharmacy has sent a concentrated solution of 25,000 units/250 mL of NS.
   a. How many mL/hr will deliver 1800 units/hr?
   b. How many hours will it take to infuse?

10. Ordered: Heparin 1000 units/hr. Your patient is on fluid restrictions. The pharmacy has sent 20,000 units/250 mL of NS.
   a. How many mL/hr will deliver 1000 units/hr?
   b. How many hours will it take to infuse?

ANSWERS ON PAGE 447

WORKSHEET
10C

IV Heparin Calculations Titrated to Kilograms

All intravenous anticoagulants are based on the PTT results. Loading (bolus) doses are individualized and are titrated to weight in kilograms. Hospital protocol is usually standardized for their institution. It is important that the nurses know what the protocol standards are and where they are located. Protocols and literature may vary, but the loading doses are usually between 70 and 100 units/kg. Infusion rates for heparin sodium also vary but are usually between 15 and 25 units/kg/hr.

Example   Ordered: IV heparin loading dose to infuse at 18 units/kg/hr. The patient weighs 210 lb.
Available: 20,000 units of heparin sodium in 1000 mL of D5W.
At what rate will you set the IV infusion pump?

Change 210 lb to kg.   210 divided by 2.2 = 95.45 = 96 kg
Multiply units/hr by the patient's weight in kg. $18 \times 96 = 1728$ units/hr.

Ratio and Proportion Method

KNOW   WANT TO KNOW
18 units : 1 kg :: x units : 96 kg
$x = 18 \times 96 = 1728$
$x = 1728$ units/hr

PROOF
$18 \times 96 = 1728$
$1 \times 1728 = 1728$

KNOW   WANT TO KNOW
20 units : 10 mL :: 1728 units : x mL
$20x = 1728$

PROOF
$1 \times 1728 = 1728$
$20 \times 86.4 = 1728$

  $x = 86.4$ mL/hr = 86 mL/hr. Set infusion pump to deliver 86 mL/hr.

1. Ordered: Heparin sodium 70 units/kg bolus loading dose. Infusion rate to run at 20 units/kg/hr. Available: 1000 mL D5W with 25,000 units of heparin. The patient weighs 176 lb.
    a. Calculate the loading dose.
    b. Calculate the units/hr based on weight.
    c. Calculate the mL/hr.

2. Ordered: 80 units/kg of heparin as a loading dose. Set infusion rate to deliver 1500 units/hr. Available: 1000 mL NS with 30,000 units of heparin. The patient weighs 160 lb.
    a. Calculate the loading dose.
    b. Calculate the mL/hr.

CLINICAL ALERT

Always have protamine sulfate available as an antidote for heparin.

ANSWERS ON PAGE 447

IV Heparin Calculations Titrated to Kilograms (Continued)

3. Ordered: Heparin sodium 90 units/kg. Infuse at 25 units/kg/hr. Available: 1000 mL 0.45% NS with 25,000 units of heparin. The patient weighs 210 lb.
   a. How many units is the loading dose?
   b. How many units/hr will the patient receive?
   c. At what rate will you set the mL/hr?

4. Ordered: Loading dose of 75 units/kg; then infuse at 20 units/kg/hr. Available: 1000 mL 0.9% NS with 50,000 units of heparin. The patient weighs 300 lb.
   a. Calculate the loading dose.
   b. How many units/hr will the patient receive?
   c. At what rate will you set the infusion device?

5. Ordered: Loading dose of heparin 75 units/kg. Infuse at 17 units/kg/hr. Available: 1000 mL D5W with 20,000 units of heparin. The patient weighs 185 lb.
   a. How many units is the loading dose?
   b. How many units/hr will the patient receive?
   c. At what rate will you set the infusion device?

6. Ordered: Loading dose of 65 units/kg. Set the infusion to run at 15 units/kg/hr. Available: 500 mL 0.45% NS with 30,000 units of heparin. The patient weighs 145 lb.
   a. How many units is the loading dose?
   b. How many units/hr will infuse?
   c. At what rate will you set the infusion device?

7. Ordered: Bolus dose of heparin at 80 units/kg. Titrate infusion to run at 1000 units/hr. Available: 1000 mL D5W with 25,000 units of heparin. The patient weighs 120 kg.
   a. Calculate the number of units for the loading dose.
   b. Calculate mL/hr to infuse 1000 units/hr.

8. Ordered: A bolus dose of heparin at 70 units/kg. Run the infusion at 18 units/kg/hr. Available: 1000 mL D5W with 30,000 units of heparin. The patient weighs 194 lb.
   a. How many units will you give as the bolus dose?
   b. How many units/hr will infuse?
   c. At what rate will you set the infusion device?

Continued

ANSWERS ON PAGE 447

WORKSHEET
10C

IV Heparin Calculations Titrated to Kilograms (Continued)

9. Ordered: A loading dose of heparin at 95 units/kg. Pharmacy has sent 1000 mL 0.9% NS with 20,000 units of heparin. Run the infusion at 20 units/kg/hr. The patient weighs 136 kg.
    a. How many units is the loading dose?
    b. How many units/hr will infuse?
    c. At what rate will you set the infusion device?

10. Ordered: Heparin 100 units/kg bolus dose. Infuse at 18 units/kg/hr. Available: 1000 mL 0.45% NS with 35,000 units of heparin. The patient weighs 108 kg.
    a. How many units is the loading dose?
    b. How many units/hr will infuse?
    c. At what rate will you set the infusion device?

Oral Anticoagulants

Oral anticoagulants such as warfarin (Coumadin) (Figure 10-4) and anisindione (Miradon) are used as prophylaxis after an episode of thrombolytic complications. They inhibit the activity of vitamin K, which is required for the activation of clotting factors. Patients receiving heparin therapy are converted to oral anticoagulants while still receiving heparin. The level of oral anticoagulants in the blood is monitored by the laboratory value of the international normalized ratio (INR). The INR standardizes the results of the prothrombin time (PT) test. The INR should be maintained at 2 to 3 for best results, depending on the illness being treated. The most common oral anticoagulant is warfarin. Other anticoagulants in use are anisindione and integrilin. Dosing for all anticoagulants is individualized. The antidote for oral anticoagulants is vitamin K, plasma, or whole blood. Foods high in vitamin K should be avoided.

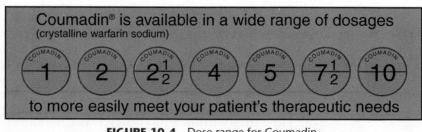

FIGURE 10-4   Dose range for Coumadin.

ANSWERS ON PAGE 449

WORKSHEET 10D

Multiple-Choice Practice

1. Ordered: Fragmin subcutaneous. Titrate to 120 international units/kg q12h × 5 days. The patient weighs 185 lb. How many international units of Fragmin will you administer for each dose?
   a. 5800 international units
   b. 1800 international units
   c. 10,080 international units
   d. 6400 international units

2. Refer to question 1. Available: 25,000 IU/mL multidose vial of Fragmin. How many milliliters of Fragmin will you give?
   a. 2.2 mL
   b. 0.4 mL
   c. 4.4 mL
   d. 0.2 mL

3. Ordered: Fragmin subcutaneous q12h titrated to kg. Titrate Fragmin to 120 international units/kg subcutaneous. The patient weighs 132 lb. How many kilograms does the patient weigh?
   a. 50 kg
   b. 120 kg
   c. 60 kg
   d. 45 kg
   How many international units of Fragmin will you prepare?
   a. 7000 international units
   b. 5000 international units
   c. 83,000 international units
   d. 7200 international units

4. Refer to question 3. How many milliliters of Fragmin will you give? Available: 10,000 IU/mL multidose vial.
   a. 0.7 mL
   b. 0.5 mL
   c. 1 mL
   d. 1.2 mL

5. Ordered: Administer a bolus of heparin sodium IV. The hospital protocol is 80 units/kg. The patient weighs 160 lb. How many units will you give?
   a. 5840 units
   b. 6620 units
   c. 4320 units
   d. 2420 units

6. Ordered: IV heparin to infuse at 18 units/kg/hr. Available: 1000 mL D5W with 20,000 units heparin. The patient weighs 175 lb. How many units/hr will the patient receive?
   a. 1220 units/hr
   b. 880 units/hr
   c. 1280 units/hr
   d. 1440 units/hr
   At what rate will you set the infusion device?
   a. 110 mL/hr
   b. 85 mL/hr
   c. 68 mL/hr
   d. 72 mL/hr

7. Ordered: Heparin drip at 40 units/kg. Available: 25,000 units of heparin in 1000 mL of D5W. The patient weighs 75 kg. At what rate will you set the infusion device?
   a. 100 mL/hr
   b. 120 mL/hr
   c. 75 mL/hr
   d. 82 mL/hr

8. Ordered: Heparin IV drip at 500 units/hr. Available: 500 mL 0.9% NS with 10,000 units of heparin. At what hourly rate will you set the infusion?
   a. 50 mL/hr
   b. 75 mL/hr
   c. 100 mL/hr
   d. 25 mL/hr

Continued

ANSWERS ON PAGE 449

WORKSHEET
10D

Multiple-Choice Practice (Continued)

9. Ordered: Fragmin subcutaneous titrated to 120 international units/kg q12h × 8 days. Begin treatment at 0800 hr. The patient weighs 220 lb. How many kg does the patient weigh?

   a. 100 kg   **b.** 120 kg   **c.** 110 kg   **d.** 60 kg

   How many international units of Fragmin will the patient receive per dose?

   a. 10,000 international units   **b.** 15,000 international units
   c. 8,000 international units   **d.** 12,000 international units

10. Refer to question 9. Available: Fragmin 10,000 international units/mL and Fragmin 25,000 international units/mL multidose vials. Which multidose vial will you use? How many mL will you give?

   a. 1 mL   **b.** 0.75 mL   **c.** 0.48 mL   **d.** 0.66 mL

CRITICAL THINKING EXERCISES

Mrs. Smith, a 76-year-old woman, was recuperating after abdominal surgery. The physician wrote an order for 2000 units heparin subcut stat. The nurse administered a 1 mL dose taken from a multidose vial labeled 20,000 units/mL. Later that day, the physician reduced the heparin order. He wrote: *Reduce heparin to 1000 units q8h.* While the nurse is preparing the 1000-unit dose from the multidose vial of 20,000 units/mL, she realizes the error when the first dose of heparin was administered.

Order:

Given:

Error(s):

Potential injuries:

Preventive measures:

Discussion
What factors contributed to the error?
How many units of heparin did Mrs. Smith receive for the first dose?
What was the potential injury?
What medication should always be on hand when a patient is receiving heparin?
Why do you think The Joint Commission does not approve of abbreviations?

1. Ordered: Heparin 4000 units subcutaneous for prophylaxis of cerebral thrombosis. Available: 5000 units/mL. How many milliliters will the patient receive?

2. Ordered: Heparin 2500 units q4h subcutaneous to prevent thrombi from recurring. Available: 10,000 units/mL vial. How many milliliters will the patient receive?

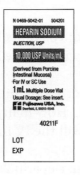

3. Ordered: Heparin 2000 units q4h for venous stasis. Available: 5000 units/mL and 10,000 units/mL. Which vial will you choose? If a tuberculin syringe is used, how many milliliters will the patient receive?

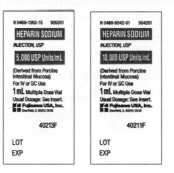

4. Ordered: Heparin 7000 units subcutaneous q8h before initiating a heparin infusion for a venous thromboembolism. Available: 5000, 10,000, and 20,000 units/mL. Which one will you choose? How many milliliters will the patient receive?

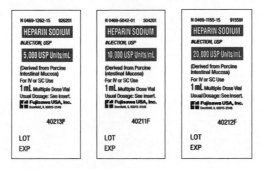

5. Ordered: Heparin 800 units subcutaneous q4h as a prophylaxis for immobility. Available: Heparin 1000 units/mL. How many milliliters will the patient receive?

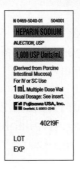

6. Ordered: 700 units/hr to infuse. Available: 20,000 units/500 mL. How many mL/hr will provide 700 units/hr? For how many hours will the IV infuse?

7. Ordered: 1500 units/hr IV for hyperlipemia. Available: 25,000 units/ 500 mL. How many mL/hr will provide 1500 units/hr? For how many hours will the IV infuse?

8. Ordered: Heparin 25,000 units IV in 24 hr for peripheral arterial embolization. Available: 1000 mL with 25,000 units of heparin sodium. How many mL/hr will give 25,000 units in 24 hr? How many units/hr will infuse?

9. Ordered: Heparin 35,000 units IV in 24 hr for atrial fibrillation. Available: 1000 mL 0.9% NS with 35,000 units of heparin sodium. How many mL/ hr will the patient receive? How many units/hr will the patient receive?

10. Ordered: Heparin 2000 units/hr IV for pulmonary emboli. Available: Heparin 20,000 units in 1000 mL 0.9% NS. How many mL/hr will be delivered via the infusion device? For how long will the IV infuse?

Refer to the Advanced Calculations section of the enclosed student CD-ROM for additional practice problems.

Children's Dosages

Objectives

- Calculate 24-hour pediatric drug doses and divided doses for specific weights.
- Calculate safe dose ranges in mg/kg, mcg/kg, and square meters of body surface area (BSA).
- Calculate reconstituted pediatric drug doses and small-volume IV flow rates for children.
- Evaluate order and safe dose range calculations.
- Make a decision:

    Give medication (within therapeutic range).

    Hold medication and clarify promptly (overdose or underdose).
- Analyze medication errors using critical thinking.

2 3 4 5 mL 6 7 8 9 10 mL

1/2 tsp 1 tsp 1 1/2 tsp 2 tsp

INTRODUCTION

Medication amounts for infants and children are usually smaller than those for average adults. The calculation and delivery of correct doses to children incorporate several steps to protect patients. With the step-by-step practice offered in this chapter, you will develop the skills, habits, and thinking processes necessary to ensure that the doses ordered are safe and to calculate accurate medication doses for at-risk patient populations.

Dosages Based on Body Weight and Surface Area

Infants and children have special medication needs because of their smaller size and weight as well as larger body-surface area (BSA) per kilogram of body weight. They have varying capabilities of drug absorption, digestion, distribution, metabolism, and excretion. It is very important for the nurse to check current references for pediatric medication orders and to double-check safe dose ranges (SDRs) to prevent errors and injury. Minute doses that require scrupulous mathematics may be ordered. Pediatric and intensive care nurses use written pediatric drug guidelines and calculators to determine weights and verify SDRs.

The two methods currently used for calculating safe pediatric doses are based on (1) *body weight* in mg/kg or mcg/kg and (2) *body surface area* in square meters (m²) using a scale called a *nomogram*.

mg/kg Method

The most *frequently* used calculation method for pediatric medication administration is *mg/kg*. References usually state the safe amount of drug in mg/kg for a 24-hour period to be given in one or more divided doses. You may also see *mcg/kg* cited for therapeutic doses when very small amounts of medication are to be given.

STEPS TO SOLVING mg/kg PROBLEMS

Step 1 *Estimate* the child's weight in kilograms by dividing the pounds in half; then *calculate* the weight in kilograms using 2.2 lb = 1 kg equivalency (divide pounds by 2.2). Use a calculator.
   a. If the child's weight is in pounds, convert the pounds directly into kilograms (one-step calculation).
   b. If the child's weight is in pounds and ounces, convert the ounces to the nearest tenth of a pound and *add* this to the total pounds. Then convert the total pounds into kilograms to the nearest tenth (two-step calculation). (Refer to page 295 for kilogram-to-pound conversions and page 26 for rounding instructions.)

Step 2 *Calculate* the safe dose range (SDR) using a calculator and current pediatric safe dose recommendations found in the drug literature or drug handbook for this weight child in mg/kg or mcg/kg.

Step 3 *Compare* and *evaluate* the 24-hr ordered amount with the recommended SDR. Be sure the comparisons are for the *same* time frame!

Step 4 If safe, *calculate* the actual dose to be administered using written ratio and proportion. If the ordered dose is *less* than or *more* than the SDR, hold the medication and clarify promptly.

Shortcut Steps

1. Weight in kg
2. SDR
3. Compare with order
4. Calculate dose if safe to give

RULE All pediatric medication administration begins with an accurate weight (Step 1) and a calculation of the SDR (Step 2).

....

Example Ordered: EryPed (erythromycin ethylsuccinate suspension) 150 mg q6h po. The infant weighs 15 lb, 6 oz today. The literature states that the SDR is 30 to 100 mg/kg per day in four divided doses for severe infections.

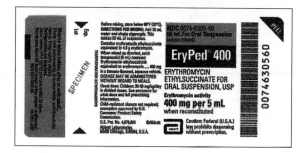

Step 1 **Estimate** the infant's weight.
a. *Pounds to kilograms:* 15 lb ÷ 2 = 7.5 kg
Calculate the actual weight.
b. **Two-step** conversion because ounces are involved.
Ounces to pounds: 6 oz ÷ 16 = 0.37 lb. Add part of pound to total pounds. The infant thus weighs 15.4 lb.
Pounds to kilograms: 15.4 lb ÷ 2.2 = 7 kg (close to estimate)

Step 2 The **SDR** recommended for children more than 1 month of age is 30 to 100 mg/kg per day po in four divided doses.
Low-range calculation: 30 mg × 7 kg = 210 mg (low SDR) per day ÷ 4
= 52.5 mg/dose
High-range calculation: 100 mg × 7 kg = 700 mg (high SDR) per day ÷ 4
= 175 mg/dose

Step 3 **Compare and evaluate:** The **SDR** recommended for this child's weight is 210 to 700 mg total q24h in four divided doses.
Ordered: 150 mg q6h or 150 mg × 4 or 600 mg total in 24 hr.

Step 4 **Decision:** Give medication. Administering 600 mg for the day is within the SDR of 210 to 700 mg in four divided doses.
Calculate the individual dose (write out and prove).

KNOW	WANT TO KNOW

400 mg : 5 mL :: 150 mg : x mL

$\dfrac{\cancel{400}}{\cancel{400}} x = \dfrac{750}{400}$ (5×150)

$x = 1.87$ or 1.9 mL

PROOF	ANSWER
$400 \times 1.87 = 748$	Give 1.9 mL
$5 \times 150 = 750$	

HINT | Review and analyze the logic of these four steps.

CLINICAL ALERT

Avoid two potential errors when converting pounds and ounces to kilograms. First, ounces must be converted to part of a pound *before* converting total pounds to kilograms; for example, 6 oz does not convert to 0.6 lb. Second, 15.4 lb does not equal 15.4 kg.

Don't forget the second step—convert the total pounds to kilograms.

ANSWERS ON PAGE 451

WORKSHEET
11A

Calculator Practice

RULE

Calculators are used in pediatric and intensive care units to determine weights and SDR. Dividing ounces by 16 will give the pound equivalent in the first step of two-step problems. Dividing or multiplying by 2.2 will give pound and kilogram equivalents.

....

1. Estimate the weights, then use a calculator to convert from pounds to kilograms or kilograms to pounds. Round to the *nearest* tenth.* Double-check all work.

    a. 14 lb (1 or 2 steps?)
        Estimate:
        Actual:

    b. 12 lb, 2 oz (1 or 2 steps?)
        Estimate:
        Actual:

    c. 10 lb
        Estimate:
        Actual:

    d. 14 kg
        Estimate:
        Actual:

    e. 10 kg
        Estimate:
        Actual:

---

* For rounding instructions, refer to p. 26.

ANSWERS ON PAGE 451

WORKSHEET
11A

Calculator Practice (Continued)

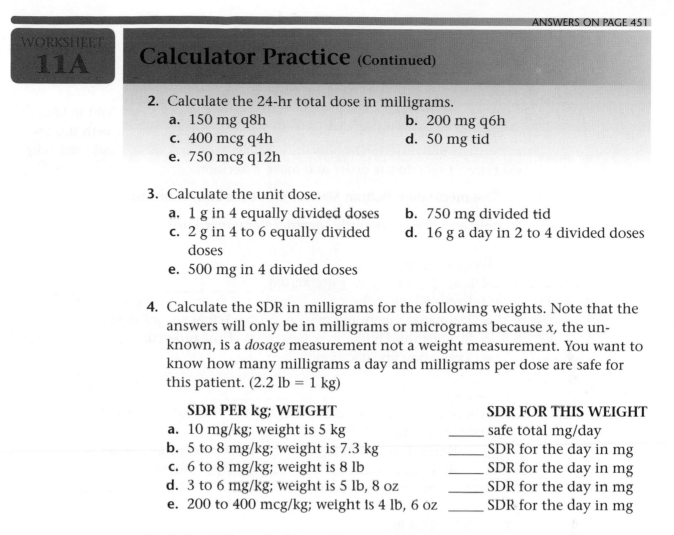

2. Calculate the 24-hr total dose in milligrams.
   a. 150 mg q8h
   b. 200 mg q6h
   c. 400 mcg q4h
   d. 50 mg tid
   e. 750 mcg q12h

3. Calculate the unit dose.
   a. 1 g in 4 equally divided doses
   b. 750 mg divided tid
   c. 2 g in 4 to 6 equally divided doses
   d. 16 g a day in 2 to 4 divided doses
   e. 500 mg in 4 divided doses

4. Calculate the SDR in milligrams for the following weights. Note that the answers will only be in milligrams or micrograms because x, the unknown, is a *dosage* measurement not a weight measurement. You want to know how many milligrams a day and milligrams per dose are safe for this patient. (2.2 lb = 1 kg)

SDR PER kg; WEIGHT	SDR FOR THIS WEIGHT
a. 10 mg/kg; weight is 5 kg	_____ safe total mg/day
b. 5 to 8 mg/kg; weight is 7.3 kg	_____ SDR for the day in mg
c. 6 to 8 mg/kg; weight is 8 lb	_____ SDR for the day in mg
d. 3 to 6 mg/kg; weight is 5 lb, 8 oz	_____ SDR for the day in mg
e. 200 to 400 mcg/kg; weight is 4 lb, 6 oz	_____ SDR for the day in mg

5. Ordered: Drug X, 50 mg tid.
   SDR: 2 to 3 mg/kg given in three divided doses. Child's weight is 18 kg.
   a. SDR for 24 hr
   b. SDR per dose
   c. Total ordered dose for day and per dose
   d. Evaluation and decision: Safe or unsafe to give? Why?

ANSWERS ON PAGE 452

WORKSHEET
11B

Children's Safe Dose Range (SDR) Practice

For each problem, use a calculator to determine the child's weight in kilograms to the nearest tenth, calculate the SDR, and compare it with the order. If the total dose for 24 hours is excessive, the unit dose is automatically excessive. Evaluate the order and make a decision.

1. Give medication (within SDR for unit dose and 24-hr dose).

2. Hold and clarify promptly (overdose or underdose).

1. Weight: 20 lb
   SDR in literature: 2 to 4 mg/kg/day
   Ordered: 50 mg daily
   a. Estimated weight in kg: b. Actual weight in kg:
   c. SDR for this child: d. Dose ordered:
   e. Evaluation and decision:

2. Weight: 33 lb
   SDR in literature: 100 to 200 mcg/kg/day in divided doses
   Ordered: 0.5 mg tid
   a. Estimated weight in kg: b. Actual weight in kg:
   c. SDR for this child: d. Dose ordered:
   e. Evaluation and decision:

3. Weight: 25.4 lb
   SDR in literature: 10 to 30 mg/kg/day in divided doses
   Ordered: 100 mg tid
   a. Estimated weight in kg: b. Actual weight in kg:
   c. SDR for this child: d. Dose ordered:
   e. Evaluation and decision:

4. Weight: 85 lb
   SDR: 10 to 15 mg/kg/day in 4 to 6 divided doses
   Ordered: 100 mg q6h
   a. Estimated weight in kg: b. Actual weight in kg:
   c. SDR for this child: d. Dose ordered:
   e. Evaluation and decision:

5. Weight 5 lb
   SDR: 10 to 20 mcg/kg/day
   Ordered: 0.03 mg four times daily
   a. Estimated weight in kg: b. Actual weight in kg:
   c. SDR for this child: d. Dose ordered:
   e. Evaluation and decision:

BSA Method (mg/m²)

The term "body surface area" refers to the total area exposed to the outside environment. The estimated BSA in square meters (m²) is derived from height and weight measurements by using a mathematical formula. It is considered the most reliable way to calculate therapeutic dosages.

This method may be used to calculate safe dosages of antineoplastic drugs, of new drugs, and of drugs for special populations such as infants, children, frail elderly patients, and patients with cancer. It may also be used to double check medication orders for safe dosage.

Nurses are not usually expected to calculate BSA. The pharmacy provides the BSA calculations. Nurses *do* have a critical responsibility to distinguish the difference in a medication order and dosage based in mg/**lb** or mg/**kg** of weight and an order based on mg/**m²** of BSA (e.g., 20 mg/kg vs 20 mg/m² vs 20 mg/lb).

Example   Child weighs 33 lb (15 kg) and has a BSA of 0.55 m².

ORDERED: 20 mg/kg   vs **ORDERED:** 20 mg/m²   vs **ORDERED** 20 mg/lb
20 mg : 1 kg ::   20 mg : 1 m² ::   20 mg : 1 lb ::
        x mg : 15 kg x mg : 0.55 x mg : 33 lb
$x = 20 \times 15 = 300$ mg $x = 20 \times 0.55 = 11$ mg $x = 20 \times 33 = 660$ mg

As seen, the doses calculated range from 11 mg to 660 mg, and depending on the unit of measurement, reflect extremely large differences. This illustrates the need to check not only the numbers but also the units of measurement.

The West nomogram in Figure 11-1 allows the user to plot the *estimated* square meters of BSA by using height and weight measurements.

Although the pharmacy usually supplies BSA calculations, the nurse has the option of estimating safe dosages easily and rapidly by using a mathematical formula and a calculator and entering the patient's height and weight data.

CALCULATING BSA (m²) USING A MATHEMATICAL FORMULA

There are two formulas for calculating BSA (m²), and both use height and weight dimensions.

A. Formula using only metric system   B. Formula using only pounds and inches

$$\sqrt{\frac{\text{Weight (kg)} \times \text{Height (cm)}}{3600}} = \text{m}^2 \text{ BSA} \qquad \sqrt{\frac{\text{Weight (lb)} \times \text{Height (in)}}{3131}} = \text{m}^2 \text{ BSA}$$

Note the differences in the divisors. The formulas must be used exactly as shown.

Directions: Use a calculator. Use the metric formula. Determine the BSA in square meters for a child with a weight of 20 kg and a height of 95 cm.

Step 1   Multiply the kilograms by centimeters first and *divide* the result by 3600 (20 × 95 = 900/3600 = 0.527)

Step 2 Obtain the *square root* of 0.527 by pushing the square root button. *Round* your answer to the *nearest* hundredth.

$$\frac{20 \times 95}{3600} = 0.527 \qquad \sqrt{0.527} = 0.725 = 0.73 \ m^2$$

Compare this answer with the West nomogram (see Figure 11-1). Create a straight line between 20 kg and 95 cm and read the result in the surface area (SA) column on the nomogram. Take care to plot the height and weight on the metric graph—the outside columns. When reading the results (m²) columns, be sure to note the value of each calibrated line on the scale at the intersection point.

You may use either the nomogram or the formula. The formula method is more accurate, and if you have a calculator on hand, it is faster.

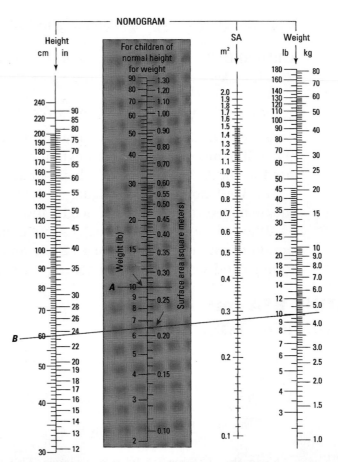

FIGURE 11-1 West nomogram for estimation of body surface area (BSA). **A,** The estimated BSA in square meters for children of normal height for weight is determined by reading the m² at the alignment point with the child's weight in pounds in the highlighted column. The red line denoted by the arrow reveals that an infant weighing 10 lb has an approximate BSA of 0.27 m². **B,** The BSA in square meters for children who are *under*weight or *over*weight (Refer to pediatric standard growth charts and development grids for normal height and weight ranges for pediatric groups.) is determined by connecting the child's plotted weight in the left column and plotted height in the right column with a straight line and reading the intersection point on the SA (surface area) column, as indicated by the arrow on the red line. This illustrates an estimated BSA of 0.28 m² for an infant of 60 cm height weighing 4.5 kg. Reading the SA column requires that height and weight be plotted in the same system of measurement, metric or pounds/inches. *(Nomogram modified with data from Berhrman RE, Kleigman RM, Jenson HB: Nelson textbook of pediatrics, ed 17, Philadelphia, 2004, Saunders.)*

ANSWERS ON PAGE 452

WORKSHEET
11C

Comparing BSA-Based (mg/m²) Dosages with mg/lb and mg/kg Orders

Use the West nomogram (page 300), highlighted section for children of normal height and weight, to obtain the BSA (m²) based on weight.

Calculate the dose to be given based on the mg/m² and dose ordered.

	WT IN lb	BSA IN m²	DOSE ORDERED	DOSE TO BE GIVEN
1.	4 lb	0.15	10 mg/m²	$10 \times 0.15 = 1.5$ mg
2.	6 lb	_____	15 mg/m²	_____
3.	10 lb	_____	5 mg/m²	_____

Calculate the dose for the same-weight children in mg/lb measurements, as illustrated in Problem 4.

	WT IN lb	DOSE ORDERED	DOSE TO BE GIVEN
4.	4 lb	10 mg/lb	$4 \times 10 = 40$ mg
5.	6 lb	15 mg/lb	_____
6.	10 lb	5 mg/lb	_____

Calculate the dose to be given in mg/kg measurements, as illustrated in Problem 9. Divide lb by 2.2 to obtain kg.

	WT IN kg (TO NEAREST TENTH)	DOSE ORDERED	DOSE TO BE GIVEN
7.	4 lb = 1.8 kg	10 mg/kg	$10 \times 1.8 = 18$ mg
8.	6 lb = _____ kg	2 mg/kg	

9. Using a calculator, obtain the BSA in m² (to the nearest hundredth for a child with a height of 60 cm and a weight of 100 kg using the appropriate BSA formula on page 299: _____

10. Using a calculator, obtain the BSA in m² for a child with a height of 70 in and weight of 12 lb using the appropriate BSA formula on page 299: _____

◆**CLINICAL ALERT**

Consider the patient safety implications when mg/m², mg/lb, and mg/kg are erroneously interchanged. This has resulted in serious errors. The nurse must understand the differences among these three terms and focus to ensure that the correct values are being used when calculating the dose.

ANSWERS ON PAGE 453

WORKSHEET
11D

Additional Children's Safe Dose Range (SDR) Practice

Estimate and calculate weights and doses. Evaluate the order. If dose is within the SDR, calculate and prove the answer.

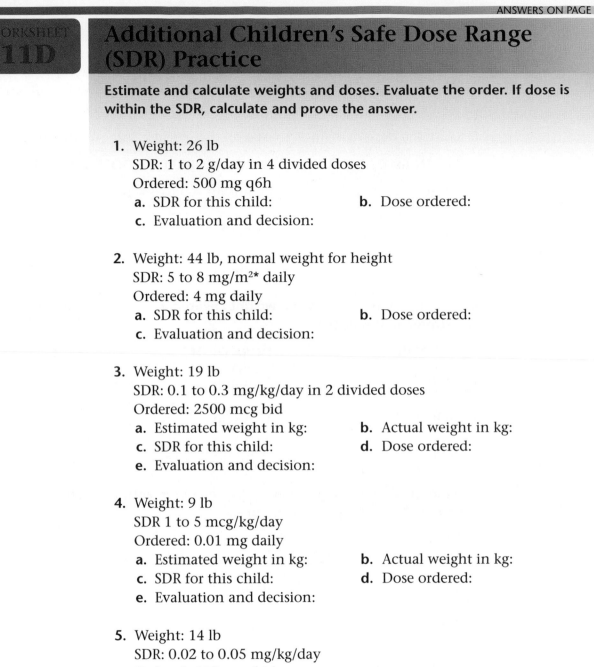

1. Weight: 26 lb
   SDR: 1 to 2 g/day in 4 divided doses
   Ordered: 500 mg q6h
   a. SDR for this child: b. Dose ordered:
   c. Evaluation and decision:

2. Weight: 44 lb, normal weight for height
   SDR: 5 to 8 mg/m²* daily
   Ordered: 4 mg daily
   a. SDR for this child: b. Dose ordered:
   c. Evaluation and decision:

3. Weight: 19 lb
   SDR: 0.1 to 0.3 mg/kg/day in 2 divided doses
   Ordered: 2500 mcg bid
   a. Estimated weight in kg: b. Actual weight in kg:
   c. SDR for this child: d. Dose ordered:
   e. Evaluation and decision:

4. Weight: 9 lb
   SDR 1 to 5 mcg/kg/day
   Ordered: 0.01 mg daily
   a. Estimated weight in kg: b. Actual weight in kg:
   c. SDR for this child: d. Dose ordered:
   e. Evaluation and decision:

5. Weight: 14 lb
   SDR: 0.02 to 0.05 mg/kg/day
   Ordered: 150 mcg bid
   a. Estimated weight in kg: b. Actual weight in kg:
   c. SDR for this child: d. Dose ordered:
   e. Evaluation and decision:

---

*For BSA conversion, refer to West nomogram on page 300.

◆ CLINICAL ALERT

Estimating the weight in kg before doing the actual calculation is a safety check for calculation errors. Estimating approximate doses of medicines is also a valuable safety check.

ANSWERS ON PAGE 454

WORKSHEET
11E

Children's Oral Medications

These medications can be given to infants and children with a dropper or in a pre-prepared oral medication syringe (Figure 11-2). Small amounts may be given to an infant in a nipple. You may need to prepare and administer these medications using an oral syringe (without a needle).

For each problem, use a calculator to determine the child's weight in kilograms or pounds if required, calculate the SDR, and compare it with the order. Evaluate the order and make a decision:

1. Give medication (within SDR for unit dose and 24-hr dose).

2. Hold and clarify promptly (overdose or underdose).

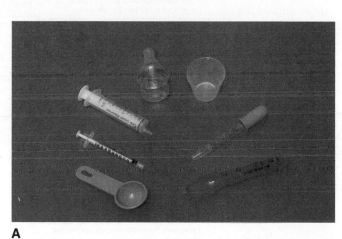

FIGURE 11-2 **A,** Acceptable devices for measuring and administering oral medication to children *(clockwise):* measuring spoon, plastic syringes, calibrated nipple, plastic medicine cup, calibrated dropper, hollow-handled medicine spoon. **B,** Pre-filled oral syringe. **C,** Calibrated droppers. *(A, From Wong DL et al: Wong's nursing care of infants and children, ed 7, St Louis, 2005, Mosby. C, From Macklin D, Chernecky C, Infortuna H: Math for clinical practice, ed 1, St Louis, 2005, Mosby.)*

A

B

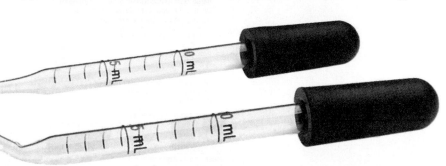

C

Continued

ANSWERS ON PAGE 454

WORKSHEET
11E

Children's Oral Medications (Continued)

For decisions 1 and 2 only, calculate the medication amount to be administered using *written ratio and proportion*. Prove your work. Do *not* calculate overdose or underdose orders. Hold them and clarify promptly.

1. Ordered: Tylenol (acetaminophen children's elixir) 160 mg po for a 4-year-old child who weighs 14 kg today. Label: 80 mg per $\frac{1}{2}$ tsp.

   a. Estimated weight in lb: **b.** Actual weight in lb:

   c. SDR for this child: **d.** Dose ordered:

   e. Evaluation and decision: **f.** Amount to be given in mL if applicable:

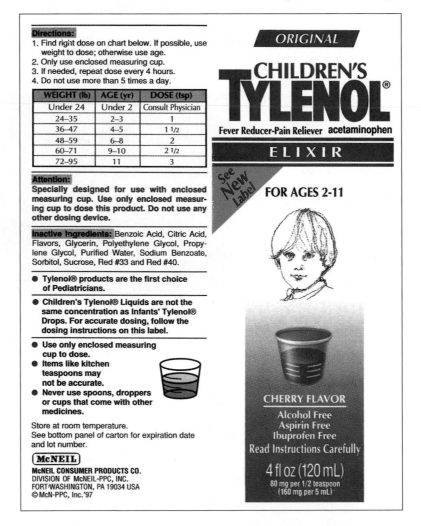

Directions:
1. Find right dose on chart below. If possible, use weight to dose; otherwise use age.
2. Only use enclosed measuring cup.
3. If needed, repeat dose every 4 hours.
4. Do not use more than 5 times a day.

WEIGHT (lb)	AGE (yr)	DOSE (tsp)
Under 24	Under 2	Consult Physician
24–35	2–3	1
36–47	4–5	1 1/2
48–59	6–8	2
60–71	9–10	2 1/2
72–95	11	3

Attention:
Specially designed for use with enclosed measuring cup. Use only enclosed measuring cup to dose this product. Do not use any other dosing device.

Inactive Ingredients: Benzoic Acid, Citric Acid, Flavors, Glycerin, Polyethylene Glycol, Propylene Glycol, Purified Water, Sodium Benzoate, Sorbitol, Sucrose, Red #33 and Red #40.

● Tylenol® products are the first choice of Pediatricians.

● Children's Tylenol® Liquids are not the same concentration as Infants' Tylenol® Drops. For accurate dosing, follow the dosing instructions on this label.

● Use only enclosed measuring cup to dose.
● Items like kitchen teaspoons may not be accurate.
● Never use spoons, droppers or cups that come with other medicines.

Store at room temperature.
See bottom panel of carton for expiration date and lot number.

McNEIL
McNEIL CONSUMER PRODUCTS CO.
DIVISION OF McNEIL-PPC, INC.
FORT WASHINGTON, PA 19034 USA
©McN-PPC, Inc.'97

ORIGINAL
CHILDREN'S TYLENOL®
Fever Reducer-Pain Reliever acetaminophen
ELIXIR
See New Label
FOR AGES 2-11
CHERRY FLAVOR
Alcohol Free
Aspirin Free
Ibuprofen Free
Read Instructions Carefully
4 fl oz (120 mL)
80 mg per 1/2 teaspoon
(160 mg per 5 mL)

CLINICAL ALERT

Avoid mixing medicines in essential foods such as formula or milk. A changed taste may result in long-term refusal of that food. The medicine may be followed immediately with formula, milk, or a popsicle as the diet permits.

ANSWERS ON PAGE 454

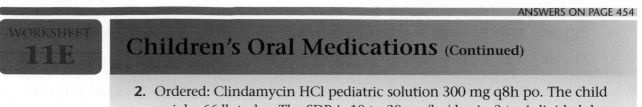

WORKSHEET
11E

Children's Oral Medications (Continued)

2. Ordered: Clindamycin HCl pediatric solution 300 mg q8h po. The child weighs 66 lb today. The SDR is 10 to 30 mg/kg/day in 3 to 4 divided doses.
   a. Estimated weight in kg:
   b. Actual weight in kg:
   c. SDR for this child:
   d. Dose ordered:
   e. Evaluation and decision:
   f. Amount to be given in mL if applicable:

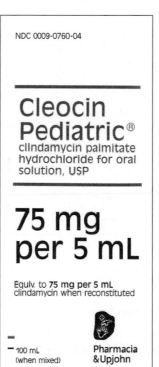

NDC 0009-0760-04

Cleocin Pediatric®
clindamycin palmitate hydrochloride for oral solution, USP

75 mg per 5 mL

Equiv. to **75 mg per 5 mL** clindamycin when reconstituted

— 100 mL
(when mixed)

Pharmacia & Upjohn

⬡ **CLINICAL ALERT**

Differentiate elixirs and concentrated drops from oral suspensions. Elixirs contain alcohol for flavoring. Suspensions contain solids that must be dispersed in the liquid by shaking or stirring. Concentrated drops contain a greater amount of drug in a smaller volume of liquid than ordinary drops. They need to be shaken prior to administration.

Continued

ANSWERS ON PAGE 454

WORKSHEET
11E

Children's Oral Medications (Continued)

3. Ordered: Tegretol (carbamazepine) oral suspension 0.25 g po tid. The SDR for maintenance in a child over 12 years of age is 400 to 800 mg/day in 3 to 4 divided doses.
   a. SDR for this child:
   b. Dose ordered in mg:
   c. Evaluation and decision:
   d. Amount to be given if applicable:

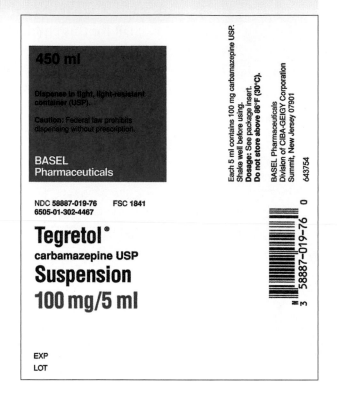

4. Ordered: Leucovorin calcium 5 mg q6h po. The child weighs 24 lb and has normal weight and height. The SDR according to the literature is 10 mg/m² q6h for 72 hr. For BSA calculation, refer to the West nomogram on page 300. The BSA is determined by pounds, not kilograms.
   a. SDR for this child:
   b. Dose ordered:
   c. Evaluation and decision:
   d. Amount to be given if applicable:

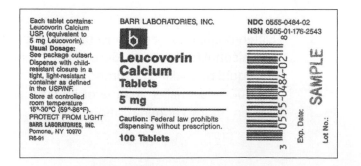

ANSWERS ON PAGE 454

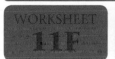

Children's Oral Medications (Continued)

5. Ordered: Amoxil 180 mg q8h po for a child who weighs 27 lb. The SDR is 40 mg/kg/day in 3 divided doses.

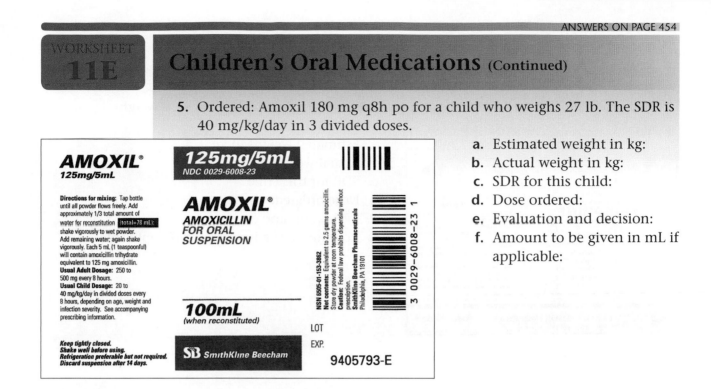

a. Estimated weight in kg:

b. Actual weight in kg:

c. SDR for this child:

d. Dose ordered:

e. Evaluation and decision:

f. Amount to be given in mL if applicable:

ANSWERS ON PAGE 455

Children's Subcutaneous and Intramuscular Medications

For each problem, use a calculator to determine the child's weight in kg to the nearest tenth, calculate the SDR, and compare It with the order. Evaluate the order and make a decision:

1. **Give medication (within SDR for unit dose and 24-hr dose).**

2. **Hold and clarify promptly (overdose or underdose).**

For decisions 1 and 2 only, calculate the medication amount to be administered using *written ratio and proportion*. **Double-check and prove your work. Do** *not* **calculate overdose orders.**

1. Ordered: Meperidine HCl 30 mg IM preoperatively for a child who weighs 32 lb, 5 oz. The SDR is 1 to 2.2 mg/kg.

   a. Estimated weight in kg:

   b. Actual weight in kg:

   c. SDR for this child:

   d. Dose ordered:

   e. Evaluation and decision:

   f. Volume to be administered if applicable:

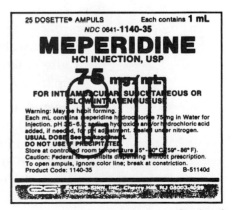

Continued

ANSWERS ON PAGE 455

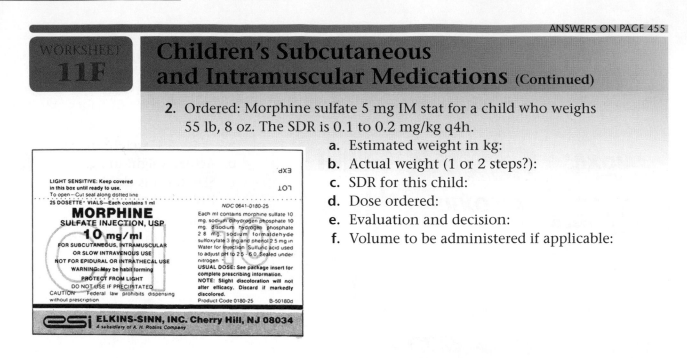

WORKSHEET 11F

Children's Subcutaneous and Intramuscular Medications (Continued)

2. Ordered: Morphine sulfate 5 mg IM stat for a child who weighs 55 lb, 8 oz. The SDR is 0.1 to 0.2 mg/kg q4h.

a. Estimated weight in kg:

b. Actual weight (1 or 2 steps?):

c. SDR for this child:

d. Dose ordered:

e. Evaluation and decision:

f. Volume to be administered if applicable:

Morphine label:

LIGHT SENSITIVE: Keep covered in this box until ready to use. To open—Cut seal along dotted line

EXP

LOT

25 DOSETTE · VIALS—Each contains 1 ml

NDC 0641-0180-25

MORPHINE
SULFATE INJECTION, USP

10 mg/ml

FOR SUBCUTANEOUS, INTRAMUSCULAR OR SLOW INTRAVENOUS USE

NOT FOR EPIDURAL OR INTRATHECAL USE

WARNING: May be habit forming

PROTECT FROM LIGHT

DO NOT USE IF PRECIPITATED

CAUTION   Federal law prohibits dispensing without prescription

Each ml contains morphine sulfate 10 mg, sodium dihydrogen phosphate 10 mg, disodium hydrogen phosphate 2 8 mg, sodium formaldehyde sulfoxylate 3 mg and phenol 2 5 mg in Water for Injection Sulfuric acid used to adjust pH to 2 5 - 6 0. Sealed under nitrogen

USUAL DOSE: See package insert for complete prescribing information.

NOTE: Slight discoloration will not alter efficacy. Discard if markedly discolored.

Product Code 0180-25   B-50180d

ELKINS-SINN, INC. Cherry Hill, NJ 08034
A subsidiary of A. H. Robins Company

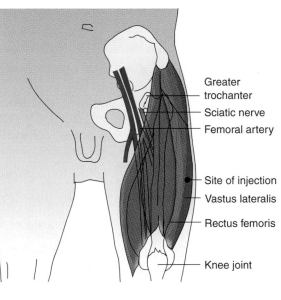

FIGURE 11-3 The mid-anterolateral thigh (vastus lateralis muscle) is the preferred site for injections in infants. *(From Lilley LL, Auker RS: Pharmacology and the nursing process, ed 3, St. Louis, 2001, Mosby.)*

Greater trochanter
Sciatic nerve
Femoral artery
Site of injection
Vastus lateralis
Rectus femoris
Knee joint

CLINICAL ALERT

Intramuscular injections are rarely ordered on a routine basis for children because of limited numbers of sites, painful physical trauma, and psychosocial implications.

The mid-anterolateral thigh is the preferred site for injections in infants (Figure 11-3) until the child has walked for a year. The ventrogluteal muscle is a preferred site after the age of 7 months. Never use the deltoid muscle in young children. Needle lengths and gauges and fluid amounts are much smaller for infants and children than for adults.*

*Refer to current pediatric clinical skills manuals.

ANSWERS ON PAGE 455

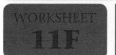

Children's Subcutaneous and Intramuscular Medications (Continued)

3. Ordered: Atropine sulfate 0.2 mg subcutaneous preoperatively for a child who weighs 17 lb, 9 oz. The SDR for a child weighing 7 to 9 kg is 0.2 mg, 30 to 60 min before surgery.

a. Estimated weight in kg:

b. Actual weight (1 or 2 steps?):

c. SDR for this child:

d. Dose ordered:

e. Evaluation and decision:

f. Volume to be administered if applicable:

NDC 0002-1675-01
20 mL   VIAL No. 419
℞ *Lilly*
POISON

ATROPINE
SULFATE
INJECTION, USP
0.4 mg per mL
CAUTION—Federal (U.S.A.) law
prohibits dispensing without
prescription.

Store at 59° to 86°F (15° to 30°C)
Usual Adult Dose—0.75 to 1.5 mL
injected subcutaneously, intramuscularly,
or slowly intravenously. See literature.
Each mL contains Atropine Sulfate,
0.4 mg with Chlorobutanol (Chloroform
Derivative) 0.5 percent.
Eli Lilly & Co., Indianapolis, IN 46285, U.S.A.
WV 6731 AMX
APPROXIMATE EQUIVALENTS
0.4 mL=0.16 mg
0.5 mL=0.2 mg
0.6 mL=0.24 mg
0.8 mL=0.32 mg
1   mL=0.4 mg
1.25 mL=0.5 mg
1.5 mL=0.6 mg
2.5 mL=1.0 mg
3.1 mL=1.25 mg
Exp. Date/Control No.

4. Ordered: Ampicillin sodium 500 mg IM q12h for a baby with septicemia weighing 7 lb. SDR is 100 to 200 mg/kg/day in two divided doses.

a. Estimated weight in kg:

b. Actual weight (1 or 2 steps?):

c. SDR for this child:

d. Dose ordered:

e. Evaluation and decision:

f. Volume to be administered if applicable:

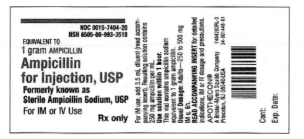

NDC 0015-7404-20
NSN 6505-00-993-3518
EQUIVALENT TO
1 gram AMPICILLIN
**Ampicillin
for Injection, USP**
Formerly known as
Sterile Ampicillin Sodium, USP
For IM or IV Use
Rx only

For IM use, add 3.5 mL diluent (read accom-
panying insert). Resulting solution contains
250 mg ampicillin per mL.
Use solution within 1 hour.
This vial contains ampicillin sodium
equivalent to 1 gram ampicillin.
Usual Dosage: Adults—250 to 500 mg
IM q. 6h.
READ ACCOMPANYING INSERT for detailed
indications, IM or IV dosage and precautions.
APOTHECON®
A Bristol-Myers Squibb Company
Princeton, NJ 08540 USA
7404210PL-3
34-001-448-01
Cont:
Exp. Date:

5. Ordered: Oxacillin sodium 1500 mg IM q8h for an 11-year-old child weighing 75 lb. The SDR is 50 to 100 mg/kg/day in 4 divided doses.

a. Estimated weight in kg:

b. Actual weight (1 or 2 steps?):

c. SDR for this child:

d. Dose ordered:

e. Evaluation and decision:

f. Volume to be administered if applicable:

NDC 0015-7979-20
EQUIVALENT TO
500 mg OXACILLIN
**OXACILLIN SODIUM
FOR INJECTION, USP**
Buffered—For IM or IV Use
CAUTION: Federal law prohibits
dispensing without prescription.

This vial contains oxacillin sodium
monohydrate equivalent to 500 mg
oxacillin and 10 mg/dibasic sodium
phosphate. • Add 2.7 mL Sterile
Water for Injection, USP • Each
1.5 mL contains 250 mg oxacillin.
Usual Dosage: Adults—250 mg to
500 mg intramuscularly every 4 to
6 hours. See circular for intravenous use.
READ ACCOMPANYING CIRCULAR
Discard solution after 3 days at
room temperature or 7 days under
refrigeration.
Manufactured by APOTHECON®
A Bristol-Myers Squibb Company
Princeton, NJ 08540
7979200BH-1
Cont:
Exp. Date:

Children's IV Medications: Reconstitution, Dilution, and Flow Rate Information

Hospital pharmacies and pediatric drug references provide directions for dilution and rates of administration of IV medications for children. The volumes are smaller than those for adults. After determining that the ordered dose is within the SDR, the nurse may have to dilute the medication in a prescribed ratio, withdraw the ordered amount, then further dilute it using a compatible IV solution, and administer it directly or by an infusion pump in a volume-control device. Devices used to administer IV medications to children are shown in Figure 11-4.

FIGURE 11-4 **A,** Electronic infusion pump with volume-control device. **B,** Gravity infusion with microdrip tubing (60 gtt/mL delivered through a needle) and volume-control device. Electronic infusion devices with volume-control devices are preferred for the administration of IV fluids to infants and children. If one of these is not available, microdrip (60-drop factor) tubing should be used with a volume-control device to prevent fluid or drug overload. Very small volumes to be delivered IV within a short period may be administered directly through a syringe or a syringe pump. **C,** Freedom 60-syringe infusion pump system. (**C,** From Repro-Med Systems, Inc., Chester NY.)

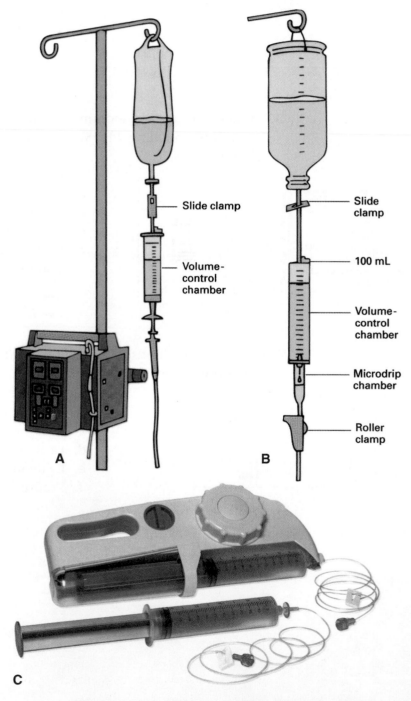

Example Ordered: Antibiotic 1 g q6h. Supplied: A powdered form of antibiotic that requires reconstitution. Pediatric directions from pharmacy: *Dilute to 100 mg/mL, withdraw ordered amount, then further dilute to 30 mL, and administer over 20 min.* The label reads 2 g.

Step 1 Dilute to 100 mg/mL.

The label reads 2 g. (Change to milligrams for dilution: 2 g = 2000 mg.)

KNOW   WANT TO KNOW

100 mg : 1 mL :: 2000 mg : x mL

PROOF
$100 \times 20 = 2000$
$1 \times 2000 = 2000$

$\dfrac{\cancel{100}}{\cancel{100}} x = \dfrac{2000}{100}$

$x = 20$ mL

Reconstitute antibiotic with 20 mL compatible solution.*

Step 2 Withdraw ordered amount (1 g).

KNOW   WANT TO KNOW

2 g : 20 mL :: 1 g : x mL

$2x = 20$

$x = 10$ mL = 1 g

PROOF
$2 \times 10 = 20$
$20 \times 1 = 20$

ANSWER
10 mL

Step 3 Place the medication in a volume-control device, adding a compatible IV solution to 30 mL. Set the flow rate. Consult a procedure book for use of volume-control devices.

Flow rate:

KNOW   WANT TO KNOW

30 mL : 20 min :: x mL : 60 min

$\dfrac{\cancel{20}}{\cancel{20}} x = \dfrac{1800}{20}$

$x = 90$ mL

PROOF
$30 \times 60 = 1800$
$20 \times 90 = 1800$

ANSWER
Set rate at 90 mL/hr for 20 min

RULES To *estimate* hourly IV flow rates for amounts to be delivered in less than 60 minutes by a pump: for **10** minutes, multiply the volume by 6 because there are six 10-minute periods in an hour; for **15** minutes, multiply the volume by 4; for **20** minutes, multiply the volume by 3; and for **30** minutes, multiply the volume by 2. This will work only for 10-, 15-, 20-, and 30-minute orders.

....

To *calculate* the setting for mL/hr on a pump for medications to be delivered in less than 1 hour, set up a ratio and proportion of milliliters to minutes. The final dilution may be made with an existing IV solution if it is compatible with the medication.

....

Example To give 10 mL in 15 min with a pump, *estimate* (10 × 4 = 40 mL/hr):

KNOW   WANT TO KNOW

10 mL : 15 min :: x mL : 60 min

$\dfrac{\cancel{15}}{\cancel{15}} x = \dfrac{600}{15}$

$x = 40$ mL

PROOF
$10 \times 60 = 600$
$15 \times 40 = 600$

ANSWER
40 mL/hr

---

*For information and practice reconstituting medications, refer to Chapter 5.

Example   Ordered: Antibiotic 250 mg q4h IV.

The label reads: *Mix (dilute) with 4.2 mL sterile water for injection to yield 5 mL of 100 mg/mL.*

Amount of ordered antibiotic to be withdrawn after mixing:

KNOW	WANT TO KNOW	PROOF	ANSWER
100 mg : 1 mL :: 250 mg : x mL		$100 \times 2.5 = 250$	2.5 mL
		$1 \times 250 = 250$	

$$\frac{\cancel{100}}{\cancel{100}} x = \frac{250}{100}$$

$$x = 2.5 \text{ mL}$$

Directions for pediatric administration: *Further dilute to 25 mL and administer over 30 minutes.*

Total volume to be administered: 25 mL.

Example   Flow rate in volume-control device, estimate ($2 \times 25 = 50$ mL/hr):

KNOW	WANT TO KNOW	PROOF	ANSWER
25 mL : 30 min :: x mL : 60 min		$25 \times 60 = 1500$	50 mL/hr
$30x = 25 \times 60$ or 1500		$30 \times 50 = 1500$	
$x = 50$ mL			

ANSWERS ON PAGE 456

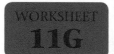
WORKSHEET **11G**

Children's IV Medications

For each problem, use a calculator to determine the child's weight in kg if required, calculate the SDR, and compare it with the order. Evaluate the order and make a decision:

1. Give medication (within SDR for unit dose 24-hr dose).

2. Hold and clarify promptly (overdose or underdose).

For directions 1 and 2 *only,* calculate the medication amount to be administered based on the label provided. Use written ratio and proportion and prove your answer even if you use a calculator to verify it. Calculate the IV pump flow rate in mL/hr if medication is to be administered for more than 5 min. Round kilograms to the nearest tenth. Prove all work.

1. Ordered: Luminal sodium 65 mg IV stat. The child's weight is 62 lb. The SDR for sedation is 1 to 3 mg/kg q24h.

   Directions: Dilute to 3 mL with sterile water for injection.
   a. Estimated weight in kg:
   b. Actual weight in kg:
   c. SDR for this child:
   d. Dose ordered:
   e. Evaluation and decision:
   f. Dose in mL to be withdrawn before dilution:

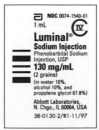

ANSWERS ON PAGE 456

WORKSHEET
11G

Children's IV Medications (Continued)

2. Ordered: Initial dose of furosemide 25 mg IV stat. The SDR is 1 mg/kg to increase gradually in 1 mg/kg increments to desired response, not to exceed 6 mg/kg. The child weighs 55 lb today.

a. Estimated weight in kg:

b. Actual weight in kg:

c. SDR for this child:

d. Dose ordered:

e. Evaluation and decision:

f. Volume to be administered
   if applicable:

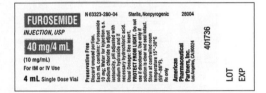

3. Ordered: Nebcin (tobramycin sulfate) 18 mg IV q8h. The child weighs 13.2 lb today. The SDR is 3 mg/kg q8h. Directions from the pharmacy state to dilute *to* 50 mL with 0.9% NaCl and administer over 60 min.

a. Estimated weight in kg:

b. Actual weight in kg:

c. SDR for this child:

d. Dose ordered:

e. Evaluation and decision:

f. Amount withdrawn from vial:

g. Flow rate in mL/hr on pump if applicable:

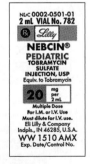

⬡ CLINICAL ALERT

> Many of the antibiotics, particularly the cephalosporins (refer to Problem 4), have very similar names, such as ceftizoxime, ceftriaxone, and cephradine. However, the uses and the SDRs are very different!

Continued

ANSWERS ON PAGE 456

WORKSHEET
11G

Children's IV Medications (Continued)

4. Ordered: Zinacef (cefuroxime sodium) IV 0.3 g q6h. The SDR is 50 to 100 mg/kg/day in divided doses q6-8h. To reconstitute for children in an intermittent infusion, dilute medication with 9 mL of compatible solution, which will make a total of 10 mL, then further dilute medication ordered *to* 20 mL of a compatible solution and administer in a volume-control device on an IV infusion pump in 30 min. The child weighs 34 lb today.

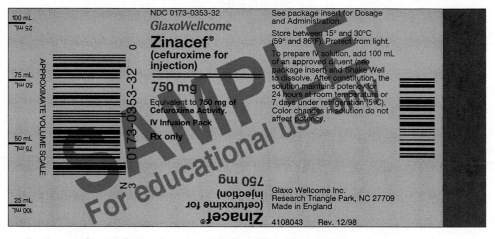

a. Estimated weight in kg: b. Actual weight in kg:
c. SDR for this child: d. Dose ordered:
e. Evaluation and decision: f. Ordered amount of medication
g. Flow rate on infusion pump in mL to be withdrawn *after first*
   after final dilution: dilution:

5. Ordered: Geopen (carbenicillin disodium) 2 g IV q6h. The SDR is 50 to 500 mg/kg q24h in divided doses every 4 to 6 hr. Dilute to 200 mg/mL with compatible solution and administer at rate of 1 g/10 min. The child weighs 26 lb.

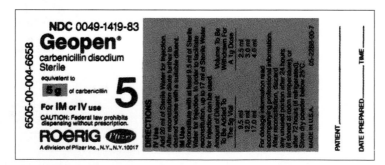

a. Estimated weight in kg:
b. Actual weight in kg:
c. SDR for this child:
d. Dose ordered:
e. Evaluation and decision:
f. Amount withdrawn after reconstitution:
g. Flow rate in mL/hr if applicable:

CLINICAL ALERT

Pediatric IV flow rates carry a high potential for errors. Consult pediatric IV drug references and pharmacy for pediatric IV dilutions and rates of administration. Note that liquids added to solids result in a higher total volume than just the amount of liquid added. Instructions to dilute *with x mL* result in more volume than instructions to dilute *to x mL*. Dilute *to* limits a total volume for the mixture. Dilute *with* is just stating the amount of liquid to be added to the solid. When in any doubt about IV dilutions and flow rates, consult the pharmacy and document the verification. The prescriber may have to be contacted too.

ANSWERS ON PAGE 458

WORKSHEET 11H

Children's Dosages

For each problem, use a calculator to determine the child's weight in kilograms to the nearest tenth, calculate the SDR, and compare it with the order. If the total dose for 24 hours is excessive, the unit dose is automatically excessive. Evaluate the order and make a decision:

1. Give the medication (within SDR for unit dose and 24-hr dose).

2. Hold and clarify promptly (overdose or underdose).

Calculate doses less than 1 mL to the nearest hundredth and doses more than 1 mL to the nearest tenth. Double-check your work and show your proof.

1. Ordered: Amoxil 100 mg tid po for a child with otitis media.
   Weight: 33 lb
   SDR: 20 mg/kg in 3 divided doses

   a. Estimated weight in kg:
   b. Actual weight in kg:
   c. SDR for this child:
   d. Dose ordered:
   e. Evaluation and decision:
   f. Amount to be administered if applicable:

Continued

ANSWERS ON PAGE 458

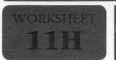

Children's Dosages (Continued)

2. Ordered: Lufyllin (dyphilline elixir) 75 mg bid for a child with asthma.
   Weight: 30 kg
   SDR: 5 mg/kg in 2 to 3 divided doses per day

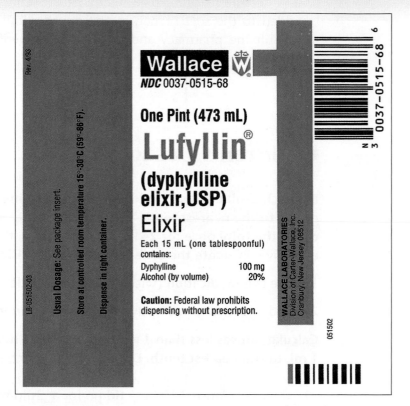

  a. SDR for this child:

  b. Dose ordered:

  c. Evaluation and decision:

  d. Amount to be administered to nearest tenth of a mL if applicable:

3. Ordered: Synthroid 0.1 mg qAM IV for a 6-year-old child with hypothyroidism.
   Weight: 49 lb
   SDR: 4 to 5 mcg/kg/day po; IV $\frac{1}{2}$ of po dose

  a. Estimated weight in kg:

  b. Actual weight in kg:

  c. SDR for this child:

  d. Dose ordered:

  e. Evaluation and decision:

  f. Amount to be administered if applicable:

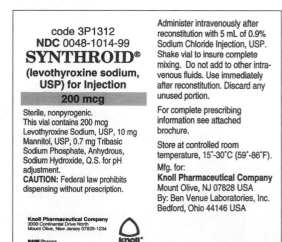

ANSWERS ON PAGE 458

Children's Dosages (Continued)

4. Ordered: Meperidine HCl 35 mg IM preoperatively.
Weight: 66 lb
SDR: 1 to 2.2 mg/kg

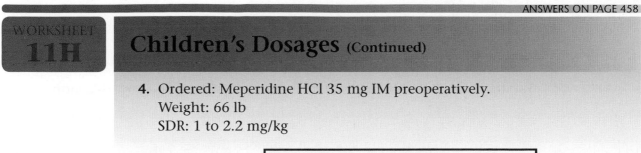

a. Estimated weight in kg:
b. Actual weight in kg:
c. SDR for this child:
d. Dose ordered:
e. Evaluation and decision:
f. Amount to be administered if applicable:

5. Ordered: Deltasone (prednisone) 30 mg/day po for a child with acute asthma.
Weight: 13.6 kg (BSA = 0.6 m^2)
SDR: 40 mg/m^2 day po

Caution: Federal law prohibits dispensing without prescription.
See package insert for complete product information.
Dispense in tight, light-resistant container.
Keep patient under close observation of a physician.
Store at controlled room temperature 20° to 25° C (68° to 77° F) [see USP].
810 362 708
Pharmacia & Upjohn Company
Kalamazoo, MI 49001, USA

NDC 0009-0193-01

Deltasone®
Tablets

prednisone tablets, USP

10 mg

100 Tablets

Lot
Exp

a. SDR for this child:
b. Dose ordered:
c. Evaluation and decision:
d. Amount to be administered if applicable:

Continued

ANSWERS ON PAGE 458

Children's Dosages (Continued)

6. Ordered: Ampicillin sodium 250 mg IV q6h for a child with a kidney infection.
   Weight: 22 lb
   SDR: 50 to 100 mg/kg/day in 4 divided doses

   Directions: Dilute 1 g vial in at least 10 mL of sterile water for injection before further dilutions. Further dilute to 20 mg/mL in D5W. Final concentration should never exceed 30 mg/mL.
   a. Estimated weight in kg:
   b. Actual weight in kg:
   c. SDR for this child:
   d. Dose ordered:
   e. Evaluation and decision:
   f. Amount to be administered if applicable:

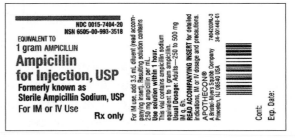

7. Ordered: Potassium chloride (KCl) 0.9 mEq to be added to each IV q8h.
   Weight: 6 lb
   SDR: Up to 3 mEq/kg/24 hr
   a. Estimated weight in kg:
   b. Actual weight in kg:
   c. SDR for this child:
   d. Dose ordered:
   e. Evaluation and decision:
   f. Dose to be added to IV:

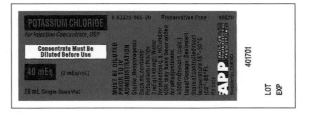

8. Ordered: Rocephin (ceftriaxone sodium) 600 mg IV q12h for a child with an infection by a *Shigella* species.
   Weight: 31 lb
   SDR: Up to 100 mg/kg/day in 2 divided doses

   Directions: Add 9.6 mL sterile water for injection to equal 100 mg/mL. Further dilute to 30 mL with compatible solution over 30 min.
   a. Estimated weight in kg:
   b. Actual weight in kg:
   c. SDR for this child:
   d. Dose ordered:
   e. Evaluation and decision:
   f. Dose to be administered after reconstitution if applicable:
   g. Flow rate in Volutrol:

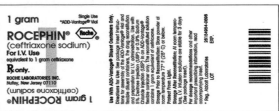

ANSWERS ON PAGE 458

WORKSHEET 11H

Children's Dosages (Continued)

9. Ordered: Acetaminophen drops 20 mg po q4h for a 3-month-old infant. Physician has verified dosage and concentrated drop preparation.

   a. Dose to be administered:

   b. Measuring device to be used:

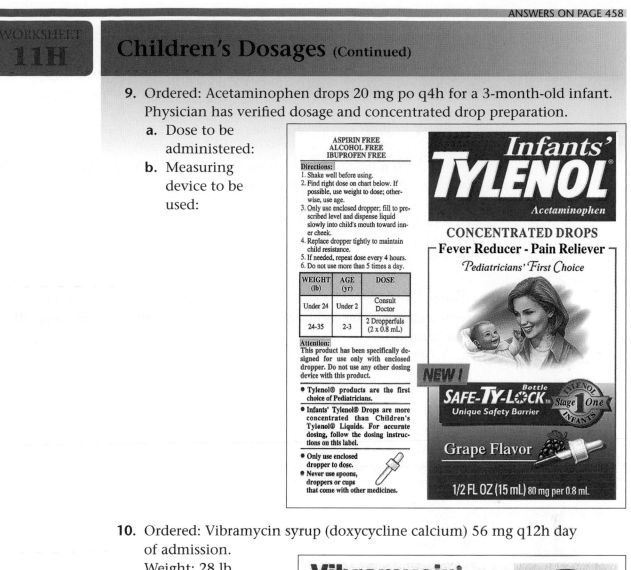

10. Ordered: Vibramycin syrup (doxycycline calcium) 56 mg q12h day of admission.

    Weight: 28 lb

    SDR: Refer to label

    a. SDR for this child:

    b. Evaluation and decision:

    c. Dose to be administered if applicable:

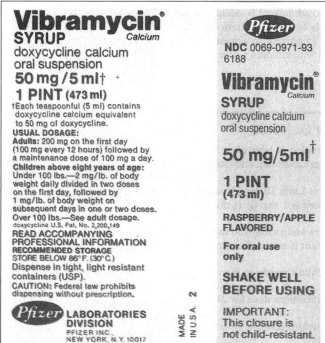

ANSWERS ON PAGE 460

WORKSHEET
11I

Multiple-Choice Practice

For the following problems, estimate kilograms, then calculate kilograms to the *nearest* tenth when a pound-to-kilogram conversion is needed and estimate the answers before solving each step.

1. Ordered: 20 mg/kg of Drug X for a child weighing 50 lb. How many milligrams of the drug will you administer to the child?
   a. 400 mg
   b. 454 mg
   c. 500 mg
   d. 1000 mg

2. Ordered: methotrexate sodium 30 mg/m² daily maintenance for a child with leukemia. The child's BSA is 1.20 m².* How much medication will you administer?
   a. 1.20 mg
   b. 30 mg
   c. 36 mg
   d. 30.12 mg

3. Ordered: 1.5 tsp of acetaminophen suspension liquid for a child with fever. How many milliliters will you administer?
   a. 5 mL
   b. 7.5 mL
   c. 8 mL
   d. 10 mL

4. Ordered: 30 mg of Drug X for a child weighing 25 lb. SDR is 2 to 5 mg/kg. Using the nursing process, what decision will you make regarding this medication order?
   a. Hold and clarify the order promptly. It is an overdose.
   b. Hold and clarify the order promptly. It is an underdose.
   c. Give the medication because the order is within the SDR.
   d. Consult with a supervisor about this order. It is unclear.

5. Ordered: Garamycin 50 mg IV q8h for a child weighing 55 lb. The SDR is 2 to 2.5 mg/kg q8h. Your decision:
   a. Give the medication. The order is within safe limits.
   b. Hold the medication. Consult with physician. The order is an overdose.
   c. Hold the medication and consult with the physician. The order is an underdose.
   d. Call the pharmacy and clarify the order.

*Note: Trailing zeros appear in BSA m² measurements. Delete them for math calculations.

ANSWERS ON PAGE 460

WORKSHEET
111

Multiple-Choice Practice (Continued)

6. Ordered: V-Cillin K 125 mg daily for a child weighing 5.5 lb. The literature states: 40 mg/kg/day in divided doses. Label states: 125 mg per 5 mL.
   Your decision:
   a. Give the medication. The order is safe.
   b. Hold the medication. Consult with a colleague.
   c. Hold the medication. Consult with physician. The order is an under-
      dose.
   d. Hold the medication and clarify with the physician promptly by tele-
      phone. The order is an overdose.

7. Ordered: Phenytoin oral suspension 15 mg bid po for a 6-kg child with
   seizures. The SDR is 5 mg/kg in 2 to 3 divided doses. Label reads: Dilantin
   pediatric suspension 30 mg/5 mL. Your decision:
   a. Hold and clarify the order with the physician. It is an overdose.
   b. The order is safe. Give 2.5 mL.
   c. Clarify the order with an experienced supervisor.
   d. The order is safe. Give 5 mL.

8. Ordered: Synthroid 0.5 mg qAM IV for a child with hypothyroidism. Label
   reads: Synthroid 200 mcg/10 mL. What is the amount to be administered?
   a. 2.0 mL
   b. 2.5 mL
   c. 20 mL
   d. 25 mL

9. Ordered: Meperidine 30 mg IM preoperatively for a child weighing 58 lb.
   SDR is 1 to 2.2 mg/kg. Label states: Meperidine HCl injection 25 mg/mL.
   What is your decision?
   a. The order is an overdose. Hold and contact physician.
   b. The order is an underdose. Hold and contact physician.
   c. The order is safe. Give 0.83 mL.
   d. The order is safe. Give 1.2 mL.

10. Ordered: Ampicillin suspension 250 mg po q8h. Weight is 30 lb. SDR is
    25 to 50 mg/kg/day po in 4 divided doses. The label reads: 125 mg/5 mL.
    What is your decision?
    a. The order is safe. Give 10 mL.
    b. The order is an overdose. Hold and contact physician.
    c. The order is an underdose. Hold and contact physician.
    d. Give 5 mL and contact the physician.

**Refer to the Pediatric Calculations section of the enclosed student
CD-ROM for additional practice problems.**

CRITICAL THINKING EXERCISES

Baby Louise is in your unit with a diagnosis of congestive heart failure secondary to a congenital heart defect. She weighs 8.4 kg at age 18 months. Her orders include lanoxin 0.05 mg po bid and furosemide 2 mg/kg po stat. The orders include temporary fluid restriction to 500 mL per 24-hr period.

On hand is digoxin elixir 50 mcg/mL. Given this AM by the night nurse: 5 mL.

On hand is furosemide oral solution 10 mg/mL. Given this AM by the reporting nurse: 2 mL.

During report, the nurse tells you that the intake exceeded 500 mL for the past 24 hours by 120 mL because the baby wouldn't take the medicine without a lot of juice. Is there a problem with mathematics? What error in concepts of arithmetic rounding might have led to one of the problems? Which knowledge bases are insufficient?

Medication error(s) and possible causes:

Fluid intake error:

Potential injuries:

Nursing actions:

Recommendations for the nurse and for patient safety if you were on a hospital committee studying these incidents:

CHAPTER 11 **Final**

ANSWERS ON PAGE 463

Use a calculator to determine the child's weight in kilograms (to the nearest tenth) and the SDR for each child. Evaluate the order and make a decision.

1. Give medication (within SDR for unit dose and 24-hr dose).

2. Hold and clarify promptly (overdose or underdose).

If the order is to be carried out, use written ratio and proportion to calculate doses, and show your proof.*

1. Ordered: Cephalexin 200 mg oral suspension four times daily po for Johnny who has a streptococcal infection of the throat and a history of allergy to penicillin. The SDR is 25 to 50 mg/kg/day in 4 divided doses. The child weighs 42 lb today.
   a. Estimated weight in kg:
   b. Actual weight in kg:
   c. SDR for this child:
   d. Dose ordered:
   e. Evaluation and decision:
   f. Dose to be administered if applicable:

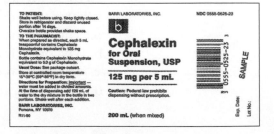

*Calculate amounts *less* than 1 mL to the nearest hundredth and *greater* than 1 mL to the nearest tenth. Calculate flow rates in mL/hr for the IV infusion pump that will be used.

2. Johnny's mother returns to the office with him 3 days after the initial visit because he has a generalized pruritic rash. His practitioner changes his antibiotic order to erythromycin oral suspension 175 mg four times daily po. The SDR is 30 to 50 mg/kg/day divided q6h. Johnny still weighs 42 lb.

   a. Actual weight in kg:

   b. SDR for this child:

   c. Dose ordered:

   d. Evaluation and decision:

   e. Dose to be administered:

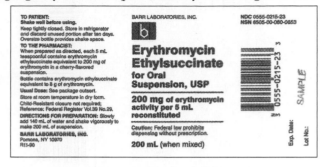

3. Also ordered for Johnny's pruritis is Benadryl Allergy Liquid (diphenhydramine HCl) 25 mg tid and at bedtime × 3 days. Johnny is 6 years old. Read the label and make your decision.

   a. Safe daily dose maximum for this child:

   b. Dose ordered for 24 hr:

   c. Evaluation and decision:

   d. Dose to be administered:

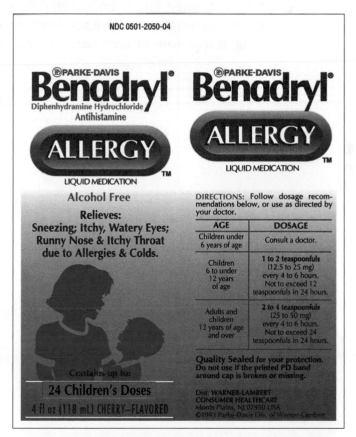

---

4. Ordered for Johnny's 8-year-old sister is dicloxacillin sodium capsules 500 mg q6h. The SDR is 12.5 to 25 mg/kg/day in divided doses q6h. His sister weighs 32 kg. Read the label and make your evaluation and decision.

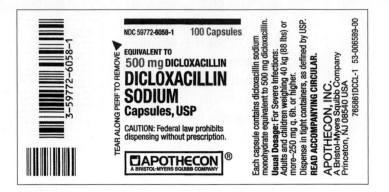

   a. SDR for this child:

   b. Dose ordered:

   c. Evaluation and decision:

   d. Dose to be administered if applicable:

5. Karen, age 3, is admitted to the hospital with a compound fracture of the femur incurred during an automobile accident. Ordered: Atropine sulfate 0.3 mg preop IM. The SDR for children weighing 12 to 16 kg is 0.3 mg 30 to 60 min before surgery. Karen weighs 35 lb.

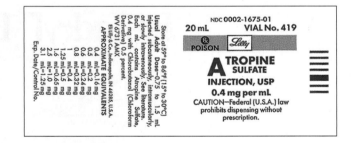

   a. Estimated weight in kg:

   b. Actual weight in kg:

   c. SDR for this child:

   d. Dose ordered:

   e. Evaluation and decision:

   f. Dose to be administered if applicable:

6. Ordered postoperatively for Karen is Amoxil oral suspension 0.5 g tid po. The SDR is 20 to 40 mg/kg in 3 divided doses. Karen weighs 35 lb.

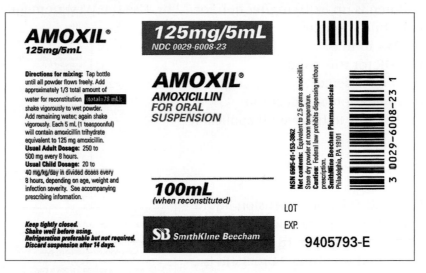

a. Estimated weight in kg:

b. Actual weight in kg:

c. SDR for this child:

d. Dose ordered:

e. Evaluation and decision:

f. Dose to be administered if applicable:

7. Also ordered for Karen postoperatively is Nebcin (tobramycin sulfate) 35 mg tid IV. The SDR is 6 to 7.5 mg/kg day in 3 divided doses. The directions from pharmacy state to dilute in 1 mg/mL and administer over 30 min via an IV infusion pump.

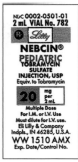

a. Actual weight in kg:

b. SDR for this child:

c. Dose ordered:

d. Evaluation and decision:

e. Dose in mL after reconstitution if applicable:

f. IV flow rate on pump:

8. Morphine sulfate 5 mg IV q4h prn pain × 48 hr is ordered for Karen. The SDR is 0.05 to 0.1 mg/kg q4h for direct IV. Directions state to dilute with 5 mL of sterile water or sterile saline for injection and administer over 5 min.

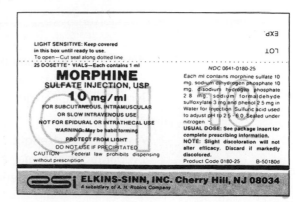

a. Actual weight in kg:

b. SDR for this child:

c. Dose ordered:

d. Evaluation and decision:

e. Dose before dilution:

9. Ordered: Leucovorin calcium 0.01 g q6h po for a child with toxic effects resulting from an antineoplastic agent. The child weighs 70 lb and has normal height for weight. The SDR for children is up to 10 mg/m² q6h for 72 hr. Use the West nomogram* to determine the BSA for this child's weight.
   a. BSA in m²:
   b. SDR for this child:
   c. Dose ordered:
   d. Evaluation and decision:
   e. Amount to be given if applicable:

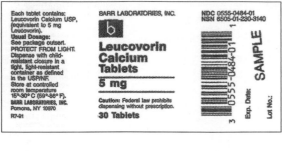

10. Ordered: Tylenol suspension liquid 240 mg for a 3-year-old child with a fever who weighs 18 kg. The SDR for a child weighing 24 to 35 lb is 1 tsp, and $1\frac{1}{2}$ tsp for a child weighing 36 to 47 lb.
    a. Estimated weight in lb:
    b. Weight in lb:
    c. SDR for this child:
    d. Dose ordered:
    e. Evaluation and decision:
    f. Dose to be administered if applicable:
    g. Measuring device to be used:

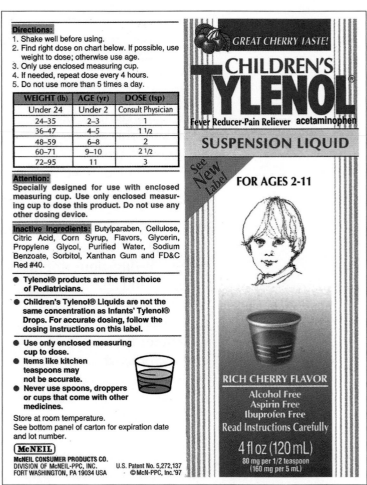

*For the West nomogram, refer to page 300.

◆ CLINICAL ALERT

Beware of medication orders for "T" and "t" and "tsp"; for example, 1 T daily or 1 tsp daily. Teaspoon and tablespoon abbreviations can easily be confused. Note that the "enclosed measuring cup" is to be used for the Tylenol product shown above.

Also, dosage strength may vary per teaspoon among infant, child, and adult preparations and may also vary among manufacturers. Call the physician and clarify the specific strength desired in milligrams or milliequivalents.

Dimensional Analysis

Objectives

- Set up problems in the correct format using dimensional analysis.
- Convert g to mg, mg to mcg, and lb to kg.
- Calculate intramuscular doses.
- Calculate subcutaneous doses in units.
- Calculate intravenous piggyback doses in mL/hr and gtt/min.
- Calculate intravenous insulin and heparin doses.
- Titrate mg/kg/min and mcg/kg/min.

2   3   4   5 mL   6   7   8   9   10 mL

1/2 tsp   1 tsp   1 1/2 tsp   2 tsp

INTRODUCTION

In this chapter you will learn how to calculate clinical medication doses using dimensional analysis. Dimensional analysis is a fractionalized method of setting up medication calculation problems. There are four worksheets, ranging from simple to complex. The setups include conversions from one metric measurement to another, IM injections, subcutaneous insulin and heparin injections, IV gravity and infusion device calculation problems, and safe dose ranges.

Dimensional Analysis

The dimensional analysis process is similar to the ratio and proportion method. The setup is in fraction form. The entire medical calculation can be written on one line, with all of the information given. Always start with the outcome, or what you are solving for. That becomes your unknown quantity. The unknown becomes the X factor. The X factor always goes on the left so that you don't forget what you want the outcome to be.

RULE All symbols in the equation must cancel out **except the X factor symbol on the left.**

Example Convert g to mg.

800 mg = ? g

REMEMBER Put the symbol that you are solving for on the left. All matching symbols must be canceled, and the remaining symbol will be the X symbol.

$$\text{X g} = \underset{\text{KNOW}}{\frac{1\,\text{g}}{1000\,\cancel{\text{mg}}}} \times \underset{\text{WANT TO KNOW}}{\frac{800\,\cancel{\text{mg}}}{1}} = \frac{800}{1000} = 0.8\,\text{g}$$

Both mg symbols are able to be canceled, and the remaining symbol is g. In order for the mg symbols to be canceled out, one symbol has to be in the numerator and one in the denominator.

Example Convert lb to kg.

155 lb = ? kg

The unknown is kg, which goes on the left.

$$\text{X kg} = \underset{\text{KNOW}}{\frac{1\,\text{kg}}{2.2\,\cancel{\text{lb}}}} \times \underset{\text{WANT TO KNOW}}{\frac{155\,\cancel{\text{lb}}}{1}} = 70.5\,\text{kg}$$

Note that the lb symbols are in the numerator and the denominator and are therefore able to be canceled out, leaving the kg symbol remaining.

This example will use the conversion factor to determine how many mL to give.

328

Example   Ordered: Ampicillin 300 mg IM q8h

This example will use the conversion factor to determine how many mL to give.

Available: Ampicillin 1 g/2 mL
How many milliliters will you give?

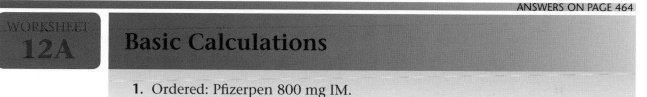

$$ \text{X mL} = \frac{2 \text{ mL}}{1 \text{ g}} \times \frac{1 \text{ g}}{1000 \text{ mg}} = \frac{300 \text{ mg}}{1} = \frac{600}{1000} = 0.6 \text{ mL} $$

Note that the mg and the g cancel out and the remaining symbol is mL.

Can you see the similarity to the ratio and proportion method?

ANSWERS ON PAGE 464

WORKSHEET 12A

Basic Calculations

1. Ordered: Pfizerpen 800 mg IM.
    Available: Pfizerpen one million units. After reconstitution with 1.8 mL of sterile water, each milliliter will contain 500 mg.
    How many milliliters will you give?

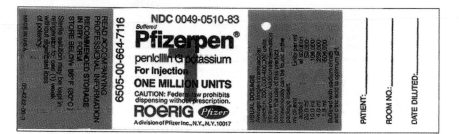

2. Ordered: Cimetidine tablets 0.8 g four times daily.
    Available: 400 mg/tab.
    How many tablets will you give?

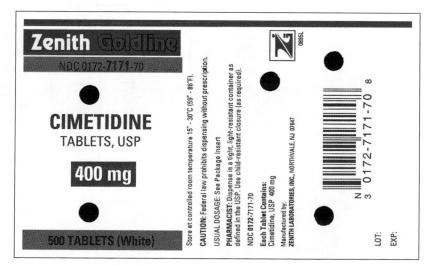

Continued

ANSWERS ON PAGE 464

WORKSHEET 12A

Basic Calculations (Continued)

3. The IV is infusing at 125 mL/hr. The drop factor is 20 gtt/mL.
   At how many drops per minute will you regulate the IV?

4. Ordered: 1.5 mg Dilaudid (hydromorphone) IM q4h prn for pain.
   Available: Dilaudid subcutaneous 2 mg/mL.
   How many milliliters will you give?

5. Ordered: Erythromycin sulfate 250 mg po q6h.
   Available: After reconstitution, there will be 200 mg/5 mL.
   How many milliliters will you give?

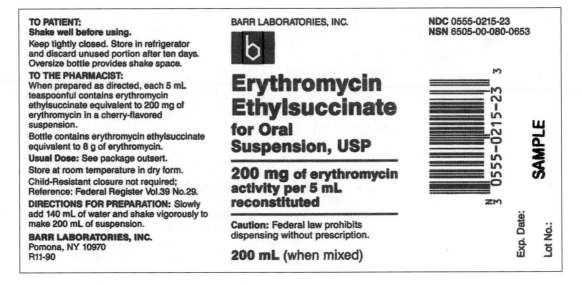

6. Ordered: 750 mg Lorabid po q12h.
   Available: Lorabid 200 mg/5 mL.
   How many milliliters will you give?

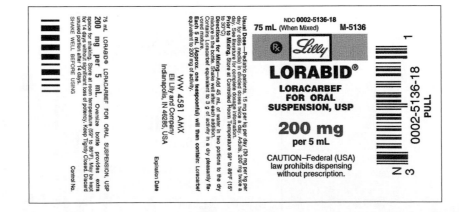

ANSWERS ON PAGE 464

WORKSHEET 12A

Basic Calculations (Continued)

7. Ordered: 8 mg morphine subcutaneous every 3 to 4 hr for pain.
   Available: morphine sulfate 10 mg/mL ampule.
   How many mL will you give?

8. Ordered: Solu-Cortef 300 mg IM q8h.
   Available: Solu-Cortef 250 mg/2 mL.
   How many milliliters will you give?

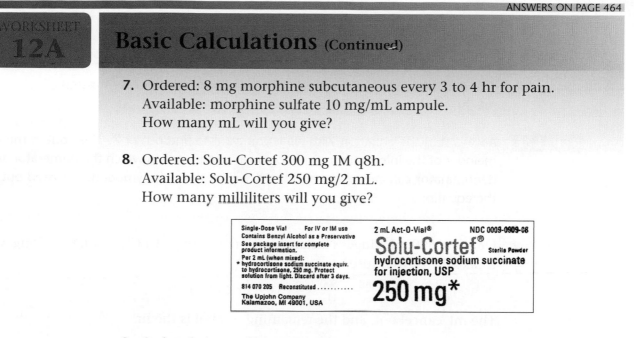

9. Ordered: Ampicillin 400 mg IM q6h.
   Available: Ampicillin for injection 1 g. After reconstitution, each milliliter contains 250 mg.
   How many milliliters will you give?

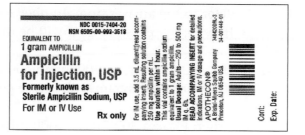

10. Ordered: Cefadyl 700 mg IM q6h.
    Available: 1 g. Each 1.2 mL = 500 mg.
    How many milliliters will you give?

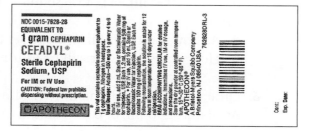

ANSWERS ON PAGE 465

WORKSHEET
12B

IV Calculations

This worksheet gives you practice in calculating the IV rate for units/hr, mL/hr, mg/hr, mEq/hr, and hours to infuse.

RULE Always start the equation with what you want to find out or X. Then put in the remainder of the information given to you in a sequence in which the numerator and denominator can cancel out and the X will be the only symbol not crossed out in the equation.

Example Ordered: 500 mL Ringer's lactate solution to infuse at 112 mL/hr. How long will it take the IV to infuse?

$$X \text{ hr} = \frac{1 \text{ hr}}{112 \text{ mL}} \times \frac{500 \text{ mL}}{1} = \frac{500}{112} = 4.46 = 4 \text{ hr } 28 \text{ min}$$

The mL cancel out, and the remaining symbol is the hr.

1. Ordered: 20,000 units heparin sodium in 1000 mL of 0.9% saline.
   Infuse at 1000 units/hr.
   For how many mL/hr will you set the IV infusion device?

2. Refer to the answer from number 1 to answer this question.
   How many units per hour will be infused?

3. Ordered: Dopamine 400 mg in 500 mL to infuse at 60 mL/hr.
   How many milligrams will infuse per hour?

4. Order: Pitocin 30 units in 1000 mL of normal saline (NS). Infuse at 2 units/hr.
   For how many mL/hr will you set the IV infusion device?

5. Ordered: 50 units Humulin R insulin to infuse in 24 hr. The pharmacy has sent 1000 mL of 0.45% sodium chloride with 50 units of Humulin insulin.
   a. At how many mL/hr will you set the IV infusion device?
   b. How many units/hr will be infused?

6. Ordered: 30 units Humulin R insulin IV to infuse in 12 hr.
   Available: 250 mL of 0.9% sodium chloride with 30 units of Humulin insulin.
   a. How many mL/hr will you set the IV infusion device?
   b. How many units/hr will be infused?

7. Ordered: 300 mg aminophylline IV in 250 mL of 0.9% sodium chloride to infuse in 8 hr.
   a. How many milliliters will infuse in 1 hr?
   b. How many mg/hr will be infused?

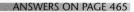

ANSWERS ON PAGE 465

WORKSHEET
12B

IV Calculations (Continued)

8. Ordered: 1000 mL Ringer's lactate solution with 20 mEq of KCl IV to infuse in 12 hr.
   a. For how many mL/hr will you set the IV infusion device?
   b. How many milliequivalents will infuse per hr?

9. Ordered: 1000 mL D5W to infuse IV at 20 gtt/min. The drop factor is 15 gtt/mL.
   How many hours will it take to infuse 1000 mL?

10. Ordered: 1000 mL D5W IV to infuse at 120 mL/hr.
    How many hours will it take to infuse?

ANSWERS ON PAGE 466

WORKSHEET
12C

Additional IV Calculations

This worksheet gives you practice in calculating units/hr, drops/min, mcg/min, mL/hr, and safe dose ranges (SDRs).

Example   Ordered: Cephalexin 150 mg oral suspension four times daily.
Available: Cephalexin 125 mg/5 mL. The SDR is 25 to 50 mg/kg/day in 4 divided doses. The child weighs 38 lb.

   a. What is the low dose range for 1 day?

$$\text{X mg/kg/day} = \underset{\text{KNOW}}{\frac{1 \text{ kg}}{2.2 \text{ lb}}} \times \underset{\text{WANT TO KNOW}}{\frac{38 \text{ lb}}{1} \times \frac{25 \text{ mg}}{1 \text{ kg}}} = \frac{950}{2.2} = 431.8 = 432 \text{ mg/kg/day}$$

   b. What is the high dose range for 1 day?

$$\text{X mg/kg/day} = \underset{\text{KNOW}}{\frac{1 \text{ kg}}{2.2 \text{ lb}}} \times \underset{\text{WANT TO KNOW}}{\frac{38 \text{ lb}}{1} \times \frac{50 \text{ mg}}{1 \text{ kg}}} = \frac{1900}{2.2} = 863.6 = 864 \text{ mg/kg/day}$$

   c. Is this a safe dose?

$$\text{X mg} = \underset{\text{HAVE}}{\frac{150 \text{ mg}}{1 \text{ dose}}} \times \underset{\text{WANT TO HAVE}}{\frac{4 \text{ doses}}{1}} = 600 \text{ mg/day}$$

   d. How many milliliters will you give per dose?

$$\text{X mL/dose} = \underset{\text{HAVE}}{\frac{5 \text{ mL}}{125 \text{ mg}}} \times \underset{\text{WANT TO HAVE}}{\frac{150 \text{ mg}}{1}} = \frac{750}{125} = 6 \text{ mL}$$

1. A peripheral parenteral nutrition solution of 1350 mL is infusing at 112 mL/hr.
   How many hours will it take to infuse?   *Continued*

ANSWERS ON PAGE 466

WORKSHEET 12C

Additional IV Calculations (Continued)

2. Ordered: 500 mL D5W to infuse in 2 hr by gravity flow. The drop factor is 10.
   At how many gtt/min will you regulate the IV?

3. Ordered: 2000 mL IV fluids to infuse in 24 hr.
   How many mL/hr will infuse?

4. Ordered: 1000 mL D5W to infuse in 6 hr.
   At how many mL/hr will you set the IV infusion device?

5. Ordered: Nitroprusside sodium 30 mg in 250 mL Ringer's lactate solution IV.
   Available: 250 mL Ringer's lactate solution with 30 mg Nipride. The directions read: Infuse at 3 mcg/kg/min. The patient weighs 190 lb.
   a. How many mcg/min will be infused?
   b. Use the answer from **a** to calculate how many mL/hr will deliver the required mcg/min.
   c. If an electronic device is not available, a microdrip infusion is used. How many gtt/min will be infused?

6. Ordered: 1000 mL of 0.9% sodium chloride with 50 mEq of potassium is to be infused over 4 hr. The drop factor of the tubing is 20 gtt/mL.
   How many gtt/min will be delivered?

7. Ordered: 500 mL 0.9% normal saline to be infused in 90 min. The drop factor is 12 gtt/mL.
   How many gtt/min will be delivered?

8. Ordered: Dobutamine 200 mg in 250 mL to infuse at 5 mcg/kg/min. The patient weighs 110 kg.
   a. How many mcg/min will the patient receive?
   b. At how many mL/hr will you set the infusion device?

9. Ordered: Dopamine HCl 800 mg in 500 mL in D5W to infuse at 6 mcg/kg/min. The patient weighs 160 lb. The drop factor is microdrip.
   a. How many mcg/min will the patient receive?
   b. At how many mL/hr will you set the IV rate?

10. Ordered: 10,000 units heparin in 1000 mL 0.9% sodium chloride to infuse in 12 hr.
    a. At how many mL/hr will you set the infusion device?
    b. How many units/hr will the patient receive?

ANSWERS ON PAGE 467

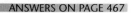

WORKSHEET
12D

More Intravenous Calculations

This worksheet provides practice in converting lb to kg, mcg/min, and titrating medication ranges to determine infusion device settings.

Example   Ordered: 3 g in 250 D5W to infuse at 100 mcg/kg/min IVPB. The patient weighs 110 kg.
At what rate will you set the infusion device?

$$mL/hr = \frac{250\,mL}{3\,g} \times \frac{1\,g}{1000\,mg} \times \frac{1\,mg}{1000\,mcg} \times \frac{100\,mcg}{1\,kg/min} \times \frac{60\,min}{1\,hr} \times \frac{110\,kg}{1} = 55\,mL/hr$$

1. Ordered: Aminophylline 30 mg/hr IVPB.
    Available: Aminophylline 250 mg in 500 mL D5W.
    At what rate should the infusion device be set?

2. Ordered: Dobutamine 10 mcg/kg/min IVPB.
    Available: 250 mg dobutamine in 250 mL D5W.
    The patient weighs 80 lb.
    a. How many mcg/min should the patient receive?
    b. At what rate should the infusion device be set?

3. Available: 50 mg of medication in 500 mL D5W. The patient weighs 75.6 kg.
    Directions: Titrate at 4 to 6 mcg/kg/min.
    a. Calculate the low and high mcg/min.
    b. Calculate the low and high mL/hr for this patient.
    c. Calculate how many mcg/min the patient will receive if the rate is set at 200 mL/hr.

4. Available: 75 mg of medication in 250 mL D5W. The patient weighs 110 kg.
    Directions: Titrate between 0.5 and 5 mcg/kg/min.
    a. Calculate the safe dose range.
    b. Calculate the flow rate to deliver the maximum safe dose.

5. Available: 50 mg of medication in 500 mL D5W. The patient weighs 120 kg.
    Directions: Titrate 0.2 to 1 mcg/kg/min.
    a. Calculate the low and high dose range.
    b. Calculate the mL/hr needed for the low and high dose range.

6. Available: 500 mg of medication in 250 mL D5W. The patient weighs 275 lb.
    Directions: Titrate IVPB to deliver 2 to 4 mcg/kg/min.
    a. What are the minimum and maximum dose ranges?
    b. Calculate the minimum and maximum mL/hr rates.

Continued

ANSWERS ON PAGE 467

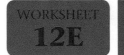

More Intravenous Calculations (Continued)

7. Available: 0.5 g of medication in 500 mL D5W. The patient weighs 100 kg.
   Directions: 5 mcg/kg/min.
   Calculate the mL/hr at which you will set the infusion device.

8. Available: 3 g of medication in 500 mL D5W. The patient weighs 84 kg.
   Directions: 100 mcg/kg/min.
   Calculate the mL/hr at which you will set the infusion device.

9. Available: 100 mg of medication in 250 mL D5W. The patient weighs 115 kg.
   Directions: 6 mcg/kg/min.
   Calculate the mL/hr at which you will set the infusion device.

10. Available: 5 g of medication in 1000 mL of D5W. The patient weighs 88.4 kg.
    Directions: 100 mcg/kg/min.
    Calculate the mL/hr at which you will set the infusion device.

ANSWERS ON PAGE 468

WORKSHEET
12E

Multiple-Choice Practice

This worksheet combines various types of calculations. Use the dimensional analysis method to calculate the answers.

1. Calculate the safe dose for a child weighing 5 kg. The safe dosage is 10 mg/kg.
   a. 0.2 mg   **b.** 0.5 mg   **c.** 50 mg   **d.** 2 mg

   The order is for a one-time dose of 25 mg. Is this a safe dose?
   a. Yes   **b.** No

2. The medication label reads 6 to 8 mg/kg. The baby weighs 8 lb.
   How many kilograms does the baby weigh?
   a. 4.5 kg   **b.** 16 kg   **c.** 6.6 kg   **d.** 3.6 kg

   Calculate the low end of the dose range.
   a. 24 mg   **b.** 22 mg   **c.** 36 mg   **d.** 12 mg

   Calculate the high end of the dose range.
   a. 29 mg   **b.** 26 mg   **c.** 32 mg   **d.** 35 mg

3. Ordered: Tylenol elixer 240 mg for a 5-year-old child who weighs 16 kg.
   Available: 80 mg/2.5 mL.
   How many milliliters will you give?
   a. 6.5 mL   **b.** 5 mL   **c.** 4 mL   **d.** 7.5 mL

4. Ordered: 600 mg of Cefadyl IM q6h.
   Available: Cefadyl 1 g. Each mL contains 0.5 g.
   How many milliliters will you give?
   a. 2.5 mL   **b.** 1.2 mL   **c.** 2.2 mL   **d.** 1.5 mL

ANSWERS ON PAGE 468

WORKSHEET
12E

Multiple-Choice Practice (Continued)

5. Ordered: 1330 mL of a parenteral nutrition solution to infuse at 112 mL/hr.
   For how many hours will the IV infuse?
   a. 10 hr 10 min   **b.** 9 hr 36 min   **c.** 11 hr 52 min   **d.** 12 hr 11 min

   If the infusion was started at 2000 hr, what time will it finish?
   a. 0800 hr   **b.** 0600 hr   **c.** 1800 hr   **d.** 0400 hr

6. Ordered: Heparin 50,000 units in 1000 mL of NS to infuse in 12 hr.
   At how many mL/hr will you set the infusion device?
   a. 83 mL/hr   **b.** 100 mL/hr   **c.** 33 mL/hr   **d.** 10 mL/hr

   How many units per minute will infuse?
   a. 24 units/min   **b.** 110 units/min
   c. 56 units/min   **d.** 69 units/min

7. Ordered: Erythromycin oral suspension 200 mg q4h. The child weighs 40 lb.
   Available: Erythromycin oral suspension 200 mg/5 mL.
   The SDR is 30 to 50 mg/kg/day in 4 divided doses.
   How many kilograms does the child weigh?
   a. 18 kg   **b.** 16.8 kg   **c.** 20 kg   **d.** 22 kg

   What is the low dosage for this child?
   a. 300 mg   **b.** 400 mg   **c.** 540 mg   **d.** 450 mg

   What is the high dosage for this child?
   a. 1000 mg   **b.** 650 mg   **c.** 900 mg   **d.** 700 mg

8. Ordered: 40 units Humulin insulin IV in 500 mL 0.9% sodium chloride to infuse at 3 units/hr.
   How many mL/hr will deliver 3 units/hr?
   a. 32 mL/hr   **b.** 18 mL/hr   **c.** 28 mL/hr   **d.** 38 mL/hr

9. Ordered: Heparin 20,000 units in 500 mL D5W to infuse at 0.5 units/kg/min. The patient weighs 195 lb. The drop factor is microdrip.
   How many kilograms does the patient weigh?
   a. 100 kg   **b.** 95 kg   **c.** 78 kg   **d.** 89 kg

   How many units per minute will infuse?
   a. 22 units/min   **b.** 45 units/min
   c. 78 units/min   **d.** 18 units/min

   At how many mL/hr will you set the infusion device?
   a. 54 mL/hr   **b.** 42 mL/hr   **c.** 68 mL/hr   **d.** 108 mL/hr

10. Ordered: 1000 mL Ringer's lactate solution with 60,000 units of heparin to infuse at the rate of 5000 units per hour.
    For how many mL/hr will you set the infusion device?
    a. 44 mL/hr   **b.** 83 mL/hr   **c.** 92 mL/hr   **d.** 100 mL/hr

CHAPTER 12   **Final**

ANSWERS ON PAGE 469

1. Ordered: 750 mg IM q8h.
   Available: Keflin 1 g/mL.
   How many milliliters will you give?

2. Ordered: 400 mg IM q12h.
   Available: 0.5 g/2 mL.
   How many milliliters will you give?

3. Ordered: 100 mg IM q12h.
   Available: 0.075 g/mL.
   How many milliliters will you give?

4. Ordered: 100 mg Biaxin po q8h.
   Available: Biaxin 125 mg/5 mL oral suspension.
   a. How many milliliters per dose will you give?
   b. How many milligrams will the patient receive in 24 hr?

5. Ordered: Erythromycin 250 mg tablets four times daily × 10 days.
   Available: 500 mg scored tablets.
   How many tablets are needed for 10 days?

6. Ordered: An IV bolus of heparin.
   The hospital protocol for heparin states 80 units/kg.
   The patient weighs 70 kg.
   How many units of heparin will the patient receive?

7. Ordered: Dobutamine. The patient weighs 105 lb.
   Available: 2 g in 1000 mL 0.9% NS.
   Directions: 75 mcg/kg/min.
   Calculate the mL/hr at which you will set the infusion device.

8. Ordered: Penicillin 600,000 units in 200 mL IVPB to infuse in 2 hr.
   The drop factor is 20.
   How many drops per minute will infuse?

9. Ordered: 100 mL IVPB with gentamycin 80 mg to infuse in 40 min.
   The IV tubing is microdrip.
   At how many gtt/min will you regulate the IV?

10. Ordered: Norcuron 0.5 mg tid.
    The label reads: 100 to 200 mcg/kg/day.
    The child weighs 25 lb.
    a. How many kilograms does the child weigh?
    b. What is the low end of the dose range for this child?
    c. What is the high end of the dose range for this child?
    d. Is the ordered medication within the safe dose range?

**Refer to the Methods of Calculating Dosages section on the enclosed
student CD-ROM for additional practice problems.**

Estimate reasonable answers when possible. Round kg to the *nearest* tenth. Round liquid oral and injection doses to the *nearest* tenth of a mL. Round IV flow rates to the *nearest* whole mL.

1. Ordered: Cimetidine 0.1 g po daily. Give:

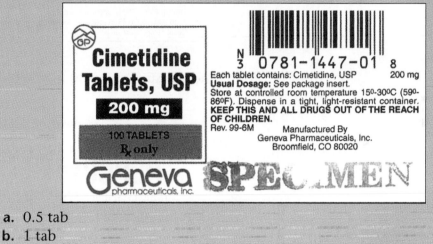

   a. 0.5 tab
   b. 1 tab
   c. 2 tab
   d. 4 tab

2. Ordered: Klonopin (clonazepam) 1 mg po stat. Give:

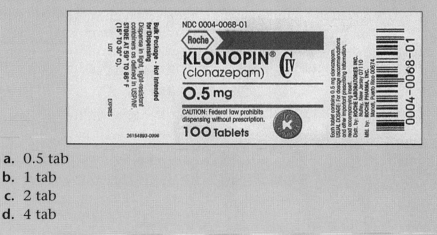

   a. 0.5 tab
   b. 1 tab
   c. 2 tab
   d. 4 tab

3. Ordered: Lanoxin 0.125 mg po daily in the AM. Give:
    a. 0.5 tab
    b. 1 tab
    c. 2 tab
    d. 4 tab

NDC 0173-0249-56

100 Tablets
(10 blisterpacks of 10 tablets each)

UNIT DOSE PACK

**LANOXIN® (digoxin)
Tablets**

Each scored tablet contains
250 mcg (0.25 mg)

See package insert for Dosage and
Administration.
Store at 25°C (77°F); excursions permitted to
15 to 30°C (59 to 86°F) [see USP Controlled
Room Temperature] in a dry place.

4. Ordered: Famotidine oral suspension 30 mg po bid. Give to the nearest
   tenth of a mL:
    a. 0.75 mL
    b. 1.5 mL
    c. 2.7 mL
    d. 3.8 mL

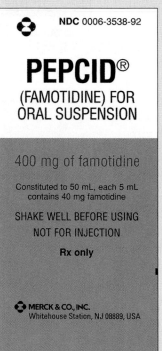

NDC 0006-3538-92

PEPCID®

(FAMOTIDINE) FOR
ORAL SUSPENSION

400 mg of famotidine

Constituted to 50 mL, each 5 mL
contains 40 mg famotidine

SHAKE WELL BEFORE USING

NOT FOR INJECTION

Rx only

MERCK & CO., INC.
Whitehouse Station, NJ 08889, USA

5. Ordered: Naloxone HCl 600 mcg IM stat. Give:

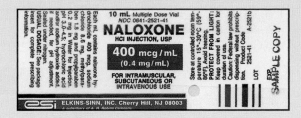

    a. 0.8 mL

    b. 1.1 mL

    c. 1.3 mL

    d. 1.5 mL

6. Ordered: Cipro (ciprofloxacin) 1.5 g po bid for a patient with an infection. Give:

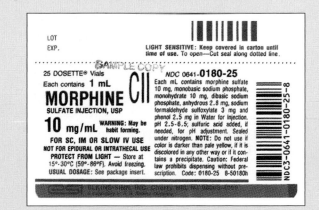

    a. 0.5 tab

    b. 1 tab

    c. 2 tab

    d. 3 tab

7. Ordered: Morphine sulfate 8 mg IM q4h prn for pain. Give:

    a. 0.6 mL

    b. 0.8 mL

    c. 1 mL

    d. 1.2 mL

8. Ordered: Glycopyrrolate 0.3 mg IM at 8 AM. Give:

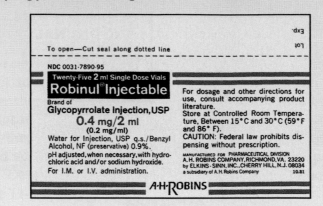

a. 0.5 mL
b. 0.7 mL
c. 1.5 mL
d. 2 mL

9. The nurse is trying to interpret a prescriber order that is illegible. What is the best action to take?
a. Ask a staff nurse who works regularly on the floor.
b. Check to see if something similar has been given before to the patient.
c. Call the pharmacy.
d. Call the prescriber.

10. Ordered: Promethazine 20 mg IM stat for nausea. Give:

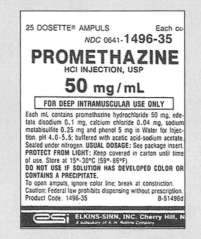

a. 0.4 mL
b. 0.5 mL
c. 0.8 mL
d. 1.2 mL

11. Ordered: Ativan (lorazepam) 5 mg IM stat for an agitated patient. Give to the nearest tenth of a mL:

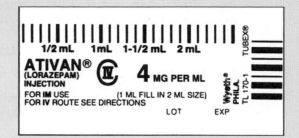

    a. 0.8 mL
    b. 1.2 mL
    c. 1.3 mL
    d. 1.4 mL

12. Ordered: 500 mg Claforan IM q8h. Available: Claforan (cefotaxime sodium) 1 g IM or IV. Follow the preparation directions. Give 500 mg with the least volume.

Strength	Diluent	Withdrawable Volume	Approx. Concentration
1 g vial (IM)	3.0 mL	3.4 mL	300 mg/mL
2 g vial (IM)	5.0 mL	6.0 mL	330 mg/mL
1 g vial (IV)	10.0 mL	10.4 mL	95 mg/mL
2 g vial (IV)	10.0 mL	11.0 mL	180 mg/mL

How many milliliters will you give the patient?
    a. 2.0 mL
    b. 1.5 mL
    c. 2.5 mL
    d. 3.0 mL

13. Ordered: Rocephin 1 g q12h IV. Available: ceftrioxone sodium (Rocephin) 1 g for IM or IV use. Directions for IV use: Reconstitute with 5 mL of normal saline solution. Mix well. Further dilute with normal saline to 50 mL and infuse in 20 to 40 minutes. What is the maximum rate in milliliters per hour you could set the infusion device?
    a. 150 mL/hr
    b. 200 mL/hr
    c. 300 mL/hr
    d. 400 mL/hr

14. Ordered: Geopen 1 g IM q8h. Available: Geopen (carbenicillin disodium) 5 g for IM or IV use. Directions for IM use: Use sterile water as diluent for injection. The medication displaces 3 mL. If you reconstitute the Geopen using 12 mL of sterile water for injection, how many doses of 1 g will you have?

Add Diluent	Volume to Be Withdrawn for 1 g Dose
9.5 mL	2.5 mL
12.0 mL	3.0 mL
17.0 mL	4.0 mL

a. 2 doses
b. 4 doses
c. 5 doses
d. 3 doses

If the first dose was given at 0700 hr on 10/20, what will be the date and time when the last dose from the vial will be given?
a. 10/22 at 0700 hr
b. 10/22 at 2000 hr
c. 10/21 at 2400 hr
d. 10/21 at 1500 hr

15. The IV is infusing at 30 gtt/min. The drop factor is 20 gtt/mL. The IV label reads 500 mL 5% dextrose and 0.45% sodium chloride. The IV had been infusing for $1\frac{1}{2}$ hours when you came on duty. How much longer does the IV have to infuse?
a. 4 hr
b. 50 min
c. 3 hr
d. $3\frac{1}{2}$ hr

16. Ordered: Monocid 600 mg IM. Available: Cefonicid 1 g for reconstitution. How many mL will you administer?

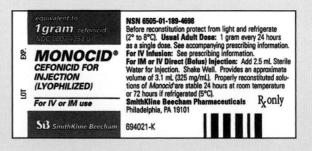

a. 1.8 mL
b. 0.7 mL
c. 1.3 mL
d. 1.5 mL

17. Ordered: IV of 1000 mL D5W to infuse at 125 mL/hr. The drop factor is 20. How many gtt/min will you set the IV to infuse?
    a. 12 gtt/min
    b. 42 gtt/min
    c. 20 gtt/min
    d. 33 gtt/min

18. Ordered: Ampicillin 1 g IV bid. Available: Ampicillin 1 g for IV use. Directions: Add 4.5 mL of sodium chloride diluent to yield 5 mL. Dilute with normal saline to 50 mL and infuse in 15 minutes. On hand you have a microdrip infusion set. At how many mL/hr will you set the IV?
    a. 100 mL/hr
    b. 150 mL/hr
    c. 200 mL/hr
    d. 250 mL/hr

19. The pharmacy standard insulin drip is 100 units of Human Regular in 250 mL of normal saline. 1 unit = 1 mL. Your patient's blood glucose level is 218 mg/dL. How many units/hr should the patient receive? Use the following chart to determine the correct insulin rate for the IV:

Blood Glucose (BG)/dL	Standard Rate in units/hr
101-140	1.0
141-180	1.5
181-220	2.0
221-260	2.5
261-300	3.0

    a. 1.5 units/hr
    b. 2.5 units/hr
    c. 3.0 units/hr
    d. 2.0 units/hr

    At what rate will you set the IV infusion device?
    a. 3 mL/hr
    b. 4 mL/hr
    c. 5 mL/hr
    d. 6 mL/hr

20. Ordered: Humulin R insulin 15 units/hr IV. Available: 250 mL of sodium chloride 0.9% with 100 units of Humulin R insulin. At how many mL/hr will you need to set the electronic infusion device?
    a. 56 mL/hr
    b. 33 mL/hr
    c. 38 mL/hr
    d. 58 mL/hr

    How many hours will it take to infuse the 250 mL?
    a. 5 hr 30 min
    b. 8 hr
    c. 9 hr 40 min
    d. 6 hr 36 min

21. Ordered: Heparin sodium 10,000 units IV in 15 hr. Available: Pharmacy has sent 1000 mL of normal saline solution with 10,000 units of heparin sodium. At how many mL/hr will you set the IV infusion device?
    a. 67 mL/hr
    b. 125 mL/hr
    c. 83 mL/hr
    d. 100 mL/hr

    If the IV described above was started at 2000 hr on 10/21, when should it be finished?
    a. 10/22 at 0900 hr
    b. 10/23 at 0200 hr
    c. 10/23 at 1000 hr
    d. 10/22 at 1100 hr

22. Ordered: Fragmin 18,000 units subcutaneous for deep venous thrombosis (DVT). Available: A 9.5 mL multidose vial of Fragmin. The label reads: 1 mL = 10,000 units. How many milliliters will you give?
    a. 1.8 mL
    b. 2 mL
    c. 1.5 mL
    d. 1.2 mL

23. A blood glucose level (BGL) of 120 mg/dL is desired. Orders for this patient are: Give 1 unit of Regular insulin for every 8 mg above 120 mg/dL. Give 1 unit of Regular insulin for each 8 g of CHO consumed. The BGL is 160 mg/dL. The amount of CHO consumed is 64 g. How many total units of insulin will the patient receive?
    a. 10 units
    b. 13 units
    c. 24 units
    d. 28 units

24. Ordered: IV heparin to infuse at 20 units/kg/hr. Available: 1000 mL D5W with 25,000 units of heparin sodium. The patient weighs 80 kg. How many units per hour will the patient receive on the electronic infusion device?

   a. 160 units
   b. 1600 units
   c. 1620 units
   d. 1640 units

   At how many mL/hr will you set the infusion device?
   a. 58 mL/hr
   b. 48 mL/hr
   c. 66 mL/hr
   d. 64 mL/hr

25. Ordered: 90 units/kg of heparin for a loading dose. Set the infusion to run at 1200 units/hr. Available: 500 mL NS with 25,000 units of heparin. The patient weighs 177 lb. How many units will you give as the loading dose?

   a. 5700 units
   b. 6900 units
   c. 7000 units
   d. 7200 units

   At how many mL/hr will you set the infusion device?
   a. 84 mL/hr
   b. 60 mL/hr
   c. 64 mL/hr
   d. 24 mL/hr

26. The patient has a TPN solution with 8.5% amino acids in 375 mL. The total volume (TV) is 1500 mL. How many grams of protein will the patient receive? Use the following formula for calculating the amino acids.

   Step 1:   % × mL = g/L

   Step 2:   g/L × TV/L × g/bag

   a. 8.5 g/bag
   b. 47.8 g/bag
   c. 478 g/bag
   d. 31.8 g/bag

27. Ordered: Methotrexate 3.3 mg/m^2 po daily for a child with lymphocytic leukemia. Child's weight is 30 lb, which is normal weight for height. Using the appropriate column in the West nomogram on page 300, calculate the dose.

   a. 12 mg
   b. 15 mg
   c. 18 mg
   d. 20 mg

28. Ordered: Dobutrex HCl to be infused at 2 mcg/kg/min in a solution of 500 mL D5W. Patient's weight: 110 lb. At how many mL/hr will the IV infusion pump be set?

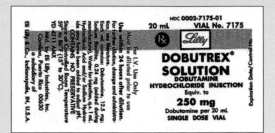

    a. 6 mL/hr
    b. 8 mL/hr
    c. 10 mL/hr
    d. 12 mL/hr

29. Ordered: Morphine sulfate 5 mg IV push for a patient in severe pain. Directions: Dilute *to* 5 mL of NS or sterile water for injection and administer over 5 minutes. Identify the correct total dose and mL/minute to inject.

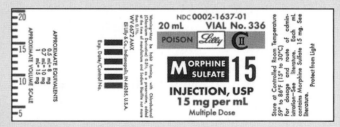

    a. Administer 5 mL at 1 mL/min.
    b. Administer 5 mL at 0.4 mL/min.
    c. Administer 6 mL at 0.4 mL/min.
    d. Administer 8 mL at 0.03 mL/min.

30. Ordered: Tobramycin sulfate 60 mg tid IV for a 40-lb child. Safe dose range (SDR): 6 to 7.5 mg/kg/day in 3 divided doses. Your decision:

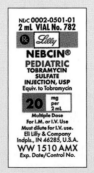

    a. Give 60 mg. The order is within the safe dose range.
    b. Hold. Contact the physician promptly and clarify. The order is an underdose.
    c. Hold. Contact the physician promptly and clarify. The order is an overdose.
    d. Hold. The order is unclear.

Estimate answers and then solve the following problems. Prove your answers.

1. Ordered: Lipitor 20 mg po daily for a patient with hypercholesterolemia. How many tablets will be administered?

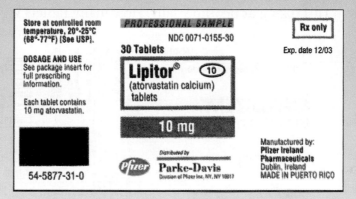

2. Ordered: Cimetidine 0.4 g bid po for a patient with a duodenal ulcer. How many tablets will be administered?

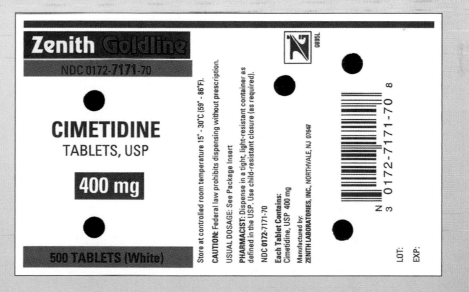

3. Ordered: Carbamazepine chewable tablet 0.2 g daily for a patient with seizures. How many tablets will be administered?

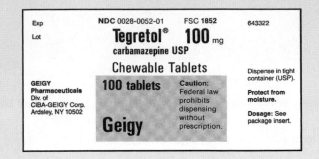

4. Ordered: Diltiazem HCl 0.24 g at bedtime daily. How many tablets will be administered?

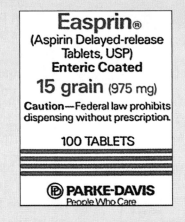

5. Ordered: Aspirin delayed-release tablet 975 mg at bedtime daily for a patient with arthritis. How many tablets will be administered?

6. Ordered: Isoniazid 0.1 g po for a patient with tuberculosis. How many tablets will be administered?

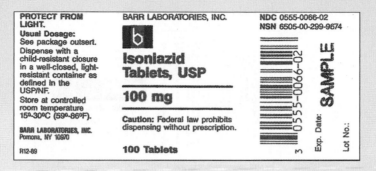

7. Ordered: Fluoxetine hydrochloride oral solution 30 mg po for a patient with anxiety. How many mL will be administered?

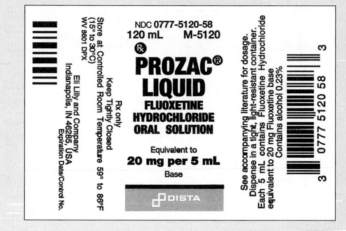

8. Ordered: Morphine sulfate 10 mg IM stat for a patient with pain. How many mL (to the nearest tenth of a mL) will be administered?

9. Ordered: Morphine sulfate 10 mg q4h prn pain; last administered according to the MAR at 0400 hr.

    Given: Morphine 10 mg at 0800 hr by Nurse A.

    Given: Morphine 10 mg at 0845 hr by Nurse B, a busy staff nurse who covered Nurse A's patient during Nurse A's break.

    Error:

    Current Actions:

    What are some ways this error might have been prevented?

10. Ordered: Codeine phosphate 25 mg IM stat for a patient with pain.
   a. How many mL (to the nearest tenth of a mL) will be administered?
   b. What is the apothecary equivalent of 30 mg noted on the label?

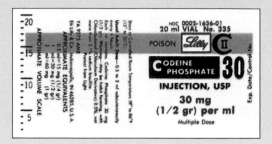

11. Ordered: Atropine sulfate 0.5 mg IV for a patient with an apical pulse 40 beats/min or below. How many mL (to the nearest tenth of a mL) will you give?

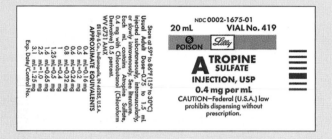

12. Ordered: Pfizerpen 400,000 units IM q8h.
   Available: Penicillin G Potassium (Pfizerpen) 5 million units for reconstitution.
   Follow the directions on the label to answer the questions.
   a. If you add 18.2 mL of diluent, how many units per milliliter will you have?
   b. How many milliliters will yield 400,000 units?
   c. If you add 8.2 mL of diluent, how many units per milliliter will you have?
   d. Use the 8.2 mL of diluent, how many milliliters will yield 400,000 units?

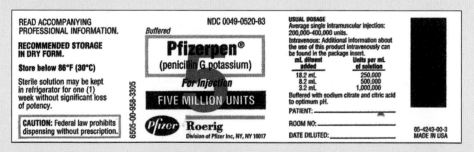

13. Ordered: Cefadyl 1 g IM q6h for cellulitis.
   a. How much diluent will you add? Shade in the syringe.
   b. How many vials will be used in 24 hr?
   c. How many mL will you give per dose?

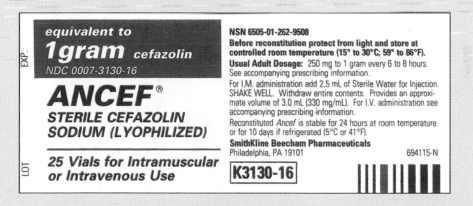

14. Ordered: Cefazolin 250 mg IM q8h.
   Available: Ancef 1 g for reconstitution.
   a. How many mL of diluent will you add?
   b. Where will the medication be stored?
   c. How many mL will you give?

15. Ordered: 2000 mL D5/Ringer's lactate solution to be infused in 24 hr. The drop factor is 15.

 a. How many gtt/min will be infused via gravity infusion?

 b. How many mL/hr will be infused by an electronic device?

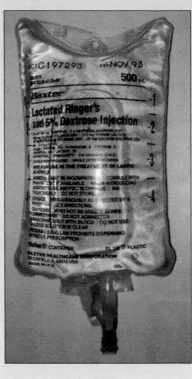

16. Ordered: Gentamicin 60 mg in 50 mL, IVPB. Infuse in 40 minutes.

 a. At how many milliliters/hr will you set the electronic infusion device?

 b. How many gtt/min will be infused by a microdrip set?

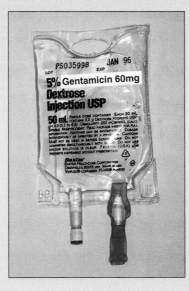

17. Ordered: 1000 mL D5NS followed by 1000 mL D5W then 500 mL NS to infuse in 24 hr. The drop factor is 10.

   a. At how many mL/hr will you set the electronic infusion device to deliver 2500 mL in 24 hr?

   b. At how many gtt/min will you regulate the IV?

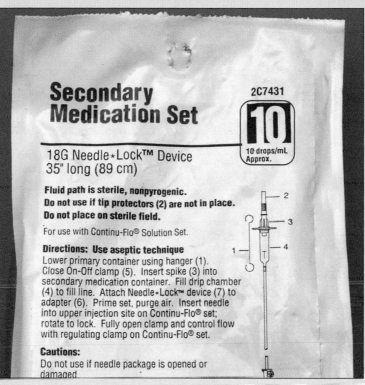

From Macklin D, Chernecky C, Infortuna H: Math for clinical practice, *ed 1*, St Louis, 2005, Mosby.

18. Your patient's blood glucose level (BGL) at 0600 hr is 176 mg/dL. According to the titration schedule, how many units of Lantus will the patient receive? Shade in the amount on the insulin syringe.

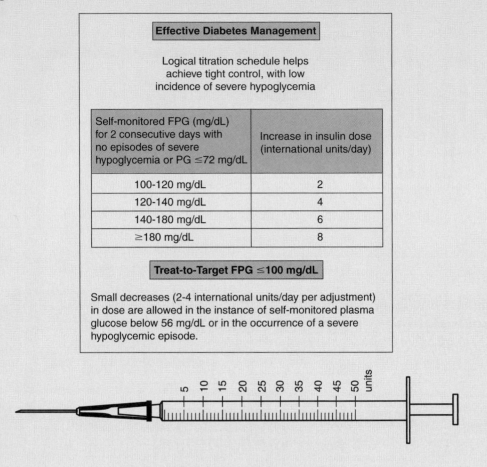

Effective Diabetes Management

Logical titration schedule helps achieve tight control, with low incidence of severe hypoglycemia

Self-monitored FPG (mg/dL) for 2 consecutive days with no episodes of severe hypoglycemia or PG ≤72 mg/dL	Increase in insulin dose (international units/day)
100-120 mg/dL	2
120-140 mg/dL	4
140-180 mg/dL	6
≥180 mg/dL	8

Treat-to-Target FPG ≤100 mg/dL

Small decreases (2-4 international units/day per adjustment) in dose are allowed in the instance of self-monitored plasma glucose below 56 mg/dL or in the occurrence of a severe hypoglycemic episode.

19. Ordered: Humulin R insulin 50 units in 500 mL of 0.9% NS IV to infuse at 7 units/hr. At what rate will you set the IV infusion device?

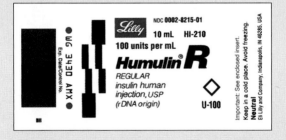

20. Ordered: The patient has consumed 35 g CHO for breakfast, 90 g CHO for lunch, and 25 g CHO for dinner. The patient weighs 270 lb.
How many total units of R has the patient received based on the units-to-CHO ratio chart?

INSULIN UNITS REQUIRED BASED ON CHO INTAKE AND WEIGHT

Weight in Pounds	Weight in Kg	Unit: grams of CHO
100-109	45.5-49.5	1:16
110-129	50-58.6	1:15
130-139	59-63.2	1:14
140-149	63.6-67.7	1:13
150-159	68.2-72.3	1:12
160-169	72.7-76.8	1:11
170-179	77.3-81.4	1:10
180-189	81.8-85.9	1:9
190-198	86.4-90	1:8
200-239	90.9-108.6	1:7
240+	109.1+	1:6

21. Ordered: Regular insulin to infuse at 3 units/hr.
Available: 250 mL NS with 40 units of insulin.
  a. At how many mL/hr will you set the electronic infusion device?
  b. The IV was started at 0830. At what hour will the IV be complete?

22. Ordered: Fragmin injection 8000 units subcutaneous q12h before surgery.
Available: A multidose vial of Fragmin (dalteparin sodium injection).
How many milliliters will you give? Shade in the amount on the syringe.

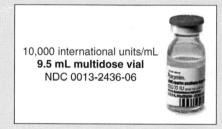

10,000 international units/mL
9.5 mL multidose vial
NDC 0013-2436-06

Used with permission from Pfizer, Inc.

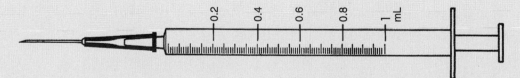

23. Ordered: Heparin sodium 1000 units/hr IV. The pharmacy has sent 1000 mL of 0.9% sodium chloride with 20,000 units of heparin sodium.
    a. At what rate will you set the infusion device?
    b. How long will it take to infuse the 20,000 units?

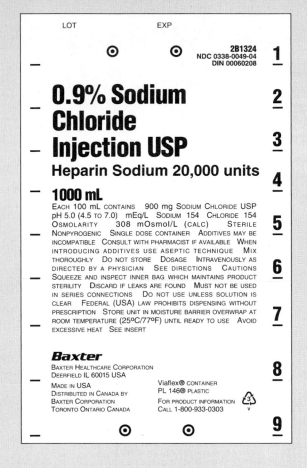

24. Ordered: Loading dose of IV heparin at 82 units/kg/min. Set infusion to run at 18 units/kg/hr. Available: 500 mL D5W with 20,000 units of heparin. The patient weighs 160 lb.
    a. How many units of heparin will you give for the bolus loading dose?
    b. How many units/hr will infuse?
    c. How many hours will it take to infuse?
    d. At what rate will you set the infusion device to deliver 18 units/kg/hr?

25. Calculate the grams of amino acids, dextrose, and lipids per bag the patient will receive. Use the following formulas on the TPN label below. The total volume is 1158 mL.

Step 1:   % × mL = g/L   **Step 2:**   g/L × TV/L = g/bag

   TPN Label
   a. Amino acid 5.5% in 300 mL
   b. Dextrose 10% in 250 mL
   c. Lipids 10% in 125 mL

26. Using the answers from Problem 24, how many kilocalories will the patient receive?

27. Ordered: Potassium Chloride (KCl) 30 mEq to be added to an IV of 500 mL D5W in ICU.
    a. How many mEq are there per milliliter in the available vial?
    b. How many mg are there per milliliter in the available vial?
    c. How many mL will be added to the IV?

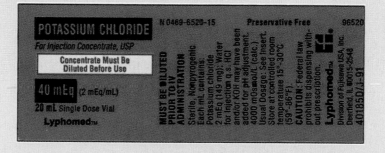

28. Ordered: Thorazine 2 mg IV push. Directions: Dilute each 25 mg (1 mL) with 24 mL of NS for IV injection. Each mL will contain 1 mg. Give at slow rate of 1 mg/min.

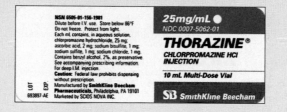

    a. Total milliliters to be injected
    b. Total time in *seconds* to be injected
    c. mL/min to be injected for how many minutes
    d. Seconds to be injected per calibration

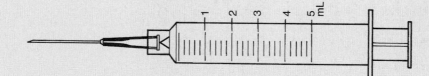

29. Ordered: Leucovorin calcium tablets 0.01 g po for a child who has delayed excretion of methotrexate. The SDR is 10 mg/m². The child's weight is 70 lb. Refer to the West nomogram on page 300 for the child's body surface area in square meters. How many milligrams are needed? How many tablets will you prepare?

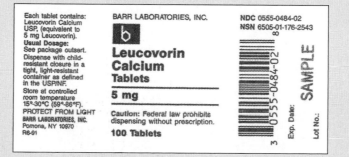

30. Ordered: Dopamine 5 mcg/kg/min. The dopamine is infusing at 30 mL/hr on an infusion device with an IV container of 200 mg/250 mL D5W. The patient weighs 176 lb.

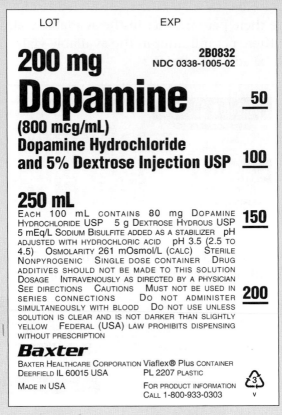

LOT   EXP

200 mg   **2B0832**
NDC 0338-1005-02

Dopamine   50
(800 mcg/mL)
Dopamine Hydrochloride
and 5% Dextrose Injection USP   100

250 mL
EACH 100 mL CONTAINS 80 mg DOPAMINE   150
HYDROCHLORIDE USP   5 g DEXTROSE HYDROUS USP
5 mEq/L SODIUM BISULFITE ADDED AS A STABILIZER   pH
ADJUSTED WITH HYDROCHLORIC ACID   pH 3.5 (2.5 TO
4.5) OSMOLARITY 261 mOsmol/L (CALC) STERILE
NONPYROGENIC SINGLE DOSE CONTAINER DRUG
ADDITIVES SHOULD NOT BE MADE TO THIS SOLUTION
DOSAGE INTRAVENOUSLY AS DIRECTED BY A PHYSICIAN   200
SEE DIRECTIONS CAUTIONS MUST NOT BE USED IN
SERIES CONNECTIONS DO NOT ADMINISTER
SIMULTANEOUSLY WITH BLOOD DO NOT USE UNLESS
SOLUTION IS CLEAR AND IS NOT DARKER THAN SLIGHTLY
YELLOW FEDERAL (USA) LAW PROHIBITS DISPENSING
WITHOUT PRESCRIPTION

Baxter
BAXTER HEALTHCARE CORPORATION Viaflex® Plus CONTAINER
DEERFIELD IL 60015 USA   PL 2207 PLASTIC
MADE IN USA   FOR PRODUCT INFORMATION
CALL 1-800-933-0303

a. How many mg/kg/hr are infusing?
b. How many mcg/hr are infusing?
c. How many mcg/kg/min are infusing?
d. Is the flow rate correct?

Answer Key

General Mathematics Self-Assessment (PAGE 1)

1. $4\frac{1}{2}$
2. $5\frac{1}{5}$
3. $\frac{25}{3}$
4. $\frac{27}{5}$
5. 88
6. 45
7. $1\frac{1}{30}$
8. $6\frac{19}{24}$
9. $\frac{8}{21}$
10. $4\frac{7}{8}$
11. $\frac{1}{18}$
12. $\frac{1}{3}$
13. $\frac{5}{6}$
14. $\frac{9}{20}$
15. $\frac{1}{30}$
16. $\frac{3}{7}$
17. 0.12
18. 3.016
19. 4.904
20. 28.708
21. 2.96
22. 0.8241
23. 0.0036
24. 1.2
25. 10.055
26. 98.095
27. 0.545
28. 9.125
29. 9.45
30. 84.2
31. $\frac{5}{1000} = \frac{1}{200}$
32. $\frac{5}{100} = \frac{1}{20}$
33. 0.17   17%
34. 0.125 $12\frac{1}{2}$%

	Decimal	Nearest Whole Number	Nearest Hundredth	Nearest Tenth
35.	0.8734	1	0.87	0.9
36.	0.842	1	0.84	0.8
37.	0.553	1	0.55	0.6
38.	0.689	1	0.69	0.7
39.	2.75	3	2.75	2.8

40. $\frac{1}{2}$ (0.5)
41. $\frac{1}{2}$ (0.5)
42. $1\frac{1}{2}$ (1.5)
43. 2
44. 2
45. 2

1 General Mathematics

1A (PAGE 5)

1. 1   2. 5   3. $3\frac{1}{4}$ 4. $1\frac{5}{9}$

5. $5\frac{2}{3}$ 6. 5   7. $2\frac{1}{4}$ 8. $1\frac{7}{8}$

9. 6   10. $6\frac{5}{6}$

1B (PAGE 5)

1. $\frac{7}{2}$ 2. $\frac{7}{6}$ 3. $\frac{33}{8}$ 4. $\frac{43}{12}$

5. $\frac{68}{5}$ 6. $\frac{49}{3}$ 7. $\frac{23}{6}$ 8. $\frac{21}{8}$

9. $\frac{63}{6}$ 10. $\frac{377}{3}$

1C (PAGE 9)

1. $$\begin{array}{r} \frac{2}{5} \\ +\frac{2}{5} \\ \hline \frac{4}{5} \end{array}$$

2. $$\begin{array}{r} \frac{4}{5}=\frac{12}{15} \\ +\frac{2}{3}=\frac{10}{15} \\ \hline \frac{22}{15}=1\frac{7}{15} \end{array}$$

3. $$\begin{array}{r} 6\frac{1}{6}=6\frac{4}{24} \\ +9\frac{5}{8}=9\frac{15}{24} \\ \hline 15\frac{19}{24} \end{array}$$

4. $$\begin{array}{r} 2\frac{1}{4}=2\frac{2}{8} \\ +3\frac{1}{8}=3\frac{1}{8} \\ \hline 5\frac{3}{8} \end{array}$$

5. $$\begin{array}{r} 1\frac{3}{4}=1\frac{30}{40} \\ +9\frac{9}{10}=9\frac{36}{40} \\ \hline 10\frac{66}{40}=11\frac{13}{20} \end{array}$$

6. $$\begin{array}{r} \frac{1}{8}=\frac{9}{72} \\ \frac{1}{4}=\frac{18}{72} \\ +\frac{3}{9}=\frac{24}{72} \\ \hline \frac{51}{72} \end{array}$$

7. $$\begin{array}{r} \frac{7}{9}=\frac{7}{90} \\ \frac{4}{5}=\frac{72}{90} \\ +\frac{9}{10}=\frac{81}{90} \\ \hline \frac{223}{90}=2\frac{43}{90} \end{array}$$

8. $$\begin{array}{r} 3\frac{1}{4} \\ +9\frac{3}{4} \\ \hline 12\frac{4}{4}=13 \end{array}$$

9. $$\begin{array}{r} 8\frac{2}{5}=8\frac{4}{10} \\ 14\frac{7}{10}=14\frac{7}{10} \\ +9\frac{9}{10}=9\frac{9}{10} \\ \hline 31\frac{20}{10}=33 \end{array}$$

10. $$\begin{array}{r} 2\frac{1}{3}=2\frac{2}{6} \\ +4\frac{1}{6}=4\frac{1}{6} \\ \hline 6\frac{3}{6}=6\frac{1}{2} \end{array}$$

1D (PAGE 11)

1. $$\begin{array}{r} \frac{2}{3}=\frac{4}{6} \\ -\frac{1}{2}=\frac{3}{6} \\ \hline \frac{1}{6} \end{array}$$

2. $$\begin{array}{r} \frac{27}{32} \\ -\frac{18}{32} \\ \hline \frac{9}{32} \end{array}$$

3. $$\begin{array}{r} 10\frac{2}{5}=10\frac{8}{20} \\ -6\frac{1}{4}=6\frac{5}{20} \\ \hline 4\frac{3}{20} \end{array}$$

4. $$\begin{array}{r} 7\frac{16}{24}=7\frac{16}{24} \\ -3\frac{1}{8}=3\frac{3}{24} \\ \hline 4\frac{13}{24} \end{array}$$

(Must borrow from the whole number.)

5.
$$6\tfrac{3}{10} = 6\tfrac{3}{10}$$
$$\underline{-\,2\tfrac{1}{5} = 2\tfrac{2}{10}}$$
$$4\tfrac{1}{10}$$

6.
$$\tfrac{7}{8} = \tfrac{21}{24}$$
$$\underline{-\,\tfrac{1}{3} = \tfrac{8}{24}}$$
$$\tfrac{13}{24}$$

7.
$$3\tfrac{5}{8}$$
$$\underline{-\,1\tfrac{3}{8}}$$
$$2\tfrac{2}{8} = 2\tfrac{1}{4}$$

8.
$$5\tfrac{3}{7} = 4\tfrac{10}{7}$$
$$\underline{-\,1\tfrac{6}{7} = 1\tfrac{6}{7}}$$
$$3\tfrac{4}{7}$$

(Must borrow from the whole number.)

9.
$$7 = 6\tfrac{4}{4}$$
$$\underline{-\,1\tfrac{3}{4} = 1\tfrac{3}{4}}$$
$$5\tfrac{1}{4}$$

10.
$$2\tfrac{7}{8} = 2\tfrac{7}{8}$$
$$\underline{-\,\tfrac{3}{4} = \tfrac{6}{8}}$$
$$2\tfrac{1}{8}$$

(Must borrow from the whole number.)

1E (PAGE 12)

1. $\dfrac{1}{5} \times \dfrac{2}{4} = \dfrac{2}{20} = \dfrac{1}{10}$

2. $\dfrac{1}{5} \times \dfrac{1}{6} = \dfrac{1}{30}$

3. $1\tfrac{3}{4} \times 3\tfrac{1}{7} = \dfrac{\cancel{7}}{4} \times \dfrac{22}{\cancel{7}} = \dfrac{22}{4} = 22 \div 4 = 5\tfrac{1}{2}$

4. $4 \times 3\tfrac{1}{3} = 4 \times \dfrac{10}{3} = \dfrac{40}{3} = 13\tfrac{1}{3}$

5. $\dfrac{2}{4} \times 2\tfrac{1}{6} = \dfrac{\cancel{2}}{4} \times \dfrac{13}{\cancel{6}} = \dfrac{13}{12} = 1\tfrac{1}{12}$

6. $5\tfrac{1}{2} \times 3\tfrac{1}{8} = \dfrac{11}{2} \times \dfrac{25}{8} = \dfrac{275}{16} = 275 \div 16 = 17\tfrac{3}{16}$

7. $\dfrac{3}{5} \times \dfrac{5}{8} = \dfrac{15}{40} = \dfrac{3}{8}$

8. $\dfrac{5}{6} \times 1\tfrac{9}{16} = \dfrac{5}{6} \times \dfrac{25}{16} = \dfrac{125}{96} = 125 \div 96 = 1\tfrac{29}{96}$

9. $\dfrac{5}{100} \times 900 = \dfrac{5}{\cancel{100}} \times \dfrac{\cancel{900}}{1} = 45$

10. $2\tfrac{1}{10} \times 4\tfrac{1}{3} = \dfrac{21}{10} \times \dfrac{13}{\cancel{3}} = \dfrac{91}{10} = 9\tfrac{1}{10}$

1F (PAGE 13)

1. $\dfrac{1}{5} \div \dfrac{1}{8} = \dfrac{1}{5} \times \dfrac{8}{1} = \dfrac{8}{5} = 1\tfrac{3}{5}$

2. $\dfrac{1}{3} \div \dfrac{1}{2} = \dfrac{1}{3} \times \dfrac{2}{1} = \dfrac{2}{3}$

3. $\dfrac{3}{4} \div \dfrac{1}{8} = \dfrac{3}{\cancel{4}} \times \dfrac{\cancel{8}}{1} = 6$

4. $\dfrac{1}{16} \div \dfrac{1}{4} = \dfrac{1}{\cancel{16}} \times \dfrac{\cancel{4}}{1} = \dfrac{1}{4}$

5. $8\tfrac{3}{4} \div 15 = \dfrac{\cancel{35}}{4} \times \dfrac{1}{\cancel{15}} = \dfrac{7}{12}$

6. $\dfrac{3}{4} \div 6 = \dfrac{\cancel{3}}{4} \times \dfrac{1}{\cancel{6}} = \dfrac{1}{8}$

7. $2 \div \dfrac{1}{5} = \dfrac{2}{1} \times \dfrac{5}{1} = 10$

8. $3\tfrac{3}{8} \div 4\tfrac{1}{2} = \dfrac{27}{8} \div \dfrac{9}{2} = \dfrac{\cancel{27}}{\cancel{8}} \times \dfrac{\cancel{2}}{\cancel{9}} = \dfrac{3}{4}$

9. $\dfrac{3}{5} \div \dfrac{3}{8} = \dfrac{\cancel{3}}{5} \times \dfrac{8}{\cancel{3}} = \dfrac{8}{5} = 1\tfrac{3}{5}$

10. $4 \div 2\tfrac{1}{8} = \dfrac{4}{1} \times \dfrac{8}{17} = \dfrac{32}{17} = 1\tfrac{15}{17}$

1G (PAGE 14)

1. $\dfrac{1}{10}$

2. $\dfrac{2}{7}$

3. $\dfrac{1}{20}$

4. $\dfrac{1}{100,000}$

5. More

6. $\dfrac{1}{5}$

7. $\dfrac{1}{150}$

8. $\dfrac{1}{250}$

9. $\dfrac{1}{9}$

10. $\dfrac{1}{200}$

1H (PAGE 16)

1. Six hundredths
2. Ninety-two thousandths
3. Five thousandths
4. One hundred and one hundredth
5. Nine ten-thousandths
6. Three thousand two hundred eighty-seven and four hundred sixty-seven thousandths
7. 0.34
8. 0.003
9. 0.0008
10. 2.017
11. 0.05
12. 4.1
13. 24.2
14. 15.01
15. 9.0002
16. 3.008
17. 100.018
18. 18.15
19. 0.055
20. 34.1

1I (PAGE 17)

Smaller:

1. 0.3	2. 0.25
3. 0.125	4. 2.07
5. 1.29	6. 0.37
7. 0.512	8. 0.094
9. 0.005	10. 1.088

Larger:

11. 0.9	12. 0.7
13. 0.58	14. 0.25
15. 0.1	16. 2.74
17. 0.31	18. 25.14
19. 0.25	20. 0.75

1J (PAGE 18)

1.	0.4 + 0.7 ――― 1.1	2.	5.030 + 2.999 ――― 8.029	3.	1.27 0.06 + 4.00 ――― 5.33	4.	15.60 0.19 + 500.00 ――― 515.79
5.	210.79 2.00 + 68.41 ――― 281.2Ø *	6.	88.60 576.46 + 79.00 ――― 744.06	7.	6.77 102.00 + 88.30 ――― 197.07	8.	79.40 68.44 + 3.00 ――― 150.84
9.	10.56 + 356.40 ――― 366.96	10.	99.70 + 293.23 ――― 392.93				

1K (PAGE 19)

1.	21.78 − 19.88 ――― 1.9Ø *	2.	98.4 − 66.5 ――― 31.9	3.	0.450 − 0.367 ――― 0.083	4.	108.56 − 5.40 ――― 103.16
5.	34.678 − 0.502 ――― 34.176	6.	7.066 − 0.200 ――― 6.866	7.	266.44 − 0.56 ――― 265.88	8.	78.567 − 6.770 ――― 71.797
9.	1.723 − 0.683 ――― 1.04Ø *	10.	0.8100 − 0.6701 ――― 0.1399				

1L (PAGE 20)

1. 0.5
    × 100
    ―――
    50.Ø   Count 1 decimal place in from the right.

2. 0.25
    × 2
    ―――
    0.5Ø

3. 3.14
    × 0.002
    ―――
    0.00628   You do not have to multiply zeros. Count 5 decimal places in from
                   the right, adding zeros where needed.

4. 2.14
    × 0.03
    ―――
    0.0642   Count 4 decimal places in from the right,
                   adding zeros as needed.

---

*Trailing zeros must be removed from answers.

5.
$$
\begin{array}{r}
36.8 \\
\times\,70.1 \\
\hline
368 \\
2578 \\
\hline
2579.68
\end{array}
$$

6.
$$
\begin{array}{r}
200 \\
\times\,0.2 \\
\hline
40.\cancel{0}
\end{array}
$$

7.
$$
\begin{array}{r}
90.1 \\
\times\,88 \\
\hline
7208 \\
7208 \\
\hline
7928.8
\end{array}
$$

8.
$$
\begin{array}{r}
2.76 \\
\times\,0.003 \\
\hline
0.00828
\end{array}
$$

9.
$$
\begin{array}{r}
54.5 \\
\times\,21 \\
\hline
545 \\
1090 \\
\hline
1144.5
\end{array}
$$

10.
$$
\begin{array}{r}
203.7 \\
\times\,28 \\
\hline
16296 \\
4074 \\
\hline
5703.6
\end{array}
$$

1M (PAGE 22)

1. $60\overline{)1.35}$

2. $20\overline{)15.6}$

3. $19\overline{)10.14}$

4. $7\overline{)60.5}$

5. $25\overline{)35.9}$

6.
$$
0.85\overline{)1.35\ 00}
$$
$$
\begin{array}{r}
1.58 \\
85 \\
\hline
50\ 0 \\
42\ 5 \\
\hline
7\ 50 \\
6\ 80 \\
\hline
70
\end{array}
$$

ANSWER: 1.6

7. $0.1\overline{)0.5}$ quotient $5.$

ANSWER: 5

8.
$$
4.8\overline{)2.0\ 40}
$$
$$
\begin{array}{r}
0.40 \\
19\ 2 \\
\hline
20
\end{array}
$$

ANSWER: 0.4

9.
$$
0.5\overline{)0.2\ 5}
$$
$$
\begin{array}{r}
0.5 \\
2\ 5
\end{array}
$$

ANSWER: 0.5

10.
$$
0.12\overline{)0.44\ 00}
$$
$$
\begin{array}{r}
3.66 \\
36 \\
\hline
8\ 0 \\
7\ 2 \\
\hline
80 \\
72 \\
\hline
8
\end{array}
$$

ANSWER: 3.7

1N (PAGE 23)

1.
$$
6.0\overline{)200.0\ 000}
$$
$$
\begin{array}{r}
3\ 3.333 \\
180 \\
\hline
20\ 0 \\
18\ 0 \\
\hline
2\ 00 \\
1\ 80 \\
\hline
2\ 00 \\
1\ 80 \\
\hline
200 \\
180
\end{array}
$$

PROOF
$$
\begin{array}{r}
33.333 \\
\times\,60 \\
\hline
1999.980
\end{array}
$$

2.
$$
6\overline{)15.06}
$$
$$
\begin{array}{r}
2.51 \\
12 \\
\hline
3\ 0 \\
3\ 0 \\
\hline
06 \\
6
\end{array}
$$

PROOF
$$
\begin{array}{r}
2.51 \\
\times\,6 \\
\hline
15.06
\end{array}
$$

3. $0.87\overline{)79.40\,000}$ → 91.264

```
        91.264
0.87 ) 79.40 000
       78 30
        1 10
          87
          23 0
          17 4
           5 60
           5 22
             380
             348
```

PROOF
```
    91.264
  ×     87
   638 848
  7301 12
  7939.968
```

4. $48\overline{)158.4}$ → 3.3

```
       3.3
48 ) 158.4
     144
      14 4
      14 4
```

PROOF
```
      48
  × 3.3
    14 4
   144
   158.4
```

5. $0.78\overline{)670.80}$ → 860.

```
          860.
0.78 ) 670.80
       624
        46 8
        46 8
```

PROOF
```
    860
  × 78
   6880
  6020
  67080
```

6. $2.43\overline{)78.60\,000}$ → 32.345

```
          32.345
2.43 ) 78.60 000
       72 9
        5 70
        4 86
          84 0
          72 9
          11 10
           9 72
           1 380
           1 215
```

PROOF
```
    32.345
  ×   243
    97 035
   1293 80
   6469 0
   7859.835
```

7. $8.2\overline{)26.7\,800}$ → 3.265

```
         3.265
8.2 ) 26.7 800
      24 6
       2 18
       1 64
        5 40
        4 92
          480
          410
```

PROOF
```
    3.265
  ×   82
   6 530
  261 20
  267.730
```

8. $5.78\overline{)266.50\,000}$ → 46.107

```
          46.107
5.78 ) 266.50 000
       231 2
        35 30
        34 68
          62 0
          57 8
           4 200
           4 046
```

PROOF
```
    46.107
  ×   578
   368 856
  3227 49
 23053 5
 26649.846
```

9. $6.5\overline{)10.8\,000}$ → 1.661

```
         1.661
6.5 ) 10.8 000
      6 5
      4 30
      3 90
        4 00
        3 90
          100
           65
```

PROOF
```
    1.661
  ×   65
   8 305
  99 66
  107.965
```

10. $10\overline{)76.530}$ → 7.653

```
        7.653
10 ) 76.530
     70
      6 5
      6 0
        53
        50
         30
         30
```

PROOF
```
    7.653
  ×   10
   76.530
```

10 (PAGE 24)

1. $\dfrac{8}{10} = \dfrac{4}{5}$ 2. $\dfrac{4}{10} = \dfrac{2}{5}$ 3. $\dfrac{25}{100} = \dfrac{1}{4}$ 4. $1\dfrac{32}{100} = 1\dfrac{8}{25}$

5. $4\dfrac{8}{100} = 4\dfrac{2}{25}$ 6. $\dfrac{5}{10} = \dfrac{1}{2}$ 7. $\dfrac{75}{100} = \dfrac{3}{4}$ 8. $\dfrac{2}{10} = \dfrac{1}{5}$

9. $\dfrac{65}{100} = \dfrac{13}{20}$ 10. $\dfrac{7}{10}$

1P (PAGE 25)

1.
$$\begin{array}{r} 0.2 \\ 5\overline{)1.0} \\ \underline{10} \end{array}$$

2.
$$\begin{array}{r} 0.666 \\ 3\overline{)2.000} \\ \underline{1\,8} \\ 20 \\ \underline{18} \\ 20 \\ \underline{18} \end{array}$$

3. $5\frac{9}{16} = 5 \times 16 + 9 = \frac{89}{16}$
$$\begin{array}{r} 5.562 \\ 16\overline{)89.000} \\ \underline{80} \\ 9\,0 \\ \underline{8\,0} \\ 1\,00 \\ \underline{96} \\ 40 \\ \underline{32} \end{array}$$

4.
$$\begin{array}{r} 0.19 \\ 100\overline{)19.00} \\ \underline{10\,0} \\ 9\,00 \\ \underline{9\,00} \end{array}$$

5.
$$\begin{array}{r} 1.285 \\ 7\overline{)9.00} \\ \underline{7} \\ 2\,0 \\ \underline{1\,4} \\ 60 \\ \underline{56} \\ 40 \\ \underline{35} \end{array}$$

6.
$$\begin{array}{r} 0.5 \\ 2\overline{)1.0} \\ \underline{10} \end{array}$$

7.
$$\begin{array}{r} 0.083 \\ 12\overline{)1.000} \\ \underline{96} \\ 40 \\ \underline{36} \end{array}$$

8.
$$\begin{array}{r} 0.75 \\ 8\overline{)6.00} \\ \underline{5\,6} \\ 40 \\ \underline{40} \end{array}$$

9.
$$\begin{array}{r} 0.075 \\ 200\overline{)15.000} \\ \underline{14\,00} \\ 1\,000 \\ \underline{1\,000} \end{array}$$

10.
$$\begin{array}{r} 2.5 \\ 8\overline{)20.0} \\ \underline{16} \\ 4\,0 \\ \underline{4\,0} \end{array}$$

1Q (PAGE 27)

	Nearest Whole Number	Nearest Tenth	Nearest Hundredth
1. 93.489	93	93.5	93.49
2. 25.43	25	25.4	25.43
3. 38.1	38	38.1	38.10
4. 57.8888	58	57.9	57.89
5. 0.0092	0	0	0.01
6. 3.144	3	3.1	3.14
7. 8.999	9	9.0	9.00
8. 77.788	78	77.8	77.79
9. 12.959	13	13.0	12.96
10. 5.7703	6	5.8	5.77

1R (PAGE 28)

	Nearest Whole Number	Nearest Tenth	Nearest Hundredth
1. $25.3 \times 4.2 =$	106	106.3	106.26
2. $9.3 \times 2.86 =$	27	26.6	26.60
3. $4.5 \times 7.57 =$	34	34.1	34.07
4. $1.3 \times 9.69 =$	13	12.6	12.60
5. $2.4 \times 5.88 =$	14	14.1	14.11
6. $8 \div 5 =$	2	1.6	1.60
7. $4.1 \div 3 =$	1	1.4	1.37
8. $5 \div 1.2 =$	4	4.2	4.17
9. $9 \div 2.2 =$	4	4.1	4.09
10. $10.2 \div 3 =$	3	3.4	3.40

1S (PAGE 30)

1. Decimal: 0.5
   Percentage: 50%

2. Fraction: $\frac{1}{2}$
   Decimal: 0.5

3. Fraction: $\frac{5}{100} = \frac{1}{20}$
   Percentage: 5%

4. Decimal: 0.083
   Percentage: 8.33%

5. Decimal: 0.003
   Percentage: 0.3%

6. Fraction: $\frac{1}{10}$
   Percentage: 10%

7. Fraction: $\frac{250}{100} = \frac{5}{2}$
   Decimal: 2.5

8. Fraction: $\frac{7}{20}$
   Percentage: 35%

9. Decimal: 0.8
   Percentage: 80%

10. Fraction: $\frac{75}{100} = \frac{3}{4}$
    Decimal: 0.75

1T (PAGE 31)

1.
$$\begin{array}{r} 1500 \\ \times\,0.02 \\ \hline 30.0\!\!\!/0\,* \end{array}$$

2.
$$\begin{array}{r} 240 \\ \times\,1.14 \\ \hline 960 \\ 240 \\ 240 \\ \hline 273.6\!\!\!/0\,* \end{array}$$

3.
$$\begin{array}{r} 50 \\ \times\,0.28 \\ \hline 400 \\ 100 \\ \hline 14.0\!\!\!/0\,* \end{array}$$

4.
$$\begin{array}{r} 200 \\ \times\,0.09 \\ \hline 18.0\!\!\!/0\,* \end{array}$$

5. $\frac{\frac{1}{2}}{100} = \frac{1}{2} \div \frac{100}{1} = \frac{1}{2} \times \frac{1}{100} = \frac{1}{200} = 200\overline{)1.000}^{\,0.005}$

$$\begin{array}{r} 9328 \\ \times\,0.005 \\ \hline 46.64\!\!\!/0\,* \end{array}$$

6. $\frac{\frac{1}{3}}{100} = \frac{1}{3} \div \frac{100}{1} = \frac{1}{3} \times \frac{1}{100} = \frac{1}{300} = 300\overline{)1.000}^{\,0.003}$
$$\begin{array}{r} 900 \\ \hline 100 \end{array}$$

$$\begin{array}{r} 930 \\ \times\,0.003 \\ \hline 2.79\!\!\!/0\,* \end{array}$$

*Trailing zeros must be removed from answers.

7.
$$\begin{array}{r} 400 \\ \times\,1.20 \\ \hline 8000 \\ 400 \\ \hline 480.0\cancel{0}\,* \end{array}$$

8.
$$\begin{array}{r} 105.80 \\ \times\,0.05 \\ \hline 5.290\cancel{0}\,* \end{array}$$

9.
$$\begin{array}{r} 520 \\ \times\,0.10 \\ \hline 52.0\cancel{0}\,* \end{array}$$

10.
$$\begin{array}{r} 40.80 \\ \times\,0.03 \\ \hline 1.224\cancel{0}\,* \end{array}$$

1U (PAGE 32)

1. **a** The other responses can be eliminated quickly because only **a** offers 3 as the whole number

2. b	3. d	4. a	5. c
6. b	7. b	8. d	9. b
10. a	11. b	12. d	13. d
14. a	15. c	16. a	17. a
18. a	19. c	20. b	

CHAPTER 1 FINAL: GENERAL MATHEMATICS (PAGE 35)

1. $6\frac{1}{4}$	2. 4	3. $\frac{51}{5}$	4. $\frac{23}{6}$
5. 20	6. 40	7. $\frac{19}{36}$	8. $10\frac{7}{8}$
9. $\frac{5}{24}$	10. 1	11. $\frac{1}{30}$	12. $\frac{10}{48} = \frac{5}{24}$
13. $\frac{24}{4} = 6$	14. $\frac{3}{4}$	15. $\frac{1}{250}$	16. $\frac{1}{3}$
17. 0.05	18. 2.017	19. 8.009	20. 60.97
21. 3.824	22. 0.1562	23. 0.00001\cancel{0}*	24. 3.5
25. 3.3\cancel{00}*	26. 91.264	27. 1.1875	28. 8.0625
29. 12.48	30. 583	31. $\frac{2}{5}$	32. $\frac{57}{200}$

*Trailing zeros must be removed from answers.

	Fraction	Decimal to Nearest Tenth	Decimal to Nearest Hundredth	Percentage
33.	$\frac{1}{3}$	0.3	0.33	33%
34.	$\frac{5}{100} = \left(\frac{1}{20}\right)$	0.1	0.05	5%
35.	$\frac{2}{5}$	0.4	0.40	40%
36.	$\frac{22}{100} = \left(\frac{11}{50}\right)$	0.2	0.22	22%
37.	$\frac{3}{8}$	0.4	0.38	38%
38.	$\frac{10}{100} = \left(\frac{1}{10}\right)$	0.1	0.10	10%
39.	$\frac{1}{12}$	0.1	0.08	8%
40.	$\frac{1}{200}$	0	0.01	$\frac{1}{2}$%
41.	$\frac{5}{16}$	0.3	0.31	31%
42.	$\frac{15}{100} = \left(\frac{3}{20}\right)$	0.2	0.15	15%
43.	$\frac{1}{4}$	0.3	0.25	25%
44.	$\frac{12}{100} = \left(\frac{3}{25}\right)$	0.1	0.12	12%
45.	$\frac{7}{9}$	0.8	0.78	78%
46.	$\frac{80}{100} = \left(\frac{4}{5}\right)$	0.8	0.80	80%
47.	$\frac{1}{6}$	0.2	0.17	17%
48.	$\frac{33}{100}$	0.3	0.33	33%
49.	$\frac{1}{250}$	0	0	$\frac{2}{5}$%
50.	$\frac{75}{100} = \left(\frac{3}{4}\right)$	0.8	0.75	75%

2 Ratio and Proportion

2A (PAGE 40)

1. $\frac{2}{4} = \frac{1}{2}$

2. $\frac{6}{8} = \frac{3}{4}$

3. $\frac{2}{500} = \frac{1}{250}$

4. $\frac{6}{1000} = \frac{3}{500}$

5. $\frac{43}{86} = \frac{1}{2}$

6. $\frac{2}{13}$

7. $\frac{8}{10} = \frac{4}{5}$

8. $\frac{1}{10}$

9. $\frac{1}{150}$

10. $\frac{4}{100} = \frac{1}{25}$

2B (PAGE 42)

1. $9 : x :: 5 : 300$

$5x = 9 \times 300$

$5x = 2700$

$\frac{\cancel{5}}{\cancel{5}} x = \frac{2700}{5} = 2700 \div 5$

$x = 540$

PROOF

$540 \times 5 = 2700$

$9 \times 300 = 2700$

2. $9 : 27 :: 300 : x$

$9x = 27 \times 300 = 8100$

$\frac{\cancel{9}}{\cancel{9}} x = \frac{8100}{9} = 8100 \div 9$

$x = 900$

PROOF

$27 \times 300 = 8100$

$9 \times 900 = 8100$

3. $\frac{1}{2} : x :: 1 : 8$

$1x = \frac{1}{2} \times 8$

$\frac{\cancel{1}}{\cancel{1}} x = \frac{1}{2} \times \frac{8}{1}$

$x = 4$

PROOF

$4 \times 1 = 4$

$\frac{1}{2} \times 8 = 4$

4. $\frac{1}{4} : 500 :: x : 1000$

$500x = \frac{1}{4} \times 1000$

$500x = \frac{1}{4} \times \frac{1000}{1} = 250$

$\frac{\cancel{500}}{\cancel{500}} x = \frac{250}{500} = 250 \div 500$

$x = 0.5$

PROOF

$500 \times 0.5 = 250$

$\frac{1}{4} \times 100 = 250$

5. $6 : 24 :: 0.75 : x$

$6x = 24 \times 0.75 = 18$

$6x = 18$

$\frac{\cancel{6}}{\cancel{6}} x = \frac{18}{6} = 18 \div 6$

$x = 3$

PROOF

$24 \times 0.75 = 18$

$6 \times 3 = 18$

6. $36 : 12 :: \frac{1}{100} : x$

$36x = 12 \times \frac{1}{100}$

$36x = \frac{12}{1} \times \frac{1}{100} = \frac{3}{25}$

$\frac{\cancel{36}}{\cancel{36}} x = \frac{3/25}{36} = \frac{3}{25} \div 36 = \frac{\cancel{3}}{25} \times \frac{1}{\cancel{36}_{12}}$

$x = \frac{1}{300}$

PROOF

$36 \times \frac{1}{300} = \frac{3}{25}$

$12 \times \frac{1}{100} = \frac{3}{25}$

7. $x : 600 :: 4 : 120$

$120x = 4 \times 600 = 2400$

$\frac{\cancel{120}}{\cancel{120}} x = \frac{240\cancel{0}}{12\cancel{0}} = 2400 \div 120$

$x = 20$

PROOF

$600 \times 4 = 2400$

$20 \times 120 = 2400$

8. $0.7 : 70 :: x : 1000$

$70x = 0.7 \times 1000 = 700$

$\frac{\cancel{70}}{\cancel{70}} x = \frac{70\cancel{0}}{7\cancel{0}} = 70 \div 7$

$x = 10$

PROOF

$70 \times 10 = 700$

$0.7 \times 1000 = 700$

9. $\frac{1}{1000} : \frac{1}{100} :: x : 60$

$$\frac{1}{100}x = \frac{1}{1000} \times 60$$

$$\frac{1}{100}x = \frac{1}{1000} \times \frac{60}{1} = \frac{1}{50} \times \frac{3}{1} = \frac{3}{50}$$

$$\frac{\cancel{1/100}}{\cancel{1/100}}x = \frac{3/50}{1/100} = \frac{3}{50} \div \frac{1}{100} = \frac{3}{50} \times \frac{100}{1} = \frac{300}{50}$$

$$x = 6$$

PROOF

$$\frac{1}{1000} \times 60 = \frac{3}{50}$$

$$\frac{1}{100} \times 6 = \frac{3}{50}$$

10. $6 : 12 :: \frac{1}{4} : x$

$$6x = 12 \times \frac{1}{4} = 3$$

$$\frac{\cancel{6}}{\cancel{6}}x = \frac{3}{6} = 3 \div 6$$

$$x = 0.5$$

PROOF

$$12 \times \frac{1}{4} = 3$$

$$6 \times 0.5 = 3$$

2C (PAGE 43)

1. $\frac{1}{2} : \frac{1}{6} :: \frac{1}{4} : x$

$$\frac{1}{2}x = \frac{1}{6} \times \frac{1}{4} = \frac{1}{24}$$

$$\frac{\cancel{1/2}}{\cancel{1/2}}x = \frac{1/24}{1/2} = \frac{1}{24} \div \frac{1}{2} = \frac{1}{24} \times \frac{2}{1}$$

$$x = \frac{1}{12}$$

PROOF

$$\frac{1}{2} \times \frac{1}{12} = \frac{1}{24}$$

$$\frac{1}{6} \times \frac{1}{4} = \frac{1}{24}$$

2. $15 : 30 :: x : 12$

$$30x = 15 \times 12$$

$$30x = 180$$

$$\frac{\cancel{30}}{\cancel{30}}x = \frac{180}{30} = 180 \div 30$$

$$x = 6$$

PROOF

$$30 \times 6 = 180$$

$$15 \times 12 = 180$$

3. $15 : x :: 1.5 : 10$

$$1.5x = 15 \times 10 = 150$$

$$\frac{\cancel{1.5}}{\cancel{1.5}}x = \frac{150}{1.5} = 150 \div 1.5$$

$$x = 100$$

PROOF

$$15 \times 10 = 150$$

$$100 \times 1.5 = 150$$

4. $6 : 12 :: 0.25 : x$

$$6x = 12 \times 0.25 = 3$$

$$\frac{\cancel{6}}{\cancel{6}}x = \frac{3}{6} = 3 \div 6$$

$$x = 0.5$$

PROOF

$$12 \times 0.25 = 3$$

$$6 \times 0.5 = 3$$

5. $300 : 5 :: x : \frac{1}{60}$

$$5x = \frac{1}{60} \times 300$$

$$5x = \frac{1}{60} \times \frac{300}{1} = 5$$

$$\frac{\cancel{5}}{\cancel{5}}x = \frac{5}{5} = 5 \div 5$$

$$x = 1$$

PROOF

$$300 \times \frac{1}{60} = 5$$

$$5 \times 1 = 5$$

6. $\frac{1}{150} : \frac{1}{200} :: 2 : x$

$$\frac{1}{150}x = \frac{1}{200} \times 2$$

$$\frac{1}{150}x = \frac{1}{200} \times \frac{2}{1} = \frac{1}{100}$$

$$\frac{\cancel{1/150}}{\cancel{1/100}}x = \frac{1/100}{1/150} = \frac{1}{100} \div \frac{1}{150} = \frac{1}{100} \times \frac{150}{1} = \frac{3}{2}$$

$$x = 1\frac{1}{2}$$

PROOF

$$\frac{1}{150} \times \frac{3}{2}(1\frac{1}{2}) = \frac{1}{100}$$

$$\frac{1}{200} \times 2 = \frac{1}{100}$$

7. $\frac{1}{200} : x :: 1 : 800$

$1x = \frac{1}{200} \times 800$

$1x = \frac{1}{200} \times \frac{800}{1} = 4$

$\frac{\cancel{1}}{\cancel{1}} x = \frac{4}{1} = 4 \div 1$

$x = 4$

PROOF

$4 \times 1 = 4$

$\frac{1}{200} \times 800 = 4$

8. $7.5 : 12 :: x : 28$

$12x = 7.5 \times 28 = 210$

$\frac{\cancel{12}}{\cancel{12}} x = \frac{210}{12} = 210 \div 12$

$x = 17.5$

PROOF

$7.5 \times 28 = 210$

$12 \times 17.5 = 210$

9. $\frac{1}{1000} : \frac{1}{100} :: x : 30$

$\frac{1}{100} x = \frac{1}{1000} \times 30$

$\frac{1}{100} x = \frac{1}{1000} \times \frac{30}{1} = \frac{3}{100}$

$\frac{\cancel{1/100}}{\cancel{1/100}} x = \frac{\cancel{3/100}}{\cancel{1/100}} = \frac{3}{100} \div \frac{1}{100} = \frac{3}{100} \times \frac{100}{1}$

$x = 3$

PROOF

$\frac{1}{1000} \times 30 = \frac{3}{100}$

$\frac{1}{100} \times 3 = \frac{3}{100}$

10. $10 : x :: 0.4 : 12$

$0.4x = 10 \times 12 = 120$

$\frac{\cancel{0.4}}{\cancel{0.4}} x = \frac{120}{0.4} = 120 \div 0.4$

$x = 300$

PROOF

$10 \times 12 = 120$

$300 \times 0.4 = 120$

2D (PAGE 43)

1. $3 : x :: 6 : 100$

$\frac{\cancel{6}}{\cancel{6}} x = \frac{300}{6}$

$x = 50$

PROOF

$3 \times 100 = 300$

$50 \times 6 = 300$

2. $3 : 24 :: 0.25 : x$

$3x = 24 \times 0.25$

$\frac{\cancel{3}}{\cancel{3}} x = \frac{6}{3}$

$x = 2$

PROOF

$3 \times 2 = 6$

$24 \times 0.25 = 6$

3. $8 : 16 :: x : 24$

$16x = 8 \times 24$

$\frac{\cancel{16}}{\cancel{16}} x = \frac{192}{16}$

$x = 12$

PROOF

$8 \times 24 = 192$

$16 \times 12 = 192$

4. $x : 600 :: 4 : 120$

$120x = 4 \times 600$

$\frac{\cancel{120}}{\cancel{120}} x = \frac{2400}{120}$

$x = 20$

PROOF

$20 \times 120 = 2400$

$600 \times 4 = 2400$

5. $5 : 3000 :: 15 : x$

$\frac{\cancel{5}}{\cancel{5}} x = \frac{45,000}{5}$

$x = 9000$

PROOF

$5 \times 9000 = 45,000$

$3000 \times 15 = 45,000$

6. $0.5 : 50 :: x : 1000$

$50x = 0.5 \times 1000$

$\frac{\cancel{50}}{\cancel{50}} x = \frac{500}{50}$

$x = 10$

PROOF

$0.5 \times 1000 = 500$

$50 \times 10 = 500$

7. $9 : 27 :: 300 : x$

$$\frac{\cancel{9}}{\cancel{9}}x = \frac{8100}{9}$$

$$x = 900$$

PROOF

$9 \times 900 = 8100$

$27 \times 300 = 8100$

8. $3 : 12 :: \frac{1}{4} : x$

$$3x = 12 \times \frac{1}{4} = \frac{12}{4} = 3$$

$$\frac{\cancel{3}}{\cancel{3}}x = \frac{\cancel{3}}{\cancel{3}}$$

$$x = 1$$

PROOF

$3 \times 1 = 3$

$12 \times \frac{1}{4} = 3$

9. $25 : x :: 75 : 3000$

$$\frac{\cancel{75}}{\cancel{75}}x = \frac{75,000}{75}$$

$$x = 1000$$

PROOF

$25 \times 3000 = 75,000$

$1000 \times 75 = 75,000$

10. $0.6 : 10 :: 0.5 : x$

$$0.6x = 10 \times 0.5 = 5$$

$$\frac{\cancel{0.6}}{\cancel{0.6}}x = \frac{5}{0.6}$$

$$x = 8.33 \text{ or } 8\frac{1}{3}$$

PROOF

$0.6 \times 8.33 = 4.998 \text{ or } 5$

$10 \times 0.5 = 5$

2E (PAGE 45)

1. | KNOW | WANT TO KNOW |
|---|---|

Bananas : Apples :: x Bananas : Apples

$6 : 9 :: x : 72$

$$9x = 6 \times 72 = 432$$

$$\frac{\cancel{9}}{\cancel{9}}x = \frac{432}{9}$$

$$x = 48 \text{ bananas}$$

PROOF

$6 : 9 :: 48 : 72$

$9 \times 48 = 432$

$6 \times 72 = 432$

2. | KNOW | WANT TO KNOW |
|---|---|

Scoops : Cups :: x Scoops : Cups

$7 : 8 :: x : 40$

$$8x = 40 \times 7 = 280$$

$$\frac{\cancel{8}}{\cancel{8}}x = \frac{280}{8}$$

$$x = 35 \text{ scoops}$$

PROOF

$7 : 8 :: 35 : 40$

$8 \times 35 = 280$

$7 \times 40 = 280$

REMEMBER Scoops : Cups :: Scoops : Cups
Apples : Bananas :: Apples : Bananas
Miles : Gallons :: Miles : Gallons

You want x to stand alone. To get x to stand alone, divide by 6. Whatever you do on one side of an equation, you must do on the other.

Obtain proof by putting your answer back into the equation in place of x. Multiply the two inside numbers, and they should equal the two outside numbers.

3. KNOW WANT TO KNOW

Scoops : Cups :: x Scoops : Cups

$4 : 6 :: x : 18$

$6x = 72$

$\dfrac{\cancel{6}}{\cancel{6}}x = \dfrac{72}{6}$

$\quad x = 12$ scoops of cocoa

PROOF

$4 : 6 :: 12 : 18$

$6 \times 12 = 72$

$4 \times 18 = 72$

4. KNOW WANT TO KNOW

4 pills : 1 day :: x pills : 21 days

$x = 4 \times 21$

$x = 84$ pills

PROOF

$4 : 1 :: 84 : 21$

$4 \times 21 = 84$

$1 \times 84 = 84$

5. KNOW WANT TO KNOW

Bushes : Trees :: x Bushes : Trees

$8 : 2 :: x : 36$

$2x = 8 \times 36 = 288$

$\dfrac{\cancel{2}}{\cancel{2}}x = \dfrac{288}{2}$

$\quad x = 144$ bushes

PROOF

$8 : 2 :: 144 : 36$

$8 \times 36 = 288$

$2 \times 144 = 288$

6. KNOW WANT TO KNOW

Cups : Day :: Cups : x Days

$4 : 1 :: 84 : x$

$4x = 84$

$\dfrac{\cancel{4}}{\cancel{4}}x = \dfrac{84}{4}$

$\quad x = 21$ days

PROOF

$4 : 1 :: 84 : 21$

$1 \times 84 = 84$

$4 \times 21 = 84$

7. KNOW WANT TO KNOW

Cups : Loaves :: Cups : x Loaves

$4 : 3 :: 24 : x$

$4x = 24 \times 3 = 72$

$\dfrac{\cancel{4}}{\cancel{4}}x = \dfrac{72}{4}$

$\quad x = 18$ loaves

PROOF

$4 : 3 :: 24 : 18$

$4 \times 18 = 72$

$3 \times 24 = 72$

8. KNOW WANT TO KNOW

3 soda : $\frac{1}{2}$ fruit juice :: x soda : 2 fruit juice

$\frac{1}{2}x = 3 \times 2$

$\dfrac{\cancel{1/2}}{\cancel{1/2}}x = \dfrac{6}{1/2} \qquad 6 \div \dfrac{1}{2} = 6 \times \dfrac{2}{1}$

$\quad x = 12$ cups soda

PROOF

$3 : \frac{1}{2} :: 12 : 2$

$3 \times 2 = 6$

$\frac{1}{2} \times 12 = 6$

9. KNOW WANT TO KNOW

4 Tbsp sugar : 1 glass :: x Tbsp sugar : 6 glasses

$x = 6 \times 4$

$x = 24$ tbsp sugar

PROOF

$4 : 1 :: 24 : 6$

$4 \times 6 = 24$

$1 \times 24 = 24$

10. KNOW WANT TO KNOW

4 cap : 1 day :: x cap : 14 days

$x = 4 \times 14$

$x = 56$ cap

PROOF

$4 : 1 :: 56 : 14$

$4 \times 14 = 56$

$1 \times 56 = 56$

2F (PAGE 46)

1. KNOW   WANT TO KNOW
200 envelopes : 1 box ::
                    4000 envelopes : x boxes
$200x = 4000$
$\frac{200}{200}x = \frac{4000}{200}$
$x = 20$ boxes
PROOF
$200 \times 20 = 4000$
$1 \times 4000 = 4000$

2. KNOW   WANT TO KNOW
10 disks : 1 package :: 300 disks : x packages
$10x = 300$
$\frac{10}{10}x = \frac{300}{10}$
$x = 30$ packages
PROOF
$10 \times 30 = 300$
$1 \times 300 = 300$

3. KNOW   WANT TO KNOW
1 computer : 18 students ::
                    x computers : 1280 students
$18x = 1280$
$\frac{18}{18}x = \frac{1280}{18}$
$x = 71.1$ or 71 computers
PROOF
$1 \times 1280 = 1280$
$18 \times 71.1 = 1279.8$ or 1280

4. KNOW   WANT TO KNOW
3 water : 2 apples :: 24 water : x apples
$3x = 48$
$\frac{3}{3}x = \frac{48}{3}$
$x = 16$ apples
PROOF
$3 \times 16 = 48$
$2 \times 24 = 48$

5. KNOW   WANT TO KNOW
6 pens : 8 pencils :: x pens : 72 pencils
$8x = 432$
$\frac{8}{8}x = \frac{432}{8}$
$x = 54$ pens
PROOF
$6 \times 72 = 432$
$8 \times 54 = 432$

6. KNOW   WANT TO KNOW
1 nurse : 6 patients :: x nurses : 36 patients
$6x = 36$
$\frac{6}{6}x = \frac{36}{6}$
$x = 6$ nurses
PROOF
$1 \times 36 = 36$
$6 \times 6 = 36$

7. KNOW   WANT TO KNOW
4 Tbsp : 8 oz water :: x Tbsp : 56 oz water
$8x = 4 \times 56 = 224$
$\frac{8}{8}x = \frac{224}{8}$
$x = 28$ Tbsp formula
PROOF
$4 \times 56 = 224$
$8 \times 28 = 224$

8. KNOW   WANT TO KNOW
2 nurses : 12 hr :: x nurses : 72 hr
$12x = 144$
$\frac{12}{12}x = \frac{124}{12}$
$x = 12$ nurses needed
PROOF
$12 \times 12 = 144$
$2 \times 72 = 144$

9. KNOW   WANT TO KNOW
8 aspirin : 1 day :: x aspirin : 14 days
$x = 8 \times 14$
$x = 112$ Aspirin tablets
PROOF
$8 \times 14 = 112$
$1 \times 112 = 112$

10. KNOW   WANT TO KNOW
5 milliliters : 1 day :: 100 milliliters : x days
$\frac{5}{5}x = \frac{100}{5}$
$x = 20$ Days
PROOF
$5 \times 20 = 100$
$1 \times 100 = 100$

2G (PAGE 47)

1. a. KNOW $\qquad$ WANT TO KNOW

10 diapers : 1 day :: 50 diapers : x days

$\frac{\cancel{10}}{\cancel{10}} x = \frac{50}{10}$

$x = 5$ days

PROOF

$10 \times 5 = 50$

$1 \times 50 = 50$

2. b. KNOW $\qquad$ WANT TO KNOW

10 syringes : 1 package ::

$\qquad$ 120 syringes : x packages

$\frac{\cancel{10}}{\cancel{10}} x = \frac{120}{10}$

$x = 12$ packages

PROOF

$10 \times 12 = 120$

$1 \times 120 = 120$

3. d. KNOW $\qquad$ WANT TO KNOW

4 tsp : 1 day :: 80 tsp : x days

$\frac{\cancel{4}}{\cancel{4}} x = \frac{80}{4}$

$x = 20$ days

PROOF

$4 \times 20 = 80$

$1 \times 80 = 80$

4. d. KNOW $\qquad$ WANT TO KNOW

3 pills : 1 day :: x pills : 21 days

$x = 3 \times 21$

$x = 63$ pills

PROOF

$3 \times 21 = 63$

$1 \times 63 = 63$

5. b. KNOW $\qquad$ WANT TO KNOW

5 mL : 1 dose :: 30 mL : x doses

$\frac{\cancel{5}}{\cancel{5}} x = \frac{30}{5}$

$x = 6$ doses

PROOF

$5 \times 6 = 30$

$1 \times 30 = 30$

6. b. KNOW $\qquad$ WANT TO KNOW

120 days : 15 depts :: x days : 1 dept

$\frac{\cancel{15}}{\cancel{15}} x = \frac{120}{15}$

$x = 8$ days

PROOF

$120 \times 1 = 120$

$15 \times 8 = 120$

7. KNOW $\qquad$ WANT TO KNOW

a. 8 patients : 1 RN :: 240 patients : x RNs

$\frac{\cancel{8}}{\cancel{8}} x = \frac{240}{8}$

$x = 30$ RNs

PROOF

$8 \times 30 = 240$

$1 \times 240 = 240$

8. KNOW $\qquad$ WANT TO KNOW

c. 4 oz : 1 portion :: x oz : 20 portions

$x = 4 \times 20$

$x = 80$ oz

PROOF

$4 \times 20 = 80$

$1 \times 80 = 80$

9. KNOW $\qquad$ WANT TO KNOW

c. $15 : 1 hr :: $450 : x hr

$\frac{\cancel{15}}{\cancel{15}} x = \frac{450}{15}$

$x = 30$ hr

PROOF

$15 \times 30 = 450$

$1 \times 450 = 450$

10. a. KNOW $\qquad$ WANT TO KNOW

1 NA : 20 beds :: x NAs : 360 beds

$\frac{\cancel{20}}{\cancel{20}} x = \frac{360}{20}$

$x = 18$ NAs

PROOF

$1 \times 360 = 360$

$20 \times 18 = 360$

CHAPTER 2 FINAL: RATIO AND PROPORTION (PAGE 49)

1. 15 supervisors
2. 25 nurses
3. 800 sheets
4. 224 patient discharges
5. $480
6. 30 CNAs
7. 5 supervisors
8. $3000 for 4 weeks
9. 21 interns
10. approximately 40 medication errors
11. 12 pills
12. 28 pills
13. 10 days
14. 64 oz
15. 8 inservice days
16. 8 doses
17. 12 people
18. 32 RNs
19. 12 guest speakers
20. 240 tablets

3 Safe Medication Administration

3A (PAGE 54)

Time	Abbreviation (if Applicable)	Time	Abbreviation (if Applicable)
before	a	after	p
before meals	ac	after meals	pc
daily	Write out daily	three times a day	tid
twice a day	bid	every other day	Write out every other day
every day	Write out every day	every 6 hours	q6h
every 4 hours	every 4 hours	every 12 hours	q12h
whenever necessary	prn	as desired, freely	ad lib (fluids and activities only)
immediately, at once	stat	bedtime	Write out bedtime
with	c̄	without	s̄

Route	Abbreviation (if Applicable)	Route	Abbreviation (if Applicable)
by mouth	po	nothing by mouth	NPO
intravenously	IV	intramuscularly	IM
sublingual	SL	subcutaneous	subcut
intradermal	ID	suppository	supp
left eye	Write out left eye	right ear	Write out right ear
nasogastric	NG	per gastrostomy tube	GT

3B (PAGE 55)

Metric Measurement Term	Metric Measurement Abbreviation
microgram(s)	mcg
milligram(s)	mg
gram(s)	g
kilogram(s)	kg
milliliter(s)	mL
milliequivalent(s)	mEq
unit	Write out unit
international unit	Write out international unit
liter	L
square meter	m^2

Other Measurement Term	Abbreviation
grain (apothecary term)	Write out grain
one-half	Write out one half
teaspoon	tsp.
tablespoon	tbs, Tbsp
pound	lb

3C (PAGE 56)

Term	Recommended Abbreviation
capsule	cap
tablet	tab
fluid	fld
solution	sol
suspension	susp
elixir	elix
teaspoon	tsp
tablespoon	tbs, Tbsp
liquid	liq
ounce	oz
double strength	DS
extended release	XR
long acting	LA
sustained release	SR
controlled release	CR

3D (PAGE 64)

1. **a.** Lopressor
   b. metoprolol tartrate USP
   c. 50 mg per tab
   d. 1000 tab
   e. 50 mg : 1 tab

2. **a.** Rifadin
   b. rifampin
   c. 150 mg per cap
   d. 30 cap
   e. 150 mg : 1 cap

3. **a.** Amoxil
   b. 78 mL
   c. 125 mg/5 mL
   d. 100 mL
   e. 125 mg : 5 mL
   f. 14 days

4. **a.** tetracycline HCl
   b. 500 mg
   c. 100 cap
   d. 500 mg : 1 cap

5. **a.** streptomycin sulfate
   b. IM only
   c. 400 mg/mL
   d. 1 g/2.5 mL
   e. Refrigerate 2° to 8° C

3E (PAGE 74)

1. Yes. Care must be taken in distinguishing this patient from other patients with the same or a similar name to avoid giving a medication to the wrong patient.

2. Yes. The patient is allergic to the intravenous iodine used in some contrast media tests and to products that contain aspirin. There are many.

3. One 24-hour day

4. Digoxin was withheld as denoted by a circle and the code "R."

5. Topical

6. Promethazine, a stat order

7. Meperidine; left arm denoted by "C."

8. 05/09/08 at 0700

9. 05/07/08 at 2000; 8 PM

10. Having both the initials and the nurse's signature identifies the nurse who administered the medication more clearly. More than one staff member may have the same initials or some initials may be illegible.

3F (PAGE 74)

1. The route is not specified.

2. The dose is not specified. Aspirin is supplied in more than one dose (e.g., 325 mg per tablet, 650 mg per tablet). The number of tablets should *not* be mentioned in the order.

3. The route is specified. Ampicillin can be administered by more than one route (PO, IM, IV).

4. The time or frequency is not specified—for example, stat, one time only, or more than one time.

5. The dose and form are not specified. Tylenol is supplied in tablet, liquid suspension, intravenous, and suppository forms and in a variety of doses targeted to infants, children, and adults.

3G (PAGE 77)

1. **b.** Correct identification of patient is always the first priority. a, c, and d would all be appropriate after the patient is identified.

2. **a.** b, c, and d would all be appropriate after the patient was assessed.

3. **a.** b is the total amount of drug in the container. c is the total volume in mL. d is the usual ordered adult dosage on the first day.

4. **d.** a, b, and c are inappropriate actions.

5. **b.** Refer to the international/military time clock on page 66.

6. **a.** b, c, and d are false statements.

7. d. A solid foundation in medication mathematics, logic, estimation of a reasonable dose as applicable during calculations, and use of reliable references and pharmacy for safe doses are more protective measures than memorized formulas for complex calculations.

8. d. The right route is usually the one that is ordered but not in this case. There is a conflict, and common sense dictates that the nurse must clarify. The patient is NPO and there must be a written order to be able to give a medication by mouth. Some medications are totally unsuitable for nasogastric tube administration, and some just obstruct the tube.

9. a. Digoxin and digitoxin have similar names but are two different medications.

10. b. Giving a medication after the expiration date, whether automatically established by the agency or written by the physician, is illegal. All other actions are appropriate.

CHAPTER 3 FINAL: SAFE MEDICATION ADMINISTRATION (PAGE 82)

1. a. Right patient
   b. Right drug
   c. Right dose
   d. Right time
   e. Right route
   f. Right documentation
   g. Right to refuse

2.

Term/Abbreviation	Meaning	Term/Abbreviation	Meaning
c̄	with	s̄	without
po	by mouth	NPO	nothing by mouth
IV	intravenous	IM	intramuscular
supp	suppository	bid	twice a day
tid	three times daily	q6h	every 6 hours
prn	whenever necessary	ad lib*	freely, as desired
ac	before meals	pc	after meals
subcut	subcutaneous	ID	intradermal
SL	sublingual	NG	nasogastric
stat	immediately	top	topical

*ad lib is used for fluids and activity but not for medications.

3.

Term	Abbreviation
milligram	mg
microgram	mcg
gram	g
kilogram	kg
liter	L
milliliter	mL

4.

Traditional Time	24-Hour Clock	24-Hour Clock	Traditional Time
12 Noon (12 PM)	1200 hours	2100 hours	9 PM
Midnight (12 AM)	2400 hours	1400 hours	2 PM
1 PM	1300 hours	0145 hours	1:45 AM
9 AM	0900 hours	0030 hours	12:30 AM
5 PM	1700 hours	1645 hours	4:45 PM

5. **a.** Generic name: acyclovir
   b. Drug form: capsule
   c. Unit dose per capsule: 200 mg
   d. Unit dose or multidose container: multidose

6. Generic name, proprietary, trade, or brand name, unit dose, form, total amount in container, recommended routes, preparation directions, storage directions, and expiration date.

7. Aspirin tablet 325 milligrams by mouth every 4 hours as needed for headache.

8. The Joint Commission's Do Not Use list contains the prohibited abbreviations that have been misinterpreted and led to medication errors.

9. If an order is unclear it should be clarified with the prescriber.

10. Decimals can be missed altogether or mistaken for the number 1.

4 Drug Measurements and Dose Calculations

4A (PAGE 88)

1. 1000 mg	2. 2000 mg	3. 500 mg	4. 1500 mg
5. 250 mg	6. 50 mcg	7. 50 mg	8. 100 mg
9. 300 mg	10. 1100 mg	11. 0.025 g	12. 5000 mcg
13. 3 g	14. 1.5 g	15. 15 g	16. 0.010 g
17. 0.1 mg	18. 0.0005 g	19. 0.0075 g	20. 0.02015 g

4B (PAGE 93)

1. KNOW   WANT TO KNOW
$1000 \text{ mg} : 1 \text{ g} :: 4 \text{ mg} : x \text{ g}$
$\frac{1000}{1000} x = \frac{4}{1000}$
$x = 0.004 \text{ g}$
PROOF
$1000 \times 0.004 = 4$
$1 \times 4 = 4$

2. KNOW   WANT TO KNOW
$1000 \text{ mg} : 1 \text{ g} :: 200 \text{ mg} : x \text{ g}$
$\frac{1000}{1000} x = \frac{200}{1000}$
$x = 0.2 \text{ g}$
PROOF
$1000 \times 0.2 = 200$
$1 \times 200 = 200$

3. KNOW   WANT TO KNOW
$1000 \text{ mg} : 1 \text{ g} :: 0.3 \text{ mg} : x \text{ g}$
$\frac{1000}{1000} x = \frac{0.3}{1000}$
$x = 0.0003 \text{ g}$
PROOF
$1000 \times 0.0003 = 0.3$
$1 \times 0.3 = 0.3$

4. KNOW   WANT TO KNOW
$1000 \text{ mg} : 1 \text{ g} :: 25 \text{ mg} : x \text{ g}$
$\frac{1000}{1000} x = \frac{25}{1000}$
$x = 0.025 \text{ g}$
PROOF
$1000 \times 0.025 = 25$
$1 \times 25 = 25$

5. KNOW   WANT TO KNOW
$1000 \text{ mg} : 1 \text{ g} :: 15 \text{ mg} : x \text{ g}$
$\frac{1000}{1000} x = \frac{15}{1000}$
$x = 0.015 \text{ g}$
PROOF
$1000 \times 0.015 = 15$
$1 \times 15 = 15$

6. KNOW   WANT TO KNOW
$1 \text{ g} : 1000 \text{ mg} :: 2.5 \text{ g} : x \text{ mg}$
$x = 1000 \times 2.5$
$x = 2500 \text{ mg}$
PROOF
$1 \times 2500 = 2500$
$1000 \times 2.5 = 2500$

7. KNOW   WANT TO KNOW
$1 \text{ g} : 1000 \text{ mg} :: 4.6 \text{ g} : x \text{ mg}$
$x = 1000 \times 4.6$
$x = 4600 \text{ mg}$
PROOF
$1 \times 4600 = 4600$
$1000 \times 4.6 = 4600$

8. KNOW   WANT TO KNOW
$1 \text{ g} : 1000 \text{ mg} :: 0.03 \text{ g} : x \text{ mg}$
$x = 1000 \times 0.03$
$x = 30 \text{ mg}$
PROOF
$1 \times 30 = 30$
$1000 \times 0.03 = 30$

9. KNOW   WANT TO KNOW
$1 \text{ g} : 1000 \text{ mg} :: 0.5 \text{ g} : x \text{ mg}$
$x = 1000 \times 0.5$
$x = 500 \text{ mg}$
PROOF
$1 \times 500 = 500$
$1000 \times 0.5 = 500$

10. KNOW   WANT TO KNOW
$1 \text{ g} : 1000 \text{ mg} :: 0.01 \text{ g} : x \text{ mg}$
$x = 1000 \times 0.01$
$x = 10 \text{ mg}$
PROOF
$1 \times 10 = 10$
$1000 \times 0.01 = 10$

11. KNOW   WANT TO KNOW
$1000 \text{ mcg} : 1 \text{ mg} :: 150 \text{ mcg} : x \text{ mg}$
$\frac{\cancel{1000}}{\cancel{1000}} x = \frac{15\cancel{0}}{100\cancel{0}}$
$x = 0.15 \text{ mg}$
PROOF
$1000 \times 0.15 = 150$
$1 \times 150 = 150$

12. KNOW   WANT TO KNOW
$1000 \text{ mcg} : 1 \text{ mg} :: 500 \text{ mcg} : x \text{ mg}$
$\frac{\cancel{1000}}{\cancel{1000}} x = \frac{50\cancel{0}}{10\cancel{0}0}$
$x = 0.5 \text{ mg}$
PROOF
$1000 \times 0.5 \text{ mg} = 500$
$1 \times 500 = 500$

13. KNOW   WANT TO KNOW
$1000 \text{ mcg} : 1 \text{ mg} :: 50 \text{ mcg} : x \text{ mg}$
$\frac{\cancel{1000}}{\cancel{1000}} x = \frac{5\cancel{0}}{100\cancel{0}}$
$x = 0.05 \text{ mg}$
PROOF
$1000 \times 0.05 = 50$
$1 \times 50 = 50$

14. KNOW   WANT TO KNOW
$1000 \text{ mcg} : 1 \text{ mg} :: 2500 \text{ mcg} : x \text{ mg}$
$\frac{\cancel{1000}}{\cancel{1000}} x = \frac{250\cancel{0}}{10\cancel{0}0}$
$x = 2.5 \text{ mg}$
PROOF
$1000 \times 2.5 = 2500$
$1 \times 2500 = 2500$

15. KNOW   WANT TO KNOW
$1000 \text{ mcg} : 1 \text{ mg} :: 3000 \text{ mcg} : x \text{ mg}$
$\frac{\cancel{1000}}{\cancel{1000}} x = \frac{300\cancel{0}}{100\cancel{0}}$
$x = 3 \text{ mg}$
PROOF
$1000 \times 3 = 3000$
$1 \times 3000 = 3000$

16. KNOW   WANT TO KNOW
$1 \text{ mg} : 1000 \text{ mcg} :: 20 \text{ mg} : x \text{ mcg}$
$x = 1000 \times 20$
$x = 20,000 \text{ mcg}$
PROOF
$1 \times 20,000 = 20,000$
$1000 \times 20 = 20,000$

17. KNOW   WANT TO KNOW
$1 \text{ mg} : 1000 \text{ mcg} :: 200 \text{ mg} : x \text{ mcg}$
$x = 1000 \times 200$
$x = 200,000 \text{ mcg}$
PROOF
$1 \times 200,000 = 200,000$
$1000 \times 200 = 200,000$

18. KNOW   WANT TO KNOW
$1 \text{ mg} : 1000 \text{ mcg} :: 5 \text{ mg} : x \text{ mcg}$
$x = 1000 \times 5$
$x = 5000 \text{ mcg}$
PROOF
$1 \times 5000 = 5000$
$1000 \times 5 = 5000$

19. KNOW   WANT TO KNOW
$1 \text{ mg} : 1000 \text{ mcg} :: 0.1 \text{ mg} : x \text{ mcg}$
$x = 1000 \times 0.1$
$x = 100 \text{ mcg}$
PROOF
$1 \times 100 = 100$
$1000 \times 0.1 = 100$

20. KNOW   WANT TO KNOW
$1 \text{ mg} : 1000 \text{ mcg} :: 0.04 \text{ mg} : x \text{ mcg}$
$x = 1000 \times 0.04$
$x = 40 \text{ mcg}$
PROOF
$1 \times 40 = 40$
$1000 \times 0.04 = 40$

21. KNOW   WANT TO KNOW
    1 kg : 1000 g :: 5.5 kg : x g
    $x = 1000 \times 5.5$
    $x = 5500$ g
    PROOF
    $1 \times 5500 = 5500$
    $1000 \times 5.5 = 5500$

22. KNOW   WANT TO KNOW
    1 kg : 1000 g :: 12 kg : x g
    $x = 1000 \times 12$
    $x = 12,000$ g
    PROOF
    $1 \times 12,000 = 12,000$
    $1000 \times 12 = 12,000$

23. KNOW   WANT TO KNOW
    1 kg : 1000 g :: 3 kg : x g
    $x = 1000 \times 3$
    $x = 3000$ g
    PROOF
    $1 \times 3000 = 3000$
    $1000 \times 3 = 3000$

24. KNOW   WANT TO KNOW
    1 kg : 1000 g :: 1.3 kg : x g
    $x = 1000 \times 1.3$
    $x = 1300$ g
    PROOF
    $1 \times 1300 = 1300$
    $1000 \times 1.3 = 1300$

25. KNOW   WANT TO KNOW
    1 kg : 1000 g :: 0.5 kg : x g
    $x = 1000 \times 0.5$
    $x = 500$ g
    PROOF
    $1 \times 500 = 500$
    $1000 \times 0.5 = 500$

26. KNOW   WANT TO KNOW
    1 L : 1000 mL :: 0.5 L : x mL
    $x = 1000 \times 0.5$
    $x = 500$ mL
    PROOF
    $1 \times 500 = 500$
    $1000 \times 0.5 = 500$

27. KNOW   WANT TO KNOW
    1 L : 1000 mL :: 1.3 L : x mL
    $x = 1000 \times 1.3$
    $x = 1300$ mL
    PROOF
    $1 \times 1300 = 1300$
    $1000 \times 1.3 = 1300$

28. KNOW   WANT TO KNOW
    1 L : 1000 mL :: 1.5 L : x mL
    $x = 1000 \times 1.5$
    $x = 1500$ mL
    PROOF
    $1 \times 1500 = 1500$
    $1000 \times 1.5 = 1500$

29. KNOW   WANT TO KNOW
    1 L : 1000 mL :: 3 L : x mL
    $x = 1000 \times 3$
    $x = 3000$ mL
    PROOF
    $1 \times 3000 = 3000$
    $1000 \times 3 = 3000$

30. KNOW   WANT TO KNOW
    1 L : 1000 mL :: 2.8 L : x mL
    $x = 1000 \times 2.8$
    $x = 2800$ mL
    PROOF
    $1 \times 2800 = 2800$
    $1000 \times 2.8 = 2800$

4C (PAGE 95)

1. **a.** 300 mg/capsule   **b.** 30 capsules

2. **a.** 175 mcg/tablet   **b.** 0.175 mg

3. **a.** 10 USP* units/mL   **b.** 10 mL

4. **a.** 250,000 units/mL   **b.** 200,000 to 400,000 units   **c.** 5 million units

5. **a.** 2 mEq/mL   **b.** 40 mEq/20 mL

6. **a.** 100 units/mL   **b.** 10 mL

7. **a.** 125 mcg   **b.** 0.125 mg

8. 1000 mL

9. 4 mEq/L†

10. 30 mg†

---

*USP refers to the *United States Pharmacopoeia,* a national listing of drugs.
†It is critical to distinguish mg from mEq on medication orders and labels. This means that the fine print must be scrutinized for critical information.

4D (PAGE 98)

1. KNOW   WANT TO KNOW
   250 mg : 1 cap :: 500 mg : x cap
   $$\frac{\cancel{250}}{\cancel{250}}x = \frac{500}{250}$$
   $$x = 2 \text{ cap}$$
   PROOF
   $250 \times 2 = 500$
   $1 \times 500 = 500$

2. KNOW   WANT TO KNOW
   175 mcg : 1 tab :: 350 mcg : x tab
   $$\frac{\cancel{175}}{\cancel{175}}x = \frac{350}{175}$$
   $$x = 2 \text{ tab}$$
   PROOF
   $175 \times 2 = 350$
   $1 \times 350 = 350$

3. KNOW   WANT TO KNOW
   0.125 mg : 1 tab :: 0.0625 mg : x tab
   $$\frac{\cancel{0.125}}{\cancel{0.125}}x = \frac{0.0625}{0.125}$$
   $$x = 0.5 \text{ or } \frac{1}{2} \text{ tab}$$
   PROOF
   $0.125 \times 0.5 = 0.0625$
   $1 \times 0.0625 = 0.0625$

4. KNOW   WANT TO KNOW
   200 mg : 5 mL :: 300 mg : x mL
   $$\frac{\cancel{200}}{\cancel{200}}x = \frac{5 \times \cancel{300}}{\cancel{200}} \text{ or } \frac{15\cancel{00}}{2\cancel{00}}$$
   $$x = 7.5 \text{ mL}$$
   PROOF
   $200 \times 7.5 = 1500$
   $5 \times 300 = 1500$

   You would use a syringe to withdraw the medication to the exact amount and then transfer it to the cup.

5. KNOW   WANT TO KNOW

80 mg : 0.8 mL :: 40 mg : x mL

$\frac{80}{80} x = \frac{32}{80}$

$x = 0.4$ mL

PROOF

$80 \times 0.4 = 32$

$0.8 \times 40 = 32$

4E (PAGE 101)

1. KNOW   WANT TO KNOW

50 mg : 1 tab :: 75 mg : x tab

$\frac{50}{50} x = \frac{75}{50}$

$x = 1.5$ tab

PROOF

$50 \times 1.5 = 75$

$1 \times 75 = 75$

2. KNOW   WANT TO KNOW

15 mg : 1 tab :: 30 mg : x tab

$\frac{15}{15} x = \frac{30}{15}$

$x = 2$ tab

PROOF

$15 \times 2 = 30$

$1 \times 30 = 30$

3. KNOW   WANT TO KNOW

300 mg : 1 tab :: 450 mg : x tab

$\frac{300}{300} x = \frac{450}{300}$

$x = 1.5$ tab

PROOF

$300 \times 1.5 = 450$

$1 \times 450 = 450$

4. KNOW   WANT TO KNOW

0.125 mg : 1 tab :: 0.25 mg : x tab

$\frac{0.125}{0.125} x = \frac{0.25}{0.125}$

$x = 2$ tab

PROOF

$0.125 \times 2 = 0.25$

$1 \times 0.25 = 0.25$

5. KNOW   WANT TO KNOW

0.1 mg : 1 tab :: 0.2 mg : x tab

$\frac{0.1}{0.1} x = \frac{0.2}{0.1}$

$x = 2$ tab

PROOF

$0.1 \times 2 = 0.2$

$1 \times 0.2 = 0.2$

6. KNOW   WANT TO KNOW

8 mEq : 5 mL :: 20 mEq : x mL

$\frac{8}{8} x = \frac{100}{8}$

$x = 12.5$ mL

PROOF

$8 \times 12.5 = 100$

$5 \times 20 = 100$

7. KNOW   WANT TO KNOW

0.01 mg : 1 tab :: 0.02 mg : x tab

$\frac{0.01}{0.01} x = \frac{0.02}{0.01}$

$x = 2$ tab

PROOF

$0.01 \times 2 = 0.02$

$1 \times 0.02 = 0.02$

8. KNOW   WANT TO KNOW

10 mg : 1 tab :: 5 mg : x tab

$\frac{10}{10} x = \frac{5}{10}$

$x = 0.5$ tab

PROOF

$10 \times 0.5 = 5$

$1 \times 5 = 5$

9. KNOW   WANT TO KNOW

400 mg : 1 tab :: 800 mg : x tab

$400 x = 800$

$x = 2$ tab

PROOF

$400 \times 2 = 800$

$1 \times 800 = 800$

10. KNOW   WANT TO KNOW

150 mg : 1 tab :: 450 mg : x tab

$\dfrac{\cancel{150}}{\cancel{150}} x = \dfrac{\cancel{450}}{\cancel{150}}$

$x = 3$ tab

PROOF

$150 \times 3 = 450$

$1 \times 450 = 450$

4F (PAGE 103)

1. Step 1:

KNOW   WANT TO KNOW

1000 mg : 1 g :: x mg : 0.5 g

$x = 1000 \times 0.5$

$x = 500$ mg

PROOF

$1000 \times 0.5 = 500$

$1 \times 500 = 500$

Step 2:

KNOW   WANT TO KNOW

500 mg : 1 tab :: 500 mg : x tab

$\dfrac{\cancel{500}}{\cancel{500}} x = \dfrac{\cancel{500}}{\cancel{500}}$

$x = 1$ tab

PROOF

$500 \times 1 = 500$

$1 \times 500 = 500$

2. Step 1:

KNOW   WANT TO KNOW

1000 mg : 1 g :: x mg : 0.3 g

$x = 1000 \times 0.3$

$x = 300$ mg

PROOF

$1000 \times 0.3 = 300$

$1 \times 300 = 300$

Step 2:

KNOW   WANT TO KNOW

100 mg : 1 cap :: 300 mg : x cap

$\dfrac{\cancel{100}}{\cancel{100}} x = \dfrac{\cancel{300}}{\cancel{100}}$

$x = 3$ cap*

PROOF

$100 \times 3 = 300$

$1 \times 300 = 300$

3. Step 1:

KNOW   WANT TO KNOW

1000 mg : 1 g :: x mg : 1 g

$x = 1000$ mg

PROOF

$1000 \times 1 = 1000$

$1 \times 1000 = 1000$

Step 2:

KNOW   WANT TO KNOW

500 mg : 1 tab :: 1000 mg : x tab

$\dfrac{\cancel{500}}{\cancel{500}} x = \dfrac{\cancel{1000}}{\cancel{500}}$

$x = 2$ tabs

PROOF

$500 \times 2 = 1000$

$1 \times 1000 = 1000$

4. Step 1:

KNOW   WANT TO KNOW

1000 mg : 1 g :: x mg : 0.3 g

$x = 1000 \times 0.3$

$x = 300$ mg

PROOF

$1000 \times 0.3 = 300$

$1 \times 300 = 300$

Step 2:

KNOW   WANT TO KNOW

300 mg : 1 cap :: 300 mg : x cap

$\dfrac{\cancel{300}}{\cancel{300}} x = \dfrac{\cancel{300}}{\cancel{300}}$

$x = 1$ cap

PROOF

$300 \times 1 = 300$

$1 \times 300 = 300$

---

*When giving more than 1 or 2 times the unit dose (more than 1 or 2 capsules), recheck the order and the math. Consult a current drug guide for the recommended dose.

5. **Step 1:**

KNOW   WANT TO KNOW

$1000 \text{ mg} : 1 \text{ g} :: x \text{ mg} : 0.6 \text{ g}$

$x = 1000 \times 0.6$

$x = 600 \text{ mg}$

PROOF

$1000 \times 0.6 = 600$

$1 \times 600 = 600$

Step 2:

KNOW   WANT TO KNOW

$600 \text{ mg} : 1 \text{ tab} :: 600 \text{ mg} : x \text{ tab}$

$\dfrac{\cancel{600}}{\cancel{600}} x = \dfrac{\cancel{600}}{\cancel{600}}$

$x = 1 \text{ tab}$

PROOF

$600 \times 1 = 600$

$1 \times 600 = 600$

4G (PAGE 105)

1. KNOW   WANT TO KNOW

$0.25 \text{ mg} : 1 \text{ tab} :: 0.5 \text{ mg} : x \text{ tab}$

$\dfrac{\cancel{0.25}}{\cancel{0.25}} x = \dfrac{0.5}{0.25}$

$x = 2 \text{ tab}$

PROOF

$0.25 \times 2 = 0.5$

$1 \times 0.5 = 0.5$

2. **Step 1:**

KNOW   WANT TO KNOW

$1000 \text{ mg} : 1 \text{ g} :: x \text{ mg} : 0.2 \text{ g}$

$x = 1000 \times 0.2$

$x = 200 \text{ mg}$

Step 2:

HAVE   WANT TO HAVE

$100 \text{ mg} : 1 \text{ cap} :: 200 \text{ mg} : x \text{ cap}$

$\dfrac{\cancel{100}}{\cancel{100}} x = \dfrac{\cancel{200}}{\cancel{100}}$

$x = 2 \text{ cap}$

PROOF

$100 \times 2 = 200$

$1 \times 200 = 200$

3. KNOW   WANT TO KNOW

$4 \text{ mg} : 5 \text{ mL} :: 6 \text{ mg} : x \text{ mL}$

$\dfrac{\cancel{4}}{\cancel{4}} x = \dfrac{30}{4}$

$x = 7.5 \text{ mL}$

PROOF

$4 \times 7.5 = 30$

$5 \times 6 = 30$

4. **Step 1:**

KNOW   WANT TO KNOW

$1000 \text{ mg} : 1 \text{ g} :: x \text{ mg} : 0.5 \text{ g}$

$x = 1000 \times 0.5$

$x = 500 \text{ mg}$

PROOF

$1000 \times 0.5 = 500$

$1 \times 500 = 500$

Step 2:

HAVE   WANT TO HAVE

$250 \text{ mg} : 1 \text{ tab} :: 500 \text{ mg} : x \text{ tab}$

$\dfrac{\cancel{250}}{\cancel{250}} x = \dfrac{\cancel{500}}{\cancel{250}}$

$x = 2 \text{ tab}$

PROOF

$250 \times 2 = 500$

$1 \times 500 = 500$

5. KNOW   WANT TO KNOW

20 mg : 5 mL :: 25 mg : x mL

$\dfrac{\cancel{20}}{\cancel{20}} x = \dfrac{125}{20}$

$\quad x = 6.25$ mL, rounded to 6.3 mL

PROOF

$20 \times 6.25 = 125$

$5 \times 25 = 125$

4H (PAGE 107)

1. **Step 1:**

   KNOW   WANT TO KNOW

   1000 mcg : 1 mg :: 125 mcg : x mg

   $\dfrac{\cancel{1000}}{\cancel{1000}} x = \dfrac{125}{1000}$

   $\quad x = 0.125$ mg

   PROOF

   $1000 \times 0.125 = 125$

   $1 \times 125 = 125$

   Step 2:

   HAVE   WANT TO HAVE

   0.125 mg : 1 tab :: 0.125 mg : x tab

   $\dfrac{\cancel{0.125}}{\cancel{0.125}} x = \dfrac{0.125}{0.125}$

   $\quad x = 1$ tab

   PROOF

   $0.125 \times 1 = 0.125$

   $1 \times 0.125 = 0.125$

2. **Step 1:**

   KNOW   WANT TO KNOW

   1000 mg : 1 g :: x mg : 0.01 g

   $x = 1000 \times 0.01$

   $x = 10$ mg

   PROOF

   1000×0.01 g $= 10$

   $1 \times 10 = 10$

   Step 2:

   HAVE   WANT TO HAVE

   5 mg : 1 tab :: 10 mg : x tab

   $\dfrac{\cancel{5}}{\cancel{5}} x = \dfrac{10}{5}$

   $\quad x = 2$ tab

   PROOF

   $5 \times 2 = 10$

   $1 \times 10 = 10$

3. **Step 1:**

   KNOW   WANT TO KNOW

   1000 mg : 1 g :: x mg : 0.2 g

   $x = 1000 \times 0.2$

   $x = 200$ mg

   PROOF

   $1000 \times 0.2 = 200$

   $1 \times 200 = 200$

   Step 2:

   HAVE   WANT TO HAVE

   100 mg : 1 cap :: 200 mg : x cap

   $\dfrac{\cancel{100}}{\cancel{100}} x = \dfrac{\cancel{200}}{\cancel{100}}$

   $\quad x = 2$ cap

   PROOF

   $100 \times 2 = 200$

   $1 \times 200 = 200$

4. **Step 1:**

   KNOW   WANT TO KNOW

   1000 mg : 1 g :: x mg : 0.05 g

   $x = 1000 \times 0.05$

   $x = 50$ mg

   PROOF

   $1000 \times 0.05 = 50$

   $1 \times 50 = 50$

   Step 2:

   HAVE   WANT TO HAVE

   25 mg : 1 tab :: 50 mg : x tab

   $\dfrac{\cancel{25}}{\cancel{25}} x = \dfrac{50}{25}$

   $\quad x = 2$ tab

   PROOF

   $25 \times 2 = 50$

   $1 \times 50 = 50$

5. **Step 1:**

KNOW   WANT TO KNOW

1000 mcg : 1 mg :: x mcg : 0.25 mg

$x = 1000 \times 0.25$

$x = 250$ mcg

PROOF

$1000 \times 0.25 = 250$

$1 \times 250 = 250$

Step 2:

HAVE   WANT TO HAVE

125 mcg : 1 tab :: 250 mcg : x tab

$\dfrac{\cancel{125}}{\cancel{125}} x = \dfrac{250}{125}$

$x = 2$ tab

PROOF

$125 \times 2 = 250$

$1 \times 250 = 250$

4I (PAGE 108)

1. KNOW   WANT TO KNOW

1000 mg : 1 g :: x mg : 0.5 g

$x = 1000 \times 0.5$

$x = 500$ mg

PROOF

$1000 \times 0.5 = 500$

$1 \times 500 = 500$

HAVE   WANT TO HAVE

250 mg : 1 tab :: 500 mg : x tab

$\dfrac{\cancel{250}}{\cancel{250}} x = \dfrac{\cancel{500}}{\cancel{250}}$

$x = 2$ tab

PROOF

$250 \times 2 = 500$

$1 \times 500 = 500$

2. KNOW   WANT TO KNOW

1000 mg : 1 g :: x mg : 0.5 g

$x = 1000 \times 0.5$

$x = 500$ mg

PROOF

$1000 \times 0.5 = 500$

$1 \times 500 = 500$

HAVE   WANT TO HAVE

250 mg : 1 cap :: 500 mg : x cap

$\dfrac{\cancel{250}}{\cancel{250}} x = \dfrac{\cancel{500}}{\cancel{250}}$

$x = 2$ capsules

PROOF

$250 \times 2 = 500$

$1 \times 500 = 500$

3. KNOW   WANT TO KNOW

1000 mg : 1 g :: x mg : 0.3 g

$x = 1000 \times 0.3$

$x = 300$ mg

PROOF

$1000 \times 0.3 = 300$

$1 \times 300 = 300$

HAVE   WANT TO HAVE

250 mg : 5 mL :: 300 mg : x mL

$\dfrac{\cancel{250}}{\cancel{250}} x = \dfrac{\cancel{1500}}{\cancel{250}}$

$x = 6$ mL

PROOF

$250 \times 6 = 1500$

$5 \times 300 = 1500$

4. KNOW   WANT TO KNOW

1000 mg : 1 g :: x mg : 1 g

$x = 1000 \times 1$

$x = 1000$ mg

PROOF

$1000 \times 1 = 1000$

$1 \times 1000 = 1000$

HAVE   WANT TO HAVE

500 mg : 1 cap :: 1000 mg : x cap

$\dfrac{\cancel{500}}{\cancel{500}} x = \dfrac{\cancel{1000}}{\cancel{500}}$

$x = 2$ cap

PROOF

$500 \times 2 = 1000$

$1 \times 1000 = 1000$

5. KNOW   WANT TO KNOW

1000 mcg : 1 mg :: x mcg : 0.2 mg

$x = 1000 \times 0.2$

$x = 200$ mcg

PROOF

$1000 \times 0.2 = 200$

$1 \times 200 = 200$

HAVE   WANT TO HAVE

100 mcg : 1 tab :: 200 mcg : x tab

$\dfrac{\cancel{100}}{\cancel{100}} x = \dfrac{200}{100}$

$x = 2$ tab

PROOF

$100 \times 2 = 200$

$1 \times 200 = 200$

4J (PAGE 112)

1. a. 3 mL
  b. tenths

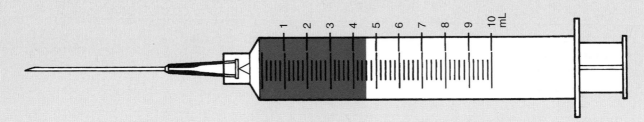

2. a. 10 mL
  b. 0.2

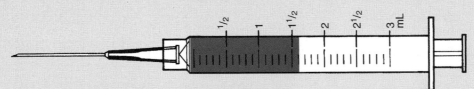

3. a. 5 mL
  b. 0.2

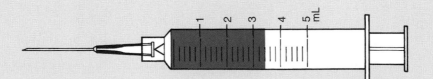

4. **a.** 3 mL

   b. tenths

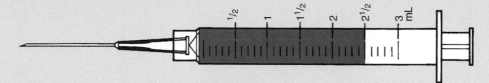

5. **a.** 1 mL

   b. hundredths

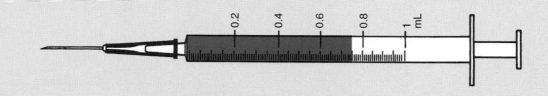

4K (PAGE 113)

1. **a.** 4 mg/mL

   b. 0.8 mL hydromorphone

   HAVE   WANT TO HAVE

   4 mg : 1 mL :: 3 mg : x mL

   $\dfrac{\cancel{4}}{\cancel{4}}x = \dfrac{3}{4}$

   x = 0.75 or 0.8 mL

   PROOF

   4 × 0.75 = 3.00

   1 × 3 = 3

   c. 5 mg/mL Compazine (prochlorperazine)

   d. HAVE   WANT TO HAVE

   5 mg : 1 mL :: 2.5 mg : x mL

   $\dfrac{\cancel{5}}{\cancel{5}}x = \dfrac{2.5}{5}$

   x = 0.5 mL

   PROOF

   5 × 0.5 = 2.5

   1 × 2.5 = 2.5

   e. 0.8 + 0.5 = 1.3 mL
   (total amount in syringe)

2. **a.** 10 mg/mL

   b. 0.6 mL morphine

   HAVE   WANT TO HAVE

   10 mg : 1 mL :: 6 mg : x mL

   $\frac{\cancel{10}}{\cancel{10}} x = \frac{6}{10}$

   $x = 0.6$ mL

   PROOF

   $10 \times 0.6 = 6$

   $1 \times 6 = 6$

   c. 25 mg/mL

   d. 1 mL promethazine

   HAVE   WANT TO HAVE

   25 mg : 1 mL :: 25 mg : x mL

   $\frac{\cancel{25}}{\cancel{25}} x = \frac{\cancel{25}}{\cancel{25}}$

   $x = 1$ mL

   PROOF

   $25 \times 1 = 25$

   $1 \times 25 = 25$

   e. 0.6 + 1 = 1.6 mL
   (total amount in syringe)

3. **a.** 75 mg/mL

   b. 0.7 mL meperidine

   KNOW   WANT TO KNOW

   75 mg : 1 mL :: 50 mg : x mL

   $\frac{\cancel{75}}{\cancel{75}} x = \frac{50}{75}$

   $x = 0.66$ or 0.7 mL

   PROOF

   $75 \times 0.66 = 49.5$

   $1 \times 50 = 50$

   c. 0.4 mg/mL

   d. 1.5 mL atropine sulfate

   KNOW   WANT TO KNOW

   0.4 mg : 1 mL :: 0.6 mg : x mL

   $0.4x = 0.6$

   $x = 1.5$ mL

   PROOF

   $0.4 \times 1.5 = 0.6$

   $1 \times 0.6 = 0.6$

   e. 0.7 + 1.5 = 2.2 mL
   (total amount in syringe)

4. a. 0.7 mL morphine sulfate

KNOW   WANT TO KNOW

15 mg : 1 mL :: 10 mg : x mL

$\dfrac{\cancel{15}}{\cancel{15}} x = \dfrac{\overset{2}{\cancel{10}}}{\underset{3}{\cancel{15}}}$ = 0.67, rounded to 0.7 mL

PROOF

15 × 0.67 = 10.05

1 × 10 = 10

b. 0.7 mL hydroxyzine

KNOW   WANT TO KNOW

50 mg : 1 mL :: 35 mg : x mL

$\dfrac{\cancel{50}}{\cancel{50}} x = \dfrac{35}{50}$

$x = 0.7$ mL

PROOF

50 × 0.7 = 35

1 × 35 = 35

c. 0.7 + 0.7 = 1.4 mL
(total amount in syringe)

5. a. 0.8 mL morphine sulfate

HAVE   WANT TO HAVE

10 mg : 1 mL :: 8 mg : x mL

$\dfrac{\cancel{10}}{\cancel{10}} x = \dfrac{8}{10}$

$x = 0.8$ mL

b. 0.5 mL Vistaril

HAVE   WANT TO HAVE

50 mg : 1 mL :: 25 mg : x mL

$\dfrac{\cancel{50}}{\cancel{50}} x = \dfrac{25}{50}$

$x = 0.5$ mL

c. 0.8 + 0.5 = 1.3 mL
(total amount in syringe)

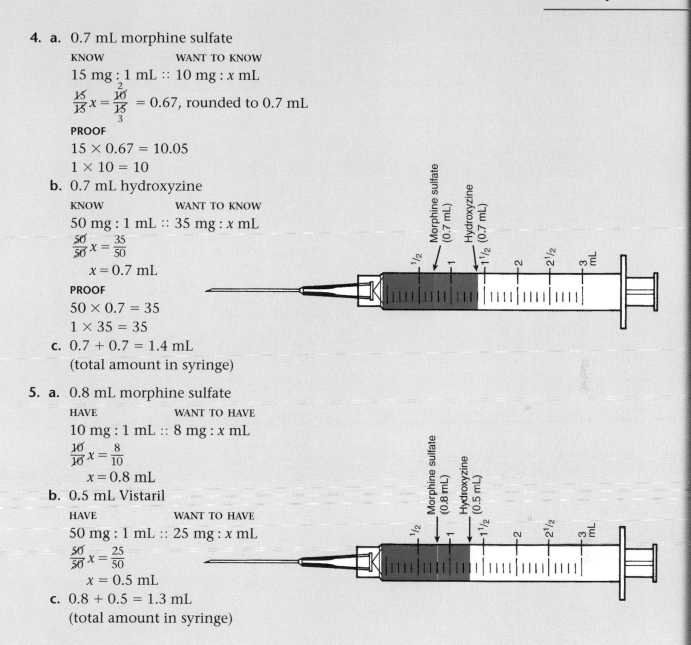

4L (PAGE 116)

1. two-step

KNOW   WANT TO KNOW
Step 1: 1000 mg : 1 g :: x mg : 0.2 g
$x = 1000 \times 0.2$ or 200 mg
PROOF
$1000 \times 0.2 = 200$
$1 \times 200 = 200$
(more)

HAVE   WANT TO HAVE
Step 2: 150 mg : 1 mL :: 200 mg : x mL
$\frac{\cancel{150}}{\cancel{150}} x = \frac{20\cancel{0}}{15\cancel{0}}$
$x = 1.3$ mL
PROOF
$150 \times 1.3 = 195$
$1 \times 200 = 200$
(rounding to 1.3 affects answer)

2. two-step

KNOW   WANT TO KNOW
Step 1: 1000 mcg : 1 mg :: 500 mcg : x mg
$\frac{\cancel{1000}}{\cancel{1000}} x = \frac{5\cancel{00}}{10\cancel{00}}$
$x = 0.5$ mg
PROOF
$1000 \times 0.5 = 500$
$1 \times 500 = 500$
(same)

HAVE   WANT TO HAVE
Step 2: 0.5 mg : 1 tab :: 0.5 mg : x tab
$\frac{\cancel{0.5}}{\cancel{0.5}} x = \frac{\cancel{0.5}}{\cancel{0.5}}$
$x = 1$ tab
PROOF
$0.5 \times 1 = 0.5$
$1 \times 0.5 = 0.5$

3. two-step

KNOW   WANT TO KNOW
Step 1: 1000 mg : 1 g :: x mg : 0.2 g
$x = 1000 \times 0.2$ or 200 mg
PROOF
$1000 \times 0.2 = 200$
$1 \times 200 = 200$
(less)

HAVE   WANT TO HAVE
Step 2: 250 mg : 2 mL :: 200 mg : x mL
$\frac{\cancel{250}}{\cancel{250}} x = \frac{40\cancel{0}}{25\cancel{0}}$
$x = 1.6$ mL
PROOF
$250 \times 1.6 = 400$
$2 \times 200 = 400$

4. one-step

HAVE   WANT TO HAVE
125 mg : 2 mL :: 75 mg : x mL
$\frac{\cancel{125}}{\cancel{125}} x = \frac{150}{125}$
$x = 1.2$ mL
PROOF
$125 \times 1.2 = 150$
$2 \times 75 = 150$
(less)

5. one-step

HAVE   WANT TO HAVE
16 mg : 1 tab :: 32 mg : x tab
$\frac{\cancel{16}}{\cancel{16}} x = \frac{32}{16}$
$x = 2$ tab
PROOF
$16 \times 2 = 32$
$1 \times 32 = 32$
(more)

6. two-step

KNOW   WANT TO KNOW
Step 1: 1000 mg : 1 g :: x mg : 0.8 g
$x = 1000 \times 0.8 = 800$ mg
PROOF
$1000 \times 0.8 = 800$
$1 \times 800 = 800$
(more)

HAVE   WANT TO HAVE
Step 2: 400 mg : 1 tab :: 800 mg : x tab
$\frac{\cancel{400}}{\cancel{400}} x = \frac{8\cancel{00}}{4\cancel{00}}$
$x = 2$ tab
PROOF
$400 \times 2 = 800$
$1 \times 800 = 800$

7. one-step

HAVE	WANT TO HAVE

300 mg : 1 mL :: 250 mg : x mL

$\dfrac{\cancel{300}}{\cancel{300}}x = \dfrac{25\cancel{0}}{30\cancel{0}}$

$x = 0.83$ or 0.8 mL

PROOF

$300 \times 0.8 = 240$

$1 \times 250 = 250$

(rounding 0.83 to 0.8 affects answer)

(less)

8. two-step

KNOW	WANT TO KNOW

Step 1: 1000 mg : 1 g :: x mg : 0.3 g

$x = 1000 \times 0.3 = 300$ mg

PROOF

$1000 \times 0.3 = 300$

$1 \times 300 = 300$

(less)

HAVE	WANT TO HAVE

Step 2: 400 mg : 1 mL :: 300 mg : x mL

$\dfrac{\cancel{400}}{\cancel{400}}x = \dfrac{3\cancel{00}}{4\cancel{00}}$

$x = 0.75$ or 0.8 mL

PROOF

$400 \times 0.8 = 320$

$1 \times 300 = 300$

(rounding 0.75 to 0.8 affects answer)

9. two-step

KNOW	WANT TO KNOW

Step 1: 1000 mcg : 1 mg :: 125 mcg : x mg

$\dfrac{\cancel{1000}}{\cancel{1000}}x = \dfrac{125}{1000}$

$x = 0.125$ mg

PROOF

$1000 \times 0.125 = 125$

$1 \times 125 = 125$

(same)

HAVE	WANT TO HAVE

Step 2: 0.125 mg : 1 tab :: 0.125 mg : x tab

$\dfrac{\cancel{0.125}}{\cancel{0.125}}x = \dfrac{\cancel{0.125}}{\cancel{0.125}}$

$x = 1$ tab

PROOF

$1 \times 0.125 = 0.125$

$0.125 \times 1 = 0.125$

10. one-step

KNOW	WANT TO KNOW

175 mcg : 1 tab :: 350 mcg : x tab

$\dfrac{\cancel{175}}{\cancel{175}}x = \dfrac{350}{175}$

$x = 2$ tab

PROOF

$175 \times 2 = 350$

$1 \times 350 = 350$

(more)

4M (PAGE 119)

1. 325 mg   5 grains*
2. 130 mg   2 grains†
3. 0.4 mg   grain $\frac{1}{150}$
4. 324 mg   grain 5
5. 30 mg   ($\frac{1}{2}$ grain/mL)

---

*Could also be written as grv.
†Could also be written as grii.

4N (PAGE 123)

1. **d.** one-step   2. **b.** one-step   3. **a.** one-step   4. **d.** one-step

5. **c.** two-step   6. **c.** two-step   7. **c.** two-step   8. **d.** two-step

9. **d.** one-step   10. **b.** two-step

CHAPTER 4 FINAL: DRUG MEASUREMENTS AND DOSE CALCULATIONS (PAGE 126)

1. 2 cap   **2.** 2 tab   **3.** 3 tab   **4.** 2 tab

5. 1 tab   **6.** 12.5 mL   **7.** 20 mL

8. 0.66 rounded to 0.7 mL

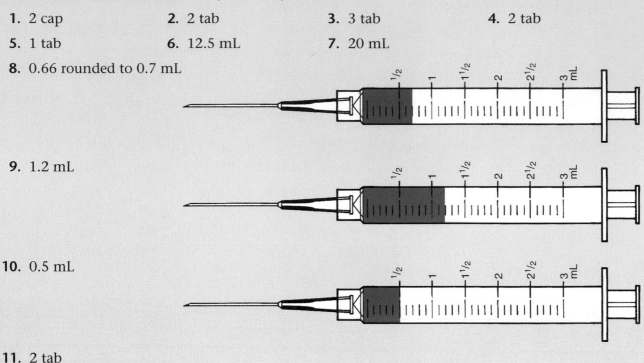

9. 1.2 mL

10. 0.5 mL

11. 2 tab

12. 3 tab. Clarify the order before giving because this amount exceeds the 1 to 2 tablets usually given to patients.

13. 2 tab

14. Give 4 tab. Clarify the order before giving because this amount exceeds the 1- to 2-unit doses usually given to patients. If the order is correct, check with the pharmacy for a different strength so that the patient will not have to take so many tablets.

15. 0.7 mL; 0.8 mL; 1.5 mL total

16. 20 mL

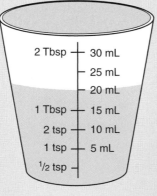

17. 2 cap

18. a. 0.5 mL   **b.** safe dose

19. 1 tab

20. 6 tab. Clarify the order before giving because this amount exceeds the 1 to 2 tablets usually given to patients.

5 Medications from Powders and Crystals: Oral and Intramuscular

5A (PAGE 137)

1. **a.** 30 mL of water in two portions.
   b. 50 mL of Lorabid in the bottle.
   c. 7.5 mL of Lorabid.

   KNOW   WANT TO KNOW
   100 mg : 5 mL :: 150 mg : x mL
   10$\emptyset x$ = 5 × 150 = 75$\emptyset$
       x = 7.5 mL yields 150 mg

   PROOF
   100 × 7.5 = 750
   5 × 150 = 750

   d. 6.6 doses per bottle

   KNOW   WANT TO KNOW
   7.5 mL : 1 dose :: 50 mL : x dose
   7.5x = 1 × 50 = 50
       x = 6.6

   PROOF
   1 × 50 = 50
   7.5 × 6.6 = 49.5 = 50

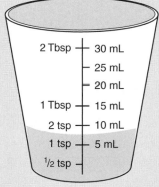

2. KNOW   WANT TO KNOW
   5 mL : 200 mg :: x mL : 500 mg
   2x = 25
   x = 12.5 mL
   PROOF
   5 × 500 = 2500
   200 × 12.5 = 2500

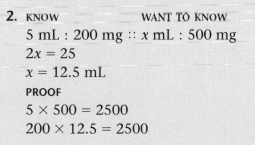

3. **a.** 1000 mg
   b. KNOW   WANT TO KNOW
   250 mg : 5 mL :: 500 mg : x mL
   25x = 5 × 50 = 250
   x = 10 mL
   PROOF
   5 × 500 = 2500
   250 × 10 = 2500

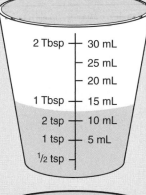

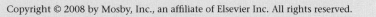

4. a. Add 90 mL of water.

   b. Amount in bottle 100 mL.

   c. Administer 8 mL.

   KNOW   WANT TO KNOW

   125 mg : 5 mL :: 200 mg : x mL

   $125x = 5 \times 200 = 1000$

   $x = 8$ mL

   PROOF

   $5 \times 200 = 1000$

   $125 \times 8 = 1000$

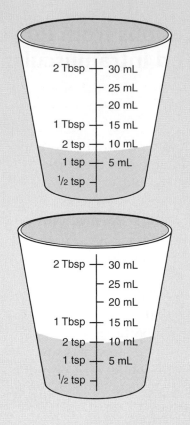

5. a. 60 mL of water in two portions.

   b. 100 mL of Lorabid.

   c. 10 mL.

   KNOW   WANT TO KNOW

   200 mg : 5 mL :: 400 mg : x mL

   $200x = 5 \times 400 = 2000$

   $x = 10$ mL

   PROOF

   $5 \times 400 = 2000$

   $200 \times 10 = 2000$

   d. 10 doses in the bottle.

   KNOW   WANT TO KNOW

   10 mL : 1 dose :: 100 mL : x dose

   $10x = 1 \times 100 = 100$

   $x = 10$

   PROOF

   $1 \times 100 = 100$

   $10 \times 10 = 100$

6. a. Add 140 mL of water.

   b. Amount in bottle: 8000 mg or 8 g.

   Step 1: KNOW   WANT TO KNOW

   200 mg : 5 mL :: x mg : 200 mL

   $5x = 200 \times 200 = 40,000$

   $5x = 40,000$

   $x = 8000$ mg in the bottle

   PROOF

   $5 \times 8000 = 40,000$

   $200 \times 220 = 40,000$

   Step 2: HAVE   WANT TO HAVE

   1 g : 1000 mg :: x g : 8000 mg

   $x = 8$ g in the bottle

   PROOF

   $1 \times 8 = 8$

   $1 \times 8 = 8$

c. Administer: 7.5 mL.

   KNOW   WANT TO KNOW

   200 mg : 5 mL :: 300 mg : x mL

   $200x = 5 \times 300$

   $x = 7.5$ mL

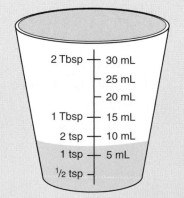

7. **a.** Add 20 mL of distilled water.
   b. 1000 mg Vancocin in the bottle.
   c. 6 mL of Vancocin.

KNOW	WANT TO KNOW

   250 mg : 5 mL :: 300 mg : x mL
   25Øx = 5 × 300 = 150Ø
   $\quad$ x = 6 mL

   PROOF
   5 × 300 = 1500
   250 × 6 = 1500

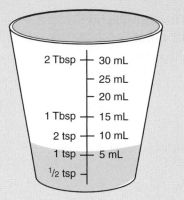

8. **a.** Add 78 mL of diluent.
   b. Amount in bottle: 2500 mg.

KNOW	WANT TO KNOW

   125 mg : 5 mL :: x mg : 100 mL
   5x = 125 × 100 = 12,500
   5x = 12,500
   $\quad$ x = 2500 mg in bottle

   PROOF
   5 × 2500 = 12,500
   125 × 100 = 12,500

   c. Amount of fluid to be given per dose: 20 mL/dose.

KNOW	WANT TO KNOW

   125 mg : 5 mL :: 500 mg : x mL
   125x = 5 × 500 = 2500
   $\quad$ x = 20 mL/dose

   PROOF
   5 × 500 = 2500
   125 × 20 = 2500

   d. Doses in bottle: 5 doses.

KNOW	WANT TO KNOW

   20 mL : 1 dose :: 100 mL : x doses
   20x = 100
   $\quad$ x = 5 doses in bottle

   PROOF
   1 × 100 = 100
   20 × 5 = 100

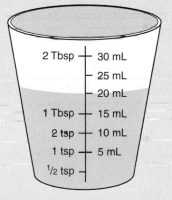

9.
KNOW	WANT TO KNOW

   125 mg : 5 mL :: 400 mg : x mL
   125x = 5 × 400 = 2000
   $\quad$ x = 16 mL

   PROOF
   5 × 400 = 2000
   125 × 16 = 2000

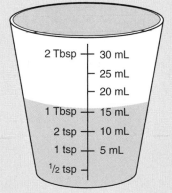

10. a. 45 mL of water in 2 portions.
   b. 75 mL of Lorabid.
   c. 5 mL = 200 mg.
   d. 15 doses in the bottle.

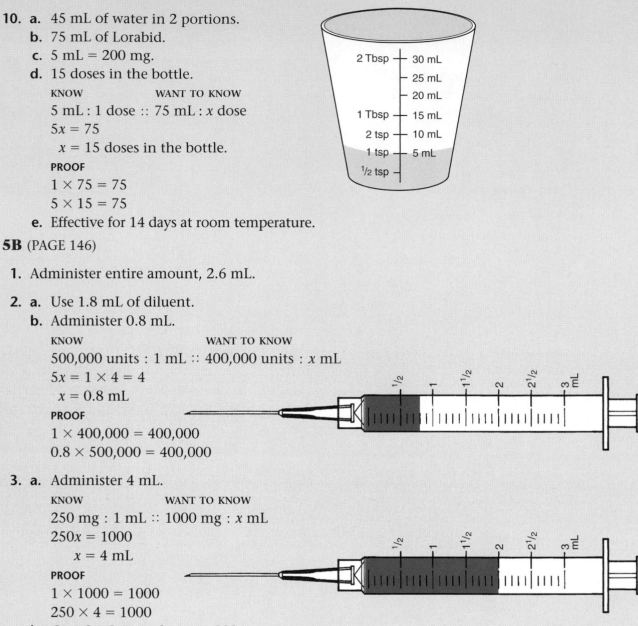

   KNOW   WANT TO KNOW
   5 mL : 1 dose :: 75 mL : x dose
   $5x = 75$
       $x = 15$ doses in the bottle.
   PROOF
   $1 \times 75 = 75$
   $5 \times 15 = 75$

   e. Effective for 14 days at room temperature.

5B (PAGE 146)

1. Administer entire amount, 2.6 mL.

2. a. Use 1.8 mL of diluent.
   b. Administer 0.8 mL.

   KNOW   WANT TO KNOW
   500,000 units : 1 mL :: 400,000 units : x mL
   $5x = 1 \times 4 = 4$
       $x = 0.8$ mL
   PROOF
   $1 \times 400,000 = 400,000$
   $0.8 \times 500,000 = 400,000$

3. a. Administer 4 mL.

   KNOW   WANT TO KNOW
   250 mg : 1 mL :: 1000 mg : x mL
   $250x = 1000$
       $x = 4$ mL
   PROOF
   $1 \times 1000 = 1000$
   $250 \times 4 = 1000$

   b. Give 2 mL in each site = 500 mg per injection.

4. Administer: 3 mL.

KNOW   **WANT TO KNOW**

$1 \text{ g} : 1000 \text{ mg} :: x \text{ g} : 500 \text{ mg}$

$1000x = 500$

$\quad x = 0.5 \text{ g}$

PROOF

$1000 \times 0.5 = 500$

$1 \times 500 = 500$

KNOW   **WANT TO KNOW**

$0.25 \text{ g} : 1.5 \text{ mL} :: 0.5 \text{ g} : x \text{ mL}$

$0.25x = 1.5 \times 0.5 = 0.75$

$\quad x = 3 \text{ mL}$

PROOF

$1.5 \times 0.5 = 0.75$

$0.25 \times 3 = 0.75$

5. a. Add 4.0 mL of diluent to yield 250,000 units/mL.

 b. KNOW   **WANT TO KNOW**

$250{,}000 \text{ units} : 1 \text{ mL} :: 300{,}000 \text{ units} : x \text{ mL}$

$250{,}000x = 300{,}000$

$25x = 30$

$\quad x = 1.2 \text{ mL}$

PROOF

$250{,}000 \times 1.2 = 300{,}000$

$1 \times 300{,}000 = 300{,}000$

 c. KNOW   **WANT TO KNOW**

$300{,}000 \text{ units} : 1 \text{ dose} :: 1{,}000{,}000 \text{ units} : x \text{ dose}$

$300{,}000x = 1{,}000{,}000$

$3x = 10$

$\quad x = 3.3 = 3 \text{ full doses in the vial}$

PROOF

$1 \times 1{,}000{,}000 = 1{,}000{,}000$

$3.3 \times 300{,}000 = 990{,}000$

6. a. Make the 500,000 units/mL

b. Administer 0.6 mL.

KNOW   WANT TO KNOW

500,000 units : 1 mL :: 300,000 units : x mL

$5x = 1 \times 3 = 3$

$x = 0.6$ mL

PROOF

$1 \times 300,000 = 300,000$

$500,000 \times 0.6 = 300,000$

Or, you may give another concentration, depending on the assessment of body mass.

a. Make the 200,000 units/mL.

b. Administer 1.5 mL.

KNOW   WANT TO KNOW

200,000 units : 1 mL :: 300,000 units : x mL

$2x = 1 \times 3 = 3$

$x = 1.5$ mL

PROOF

$1 \times 300,000 = 300,000$

$200,000 \times 1.5 = 300,000$

Or, you may give another concentration, depending on the assessment of body mass.

a. Make the 100,000 units/mL.

b. Administer 3 mL.

KNOW   WANT TO KNOW

100,000 units : 1 mL :: 300,000 units : x mL

$1x = 1 \times 3 = 3$

$x = 3$ mL

PROOF

$1 \times 300,000 = 300,000$

$100,000 \times 3 = 300,000$

7. a. Add 3 mL of sterile water for injection as the diluent.

b. 280 mg/mL is the concentration.

c. KNOW   WANT TO KNOW

280 mg : 1 mL :: 250 mg : x mL

$280x = 250$

$x = 0.892 = 0.9$ mL

PROOF

$1 \times 250 = 250$

$0.892 \times 280 = 250$

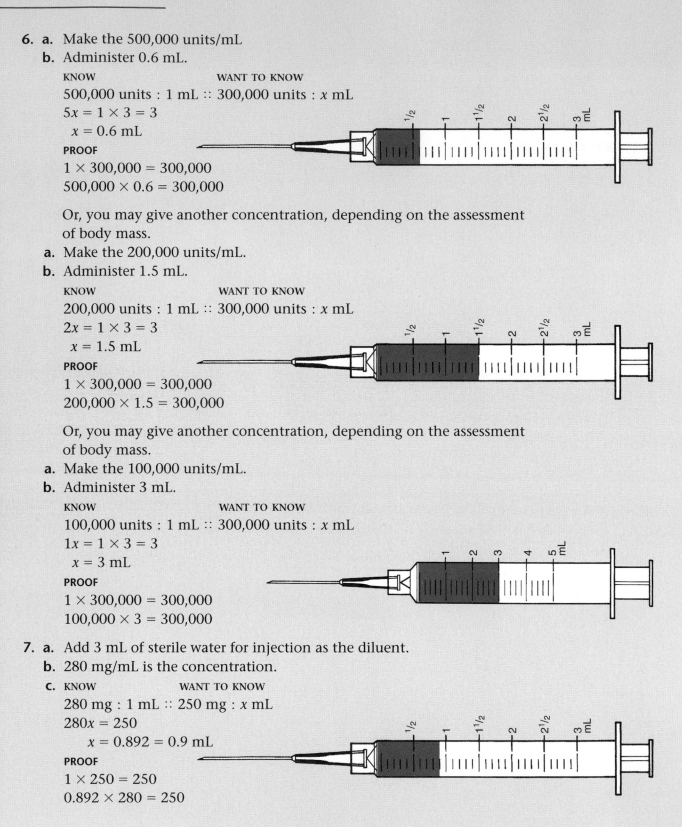

8. a. Add 1.2 mL of diluent.

    b. 1 hour

    c. 125 mg/mL

    d. KNOW   WANT TO KNOW

        125 mg : 1 mL :: 100 mg : x mL

        $125x = 100$

           $x = 0.8$ mL

        PROOF

        $125 \times 0.8 = 100$

        $100 \times 1 = 100$

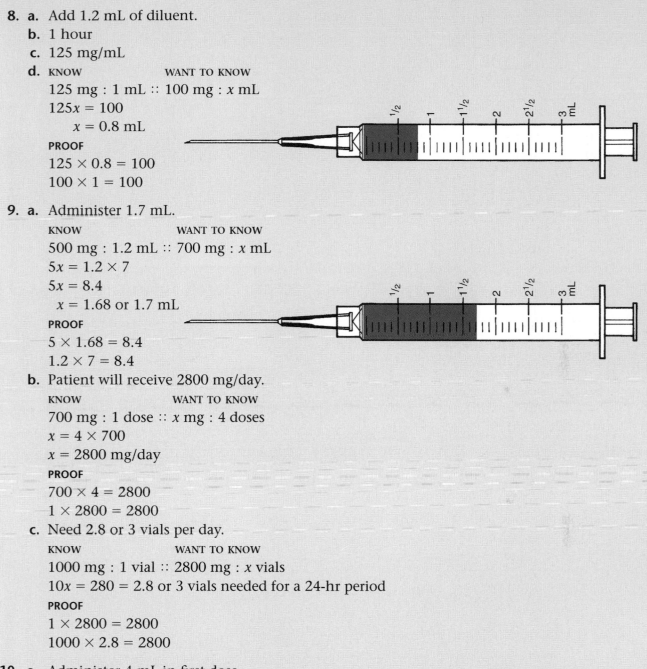

9. a. Administer 1.7 mL.

        KNOW   WANT TO KNOW

        500 mg : 1.2 mL :: 700 mg : x mL

        $5x = 1.2 \times 7$

        $5x = 8.4$

           $x = 1.68$ or 1.7 mL

        PROOF

        $5 \times 1.68 = 8.4$

        $1.2 \times 7 = 8.4$

    b. Patient will receive 2800 mg/day.

        KNOW   WANT TO KNOW

        700 mg : 1 dose :: x mg : 4 doses

        $x = 4 \times 700$

        $x = 2800$ mg/day

        PROOF

        $700 \times 4 = 2800$

        $1 \times 2800 = 2800$

    c. Need 2.8 or 3 vials per day.

        KNOW   WANT TO KNOW

        1000 mg : 1 vial :: 2800 mg : x vials

        $10x = 280 = 2.8$ or 3 vials needed for a 24-hr period

        PROOF

        $1 \times 2800 = 2800$

        $1000 \times 2.8 = 2800$

10. a. Administer 4 mL in first dose.

    b. Divide into two equal injections.

    c. Give deep intramuscularly in the right or left ventrogluteal area.

5C (PAGE 151)

1. KNOW   WANT TO KNOW

250 mg : 1 mL :: 500 mg : x mL

$250x = 500$

    $x = 2$ mL = 500 mg

PROOF

$500 \times 1 = 500$

$250 \times 2 = 500$

OR

KNOW   WANT TO KNOW

350 mg : 1 mL :: 500 mg : x mL

$350x = 1 \times 500 = 500$

    $x = 1.428 = 1.4$ mL = 500 mg

PROOF

$1 \times 500 = 500$

$350 \times 1.428 = 500$

2. a. Add 2 mL of sterile water.
  b. Have 500 mg/1.2 mL.
  c. Administer 1.2 mL.

3. a. Add 2.7 mL sterile water for injection.
  b. The reconstituted medication will yield 250 mg/1.5 mL.
  c. Refrigerated, 7 days; room temperature, 3 days.
  d. Administer 1.8 mL.

KNOW   WANT TO KNOW

250 mg : 1.5 mL :: 300 mg : x mL

$250x = 1.5 \times 300 = 450$

    $x = 1.8$ mL

PROOF

$1.5 \times 300 = 450$

$250 \times 1.8 = 450$

4. a. Add 3.5 mL diluent.
  b. The reconstituted medication will yield 250 mg/mL.
  c. Use within 1 hr as this is a very unstable medication.
  d. Administer 2 mL.

KNOW   WANT TO KNOW

250 mg : 1 mL :: 500 mg : x mL

$250x = 500$

    $x = 2$ mL

PROOF

$1 \times 500 = 500$

$250 \times 2 = 500$

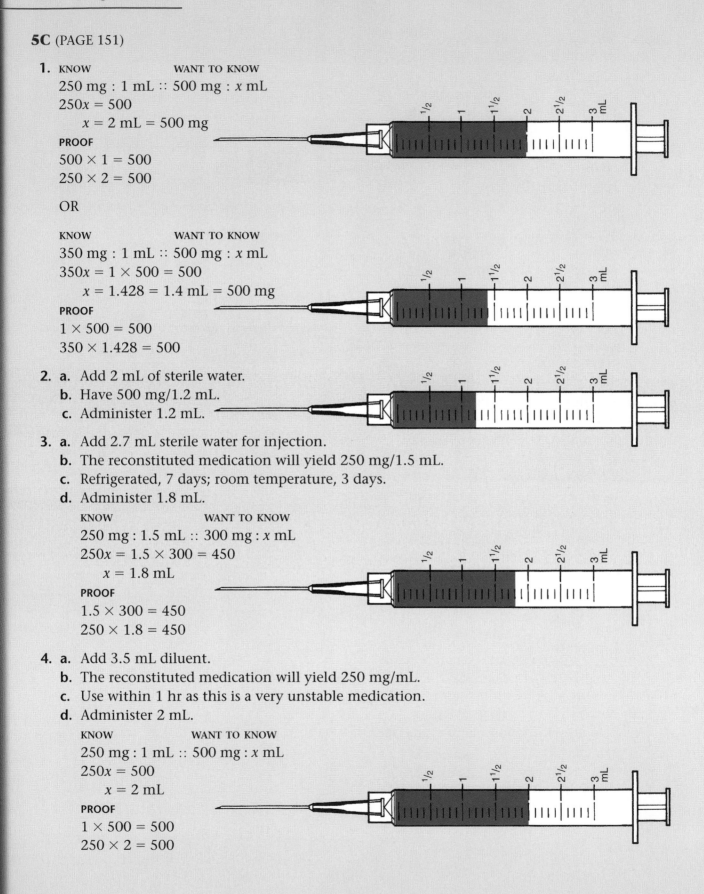

5. a. Add 2 mL of sterile water.
 b. Each dose will contain 1.2 mL = 500 mg.
 c. 3 vials needed in 24 hr.

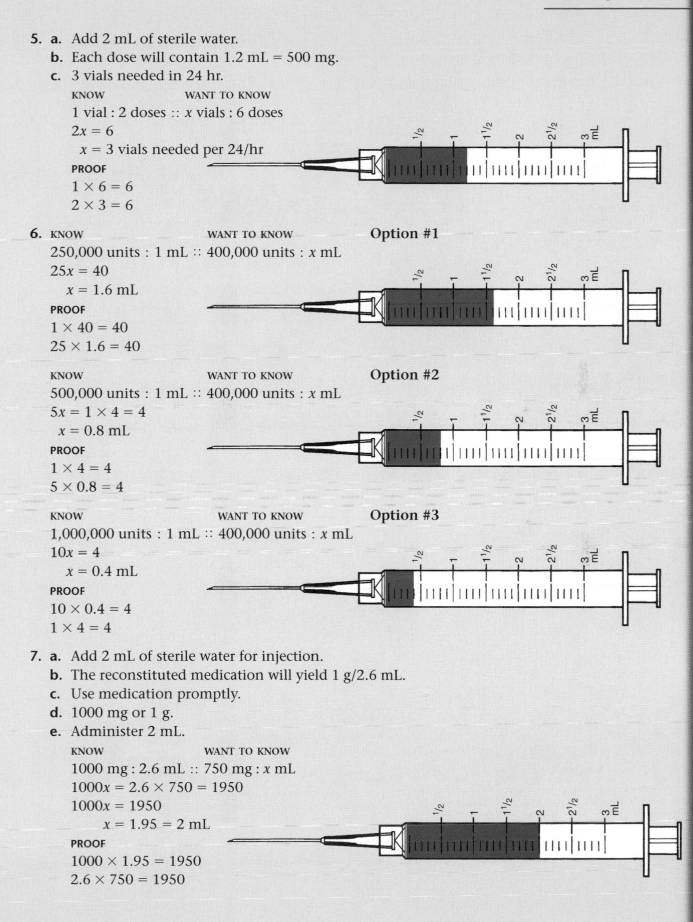

  KNOW   WANT TO KNOW
  1 vial : 2 doses :: x vials : 6 doses
  $2x = 6$
   $x = 3$ vials needed per 24/hr
  PROOF
  $1 \times 6 = 6$
  $2 \times 3 = 6$

6. KNOW   WANT TO KNOW Option #1
 250,000 units : 1 mL :: 400,000 units : x mL
 $25x = 40$
  $x = 1.6$ mL
 PROOF
 $1 \times 40 = 40$
 $25 \times 1.6 = 40$

 KNOW   WANT TO KNOW Option #2
 500,000 units : 1 mL :: 400,000 units : x mL
 $5x = 1 \times 4 = 4$
  $x = 0.8$ mL
 PROOF
 $1 \times 4 = 4$
 $5 \times 0.8 = 4$

 KNOW   WANT TO KNOW Option #3
 1,000,000 units : 1 mL :: 400,000 units : x mL
 $10x = 4$
  $x = 0.4$ mL
 PROOF
 $10 \times 0.4 = 4$
 $1 \times 4 = 4$

7. a. Add 2 mL of sterile water for injection.
 b. The reconstituted medication will yield 1 g/2.6 mL.
 c. Use medication promptly.
 d. 1000 mg or 1 g.
 e. Administer 2 mL.

  KNOW   WANT TO KNOW
  1000 mg : 2.6 mL :: 750 mg : x mL
  $1000x = 2.6 \times 750 = 1950$
  $1000x = 1950$
    $x = 1.95 = 2$ mL
  PROOF
  $1000 \times 1.95 = 1950$
  $2.6 \times 750 = 1950$

8. **a.** 500,000 units/mL.
   b. Add 1.6 mL diluent.
   c. Administer 1.5 mL.
   d. Refrigerated, 7 days.

   KNOW   WANT TO KNOW
   500,000 units : 1 mL :: 750,000 units : x mL
   $50x = 1 \times 75$
   $50x = 75$
   $\quad x = 1.5$ mL
   PROOF
   $50 \times 1.5 = 75$
   $1 \times 75 = 75$

9. If you add 4 mL of diluent

   KNOW   WANT TO KNOW
   250,000 units : 1 mL :: 400,000 units : x mL
   $25x = 40$
   $\quad x = 1.6$ mL
   PROOF
   $25 \times 1.6 = 40$
   $1 \times 40 = 40$

   If you add 1.5 mL of diluent

   KNOW   WANT TO KNOW
   500,000 units : 1 mL :: 400,000 units : x mL
   $5x = 4$
   $\quad x = 0.8$ mL
   PROOF
   $5 \times 0.8 = 4$
   $1 \times 4 = 4$

10. **a.** Add 2.7 mL of sterile water for injection.
    b. 1.5 mL/250 mg.
    c. Refrigerated, 7 days; room temperature, 3 days.
    d. 500 mg.
    e. Administer 2.7 mL.

    KNOW   WANT TO KNOW
    250 mg : 1.5 mL :: 450 mg : x mL
    $250x = 1.5 \times 450$
    $250x = 675$
    $\quad x = 2.7$ mL
    PROOF
    $250 \times 2.7 = 675$
    $1.5 \times 450 = 675$

5D (PAGE 156)

1. c. KNOW   WANT TO KNOW
4 mL : 2000 mg :: x mL :: 1000 mg
2000x = 4 × 1000 = 4000
2x = 4
x = 2 mL
PROOF
2000 × 2 = 4000
4 × 1000 = 4000

2. b. Directions read: Add 1.2 mL of diluent to yield 125 mg/mL.
d. KNOW   WANT TO KNOW
250 mg : 1 dose :: x mg : 2 doses
x = 250 × 2 = 500
x = 500 mg for 2 doses
PROOF
1 × 500 = 500
500 × 1 = 500

KNOW   WANT TO KNOW
125 mg : 1 vial :: 500 mg : x vials
125x = 1 × 500 = 500
x = 4 vials for 24 hr
PROOF
1 × 500 = 500
125 × 4 = 500

3. d. The directions read: Add 5.7 mL sterile water for injection.
b. KNOW   WANT TO KNOW
250 mg : 1.5 mL :: 500 mg : x mL
250x = 1.5 × 500 mg = 750
x = 3 mL
PROOF
1.5 × 500 = 750
250 × 3 = 750

4. b. KNOW   WANT TO KNOW
2 mL : 1 g :: x mL : 1.5 g
x = 2 × 1.5 = 3
x = 3 mL divided into 2 doses
PROOF
1 × 3 = 3
2 × 1.5 = 3

d. KNOW   WANT TO KNOW
1000 mg : 1 vial :: 3000 mg : x vials
1000x = 3000
x = 3 vials needed
PROOF
1000 × 3 = 3000
1 × 3000 = 3000

5. b. Directions read: Add 30 mL of water in 2 portions. Mix well.
b. KNOW   WANT TO KNOW
100 mg : 5 mL :: 200 mg : x mL
100x = 5 × 200 = 1000
x = 10 mL
PROOF
10 × 100 = 1000
5 × 200 = 1000

6. c. KNOW   WANT TO KNOW
2.6 mL : 1000 mg :: x mL : 500 mg
10x = 2.6 × 5 = 13
x = 1.3 mL
PROOF
2.6 × 500 = 1300
1000 × 1.3 = 1300

7. c. KNOW   WANT TO KNOW

500 mg : 1 dose :: x mg : 3 doses

$x = 500 \times 3 = 1500$

$x = 1500$ mg/24 hr

PROOF

$500 \times 3 = 1500$

$1500 \times 1 = 1500$

KNOW   WANT TO KNOW

1000 mg : 1 vial :: 1500 mg : x vials

$1000x = 1500$

     $x = 1.5$ vials

PROOF

$1 \times 1500 = 1500$

$1000 \times 1.5 = 1500$

You will need to have 2 vials on hand for 24 hr.

8. c. Directions read: Add 1.5 mL of diluent = 500,000 units/mL

d. KNOW   WANT TO KNOW

500,000 units : 1 mL ::

               400,000 units : x mL

$500,000x = 1 \times 400,000 = 400,000$

$5x = 4$

  $x = 0.8$ mL

PROOF

$0.8 \times 500,000 = 400,000$

$1 \times 400,000 = 400,000$

9. c. Add 9 mL of diluent = 400 mg/mL

a. KNOW   WANT TO KNOW

400,000 mg : 1 mL :: 500,000 mg : x mL

$400,000x = 1 \times 500,000 = 500,000$

      $4x = 5$

        $x = 1.25 = 1.3$ mL

PROOF

$1 \times 500,000 = 500,000$

$400,000 \times 1.25 = 500,000$

10. c. 330 mg : 1 mL :: 250 mg : x mL

$330x = 250$

   $x = 0.757 = 0.8$ mL

PROOF

$1 \times 250 = 250$

$0.757 \times 330 = 249.8$

CHAPTER 5 FINAL: MEDICATIONS FROM POWDERS AND CRYSTALS: ORAL AND INTRAMUSCULAR (PAGE 161)

1. Add 2 mL distilled water.

2. Administer 2 mL.

3. a. Add 3.5 mL diluent.
    b. Administer 1 mL.

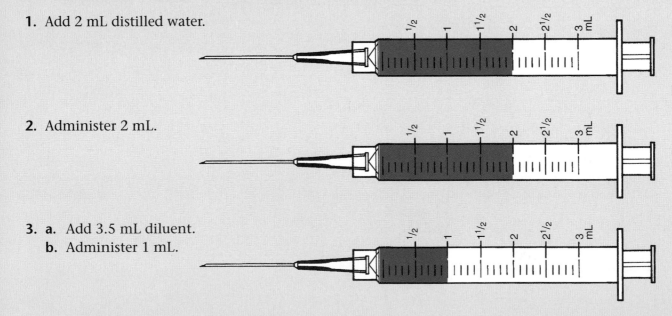

4. a. Add 2 mL of sterile water for injection.
   b. Administer 1.3 mL.

5. a. 250,000 units/mL
   b. 1.2 mL
   c. 16.6 doses in the vial

6. a. Add 9.5 mL of diluent.
   b. Give 1.9 mL IM.

7. a. Add 2.5 mL of sterile water for injection.
   b. Give 1.5 mL IM.

8. a. Add 9.6 mL of diluent to make
   100,000 units/mL. A more concentrated
   solution may be caustic to the tissue.
   b. Administer 1 mL.

9. a. Add 2.7 mL sterile water for injection.
   b. Administer 1.5 mL.

10. Administer 0.7 mL.

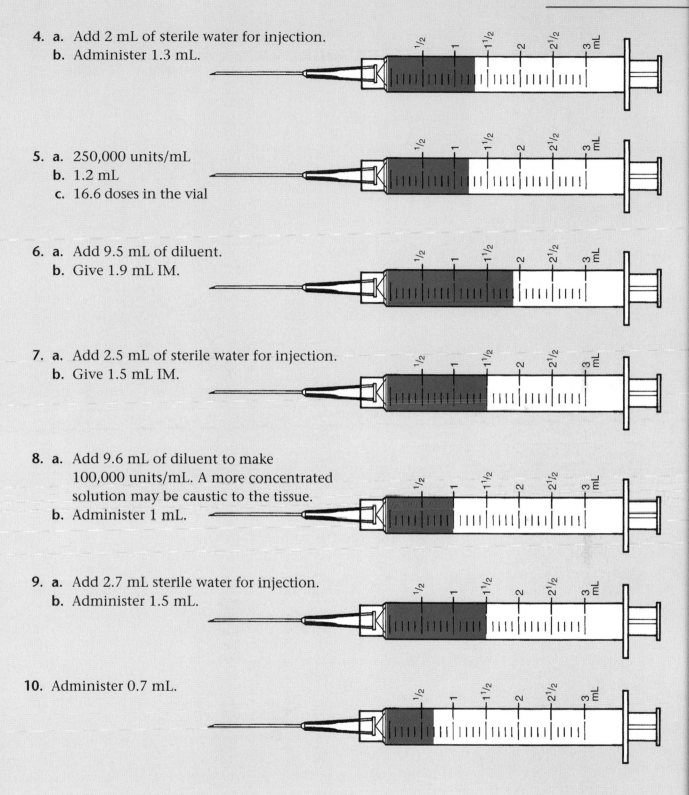

6 Basic Intravenous Calculations

6A (PAGE 172)

$$\boxed{\textbf{REMEMBER}} \quad 1 \frac{TV}{TT \text{ in hr}} = mL/hr$$

$$2 \frac{Df}{Time \text{ in min}} \times V/hr = gtt/min$$

1. Step 1: $\frac{1500}{12} = 125$ mL/hr

   Step 2: $\frac{15}{60} \times \frac{125}{1} = \frac{1}{4} \times \frac{125}{1} = 31.25$ or 31 gtt/min

2. Step 2: $\frac{60}{60} \times \frac{50}{1} = \frac{1}{1} \times \frac{50}{1} = \frac{50}{1} = 50$ gtt/min

3. Step 2: $\frac{10}{30} \times \frac{100}{1} = \frac{1}{3} \times \frac{100}{1} = \frac{100}{3} = 33.3$ or 33 gtt/min

4. Step 1: $\frac{TV}{TT} = \frac{1000}{8} = 125$ mL/hr

   Step 2: $\frac{10}{60} \times \frac{125 \text{ mL}}{1} = \frac{1}{6} \times \frac{125}{1} = \frac{125}{6} = 20.8$ or 21 gtt/min

5. Step 2: $\frac{15}{60} \times \frac{200}{1} = \frac{1}{4} \times \frac{200}{1} = \frac{200}{4} = 50$ gtt/min

6. Step 2: $\frac{\overset{1}{\cancel{20}}}{\underset{3}{\cancel{60}}} \times 150 = \frac{1}{3} \times \frac{150}{1} = \frac{150}{3} = 50$ gtt/min

7. Step 2: $\frac{10}{45} \times \frac{75}{1} = \frac{750}{45} = 16.6$ or 17 gtt/min

8. Step 2: $\frac{\overset{2}{\cancel{60}}}{\underset{3}{\cancel{90}}} \times 250 = \frac{2}{3} \times \frac{250}{1} = \frac{500}{3} = 166.6$ or 167 gtt/min

9. Step 2: $\frac{\overset{3}{\cancel{15}}}{\underset{8}{\cancel{40}}} \times 150 = \frac{3}{8} \times \frac{150}{1} = \frac{450}{8} = 56.25$ or 56 gtt/min

10. Step 1: $\frac{1500}{8} = 188$ mL/hr

    Step 2: **a.** $\frac{10}{60} \times \frac{188}{1} = \frac{1}{6} \times \frac{188}{1} = \frac{188}{6} = 31.3$ or 31 gtt/min

    b. $\frac{15}{60} = \frac{1}{4} \times \frac{188}{1} = 47$ gtt/min

6B (PAGE 173)

$$\boxed{\textbf{REMEMBER}} \quad 1\,\frac{TV}{TT\text{ in hr}} = mL/hr$$

$$2\,\frac{Df}{Time\text{ in min}} \times V/hr = gtt/min$$

1. **Step 1:** $\frac{TV}{TT} = \frac{2000}{24} = 83.3$ or 83 mL/hr

   Step 2: $\frac{\overset{1}{\cancel{15}}}{\underset{4}{\cancel{60}}} \times \frac{83}{1} = \frac{83}{4} = 20.75$ or 21 gtt/min

2. **Step 1:** $\frac{TV}{TT} = \frac{500}{4} = 125$ mL/hr

   Step 2: $\frac{\overset{1}{\cancel{15}}}{\underset{4}{\cancel{60}}} \times \frac{125}{1} = \frac{125}{4} = 31.2$ or 31 gtt/min

3. **Step 1:** $\frac{TV}{TT} = \frac{3000}{24} = 125$ mL/hr

   Step 2: $\frac{60}{60} \times \frac{125}{1} = 1 \times 125 = 125$ gtt/min

4. **Step 1:** $\frac{TV}{TT} = \frac{1500}{8} = 187.5$ or 188 mL/hr

   Step 2: $\frac{\overset{1}{\cancel{15}}}{\underset{4}{\cancel{60}}} \times \frac{188}{1} = 47$ gtt/min

5. **Step 1:** $\frac{TV}{TT} = \frac{1000}{12} = 83.3$ or 83 mL/hr

   Step 2: $\frac{\overset{1}{\cancel{60}}}{\underset{1}{\cancel{60}}} \times \frac{83}{1} = \frac{83}{1} = 83$ gtt/min

6. Start with Step 2 because we already know how many milliliters per 30 minutes.

   Step 2: $\frac{\overset{2}{\cancel{20}}}{\underset{3}{\cancel{30}}} \times \frac{100}{1} = \frac{200}{3} = 67$ gtt/min

7. **Step 1:** $\frac{TV}{TT} = \frac{2000}{24} = 83.3$ or 83 mL/hr

8. **Step 1:** $\frac{TV}{TT} = \frac{250}{10} = 25$ mL/hr

   Step 2: $\frac{\overset{1}{\cancel{60}}}{\underset{1}{\cancel{60}}} \times \frac{25}{1} = 25$ gtt/min

9. **Step 1:** $\frac{TV}{TT} = \frac{1500}{12} = 125$ mL/hr

   Step 2: $\frac{\overset{1}{\cancel{15}}}{\underset{4}{\cancel{60}}} \times \frac{125}{1} = \frac{125}{4} = 31.25$ or 31 gtt/min

10. **MEMORIZE** ✳ **Step 1:** $\frac{TV}{TT\text{ in hr}} = mL/hr$

    Step 2: $\frac{Df}{Time\text{ in min}} \times V/hr = gtt/min$

6C (PAGE 174)

$$\left(\text{ REMEMBER }\right) \quad 1\,\frac{TV}{TT\text{ in hr}} = mL/hr$$

$$2\,\frac{Df}{\text{Time in min}} \times V/hr = gtt/min$$

1. **Step 2:** $\frac{15}{30} \times \frac{100}{1} = \frac{1}{2} \times \frac{100}{1} = \frac{100}{2} = 50$ gtt/min

2. **Step 2:** $\frac{1\cancel{0}}{3\cancel{0}} \times \frac{50}{1} = \frac{50}{3} = 16.6$ or 17 gtt/min

3. **Step 1:** $\frac{TV}{TT} = \frac{1000}{6} = 166.6$ or 167 mL/hr

   Step 2: $\frac{\overset{1}{\cancel{15}}}{\underset{4}{\cancel{60}}} \times \frac{167}{1} = \frac{167}{4} = 41.75$ or 42 gtt/min

4. **Step 2:** $\frac{\overset{1}{\cancel{60}}}{\underset{1}{\cancel{60}}} \times \frac{100}{1} = 100$ gtt/min   Yes, the mL/hr is the same as the drops/min rate.

5. **Step 2:** $\frac{20}{60} \times 85 = \frac{1}{3} \times \frac{85}{1} = \frac{85}{3} = 28.3$ or 28 gtt/min

6. **Step 2:** $\frac{1\cancel{0}}{6\cancel{0}} \times 100 = \frac{100}{6} = 16.6$ or 17 gtt/min

7. **Step 1:** $\frac{TV}{TT} = \frac{1500}{24} = 62.5$ or 63 mL/hr

   Step 2: $\frac{1\cancel{0}}{6\cancel{0}} \times \frac{63}{1} = \frac{63}{3} \times 10.5 = 11$ gtt/min

8. **Step 1:** $\frac{TV}{TT} = \frac{500}{8} = 62.5$ or 63 mL/hr

   Step 2: $\frac{\overset{1}{\cancel{60}}}{\underset{1}{\cancel{60}}} \times \frac{63}{1} = 63$ gtt/min

9. **Step 2:** $\frac{\overset{1}{\cancel{15}}}{\underset{4}{\cancel{60}}} \times \frac{75}{1} = \frac{75}{4} = 18.7$ or 19 gtt/min

10. **Step 1:** $\frac{TV}{TT} = \frac{2000}{12} = 166.6$ or 167 mL/hr

    Step 2: $\frac{\overset{1}{\cancel{60}}}{\underset{1}{\cancel{60}}} \times \frac{167}{1} = 167$ gtt/min

6D (PAGE 176)

1. KNOW　　　　WANT TO KNOW
5 g : 100 mL :: x g : 1000 mL
$x = 5 \times 10 = 50$
$x = 50$ g or mL dextrose
PROOF
$5 \times 1000 = 5000$
$100 \times 50 = 5000$

KNOW　　　　WANT TO KNOW
0.9 g : 100 mL :: x g : 1000 mL
$x = 0.9 \times 10 = 9$
$x = 9$ g of sodium chloride
PROOF
$0.9 \times 1000 = 900$
$100 \times 9 = 900$

2. KNOW　　　　WANT TO KNOW
5 g : 100 mL :: x g : 500 mL
$x = 5 \times 5 = 25$
$x = 25$ g or mL of dextrose
PROOF
$5 \times 500 = 2500$
$100 \times 25 = 2500$

KNOW　　　　WANT TO KNOW
0.45 g : 100 mL :: x g : 500 mL
$x = 0.45 \times 5 = 2.25$
$x = 2.25$ g of sodium chloride
PROOF
$0.45 \times 500 = 2.25$
$100 \times 2.25 = 225$

3. KNOW　　　　WANT TO KNOW
10 g : 100 mL :: x g : 500 mL
$x = 10 \times 5 = 50$
$x = 50$ g or mL of dextrose
PROOF
$10 \times 500 = 5000$
$100 \times 50 = 5000$

KNOW　　　　WANT TO KNOW
0.9 g : 100 mL :: x g : 500 mL
$x = 0.9 \times 5$
$x = 4.5$ g or mL of sodium chloride
PROOF
$0.9 \times 500 = 450$
$4.5 \times 100 = 450$

4. KNOW　　　　WANT TO KNOW
0.9 g : 100 mL :: x g : 1000 mL
$x = 0.9 \times 10 = 9$
$x = 9$ g or mL of sodium chloride
PROOF
$0.9 \times 1000 = 900$
$9 \times 100 = 900$

5. KNOW　　　　WANT TO KNOW
0.45 g : 100 mL :: x g : 500 mL
$x = 0.45 \times 5 = 2.25$
$x = 2.25$ g or mL of sodium chloride
PROOF
$0.45 \times 500 = 225$
$100 \times 2.25 = 225$

6. KNOW　　　　WANT TO KNOW
5 g : 100 mL :: x g : 1000 mL
$x = 5 \times 10 = 50$
$x = 50$ g or mL of dextrose
PROOF
$5 \times 1000 = 500$
$100 \times 50 = 5000$

7. KNOW   WANT TO KNOW
   5 g : 100 mL :: x g : 500 mL
   $x = 5 \times 5 = 25$
   $x = 25$ g or mL of dextrose
   PROOF
   $100 \times 25 = 2500$
   $5 \times 500 = 2500$

8. KNOW   WANT TO KNOW
   600 mg : 100 mL :: x mg : 1000 mL
   $x = 10 \times 600 = 6000$
   $x = 6000$ mg of sodium chloride in 1000 mL
   PROOF
   $600 \times 1000 = 600,000$
   $100 \times 6000 = 600,000$

   KNOW   WANT TO KNOW
   1 g : 1000 mg :: x g : 6000 mg
   $x = 6 \times 1 = 6$
   $x = 6$ g of sodium chloride in 1000 mL
   PROOF
   $1 \times 6000 = 6000$
   $6 \times 1000 = 6000$

9. KNOW   WANT TO KNOW
   5 g : 100 mL :: x g : 1000 mL
   $x = 5 \times 10 = 50$
   $x = 50$ g or mL of dextrose
   PROOF
   $5 \times 1000 = 5000$
   $100 \times 50 = 5000$

   KNOW   WANT TO KNOW
   0.9 g : 100 mL :: x g : 1000 mL
   $x = 0.9 \times 10 = 9$
   $x = 9$ g or mL of sodium chloride
   PROOF
   $100 \times 9 = 900$
   $0.9 \times 1000 = 900$

10. KNOW   WANT TO KNOW
   5 g : 100 mL :: x g : 500 mL
   $x = 5 \times 5 = 25$
   $x = 25$ g or mL of dextrose
   PROOF
   $5 \times 500 = 2500$
   $100 \times 25 = 2500$

   KNOW   WANT TO KNOW
   0.45 g : 100 mL :: x g : 500 mL
   $x = 0.45 \times 5 = 2.25$
   $x = 2.25$ g or mL of sodium chloride
   PROOF
   $0.45 \times 500 = 225$
   $100 \times 2.25 = 225$

6E (PAGE 181)

1. $\dfrac{\text{Total volume}}{\text{Total time}} = \text{mL/hr}$

   $\dfrac{1500 \text{ mL}}{4 \text{ hr}} = 375 \text{ mL/hr}$

2. KNOW   WANT TO KNOW
   125 mL : 1 hr :: 1000 mL : x hr
   $125x = 1000$
   $x = 8$ hr

   The IV will be completed by 1700 hours.
   PROOF
   $1 \times 1000 = 1000$
   $125 \times 8 = 1000$

3. HAVE   WANT TO HAVE
   1000 mL : 6 hr :: x mL : 1 hr
   $6x = 1000$
   $x = 166.6 = 167$ mL/hr
   PROOF
   $1000 \times 1 = 1000$
   $6 \times 166.6 = 999.96$

4. $\dfrac{\text{Total volume}}{\text{Total time}} = \text{mL/hr}$

   $\dfrac{1000 \text{ mL}}{8 \text{ hr}} = 125 \text{ mL/hr}$

   The IV was started at 0715 + 8 = 1515 for the hour of completion.

5. KNOW   WANT TO KNOW

$5 \text{ g} : 100 :: x \text{ g} : 125 \text{ mL}$

$100x = 5 \times 125 = 625$

$\qquad x = 6.25 \text{ g/hr}$

PROOF

$5 \times 125 = 625$

$100 \times 6.25 = 625$

6. HAVE   WANT TO HAVE

$30 \text{ mL} : 1 \text{ hr} :: 250 \text{ mL} : x \text{ hr}$

$30x = 250$

$\qquad x = 8.33 \text{ hr}$

Convert $0.33 \times 60 \text{ min} = 19.8 = 20 \text{ min}$
The IV will take 8 hr and 20 min to infuse.
The IVPB was started at 1330 hr + 8 hr
20 min = 2150 for the hour of completion.

PROOF

$1 \times 250 = 250$

$8.33 \times 30 = 249.9$

7. HAVE   WANT TO HAVE

$500 \text{ mL} : 4 \text{ hr} :: x \text{ mL} : 1 \text{ hr}$

$4x = 500 \times 1 = 500$

$\qquad x = 125 \text{ mL/hr}$

PROOF

$500 \times 1 = 500$

$4 \times 125 = 500$

8. HAVE   WANT TO HAVE

$40 \text{ mL} : 1 \text{ hr} :: 500 \text{ mL} : x \text{ hr}$

$40x = 500$

$\qquad x = 12.5 \text{ hr}$

IV started at 2100 hr + 12.5 hr (12 hr
30 min) = 0930 for the hour of completion.

PROOF

$1 \times 500 = 500$

$40 \times 12.5 = 500$

9. HAVE   WANT TO HAVE

$200 \text{ mL} : 3 \text{ hr} :: x \text{ mL} : 1 \text{ hr}$

$3x = 200$

$\qquad x = 66.66 = 67 \text{ mL/hr}$

OR

$$\frac{\text{Total volume}}{\text{Total time}} = \text{mL/hr}$$

$$\frac{200 \text{ mL}}{3 \text{ hr}} = 66.66 = 67 \text{ mL/hr}$$

PROOF

$200 \times 1 = 200$

$66.66 = 199.98$

10. $\dfrac{\text{Total volume}}{\text{Total time}} = \text{vol/hr}$

$\dfrac{500 \text{ mL}}{4 \text{ hr}} = 125 \text{ mL/hr}$

6F (PAGE 189)

1. a. $\dfrac{\overset{2}{\cancel{60}}}{\underset{1}{\cancel{30}}} \times 100 = 200 \text{ gtt/min}$

b. The infusion device will be set at
200 mL/hr.

KNOW   WANT TO KNOW

$100 \text{ mL} : 30 \text{ min} :: x \text{ mL} : 60 \text{ min}$

$30x = 100 \times 60 = 6000$

$30x = 600\cancel{0}$

$\qquad x = 200 \text{ mL/hr}$

2. KNOW   WANT TO KNOW

$100 \text{ mL} : 60 \text{ min} :: x \text{ mL} : 60 \text{ min}$

$60x = 6000$

$\qquad x = 100 \text{ mL/hr}$

PROOF

$100 \times 60 = 6000$

$60 \times 100 = 6000$

3. KNOW WANT TO KNOW
150 mL : 60 min :: 250 mL : x min
$150x = 250 \times 60 = 15,000$
$x = 100$ min $= 1.6$ hr $= 1$ hr 36 min
PROOF
$100 \times 150 = 15,000$
$250 \times 60 = 15,000$

4. a. KNOW WANT TO KNOW
50 mL : 20 min :: x mL : 60 min
$20x = 50 \times 60 = 3000$
$x = 150$ mL/hr
PROOF
$20 \times 150 = 3000$
$50 \times 60 = 3000$

b. $\dfrac{15}{20} \times \dfrac{50}{1} = \dfrac{\overset{3}{\cancel{15}}}{\underset{4}{\cancel{20}}} \times \dfrac{50}{1} = \dfrac{150}{4}$
$= 37.5$ or 38 gtt/min

5. a. $\dfrac{15}{60} \times \dfrac{100}{1} = \dfrac{1}{4} \times \dfrac{100}{1} = \dfrac{100}{4} = 25$ gtt/min

b. 100 mL : 60 min :: x mL : 60 min
$60x = 100 \times 60 = 6000$
$60x = 6000$
$x = 100$ mL/hr
PROOF
$100 \times 60 = 6000$
$60 \times 100 = 6000$

6. a. KNOW WANT TO KNOW
50 mL : 30 min :: x mL : 60 min
$30x = 50 \times 60 = 3000$
$x = 100$ mL/hr
PROOF
$30 \times 150 = 3000$
$50 \times 60 = 3000$

b. $\dfrac{60}{30} \times \dfrac{50}{1} = \dfrac{\overset{2}{\cancel{60}}}{\underset{1}{\cancel{30}}} \times \dfrac{50}{1} = 100$ gtt/min

7. a. $\dfrac{\overset{2}{\cancel{60}}}{\underset{3}{\cancel{90}}} \times 200 = \dfrac{400}{3} = 133$ gtt/min

OR
200 mL : 90 min :: x mL : 60 min
$90x = 200 \times 60 = 12,000$
$9\cancel{0}x = 12,00\cancel{0}$
$x = 133$ mL/hr

b. Set infusion device for 133 mL/hr.

8. Step 1: $\dfrac{1000}{12} = 83.3$ or 83 mL/hr

a. Step 2: $\dfrac{\overset{1}{\cancel{15}}}{\underset{4}{\cancel{60}}} \times 83 = \dfrac{83}{4}$
$= 20.8$ or 21 gtt/min

b. The infusion device will be set at 83 mL/hr.

KNOW WANT TO KNOW
c. 0.9 g : 100 mL :: x g : 1000 mL
$x = 0.9 \times 10 = 9$
$x = 9$ g of sodium chloride (solute)
PROOF
$0.9 \times 1000 = 900$
$100 \times 9 = 900$

9. a. Step 1: $\frac{TV}{TT} = \frac{2000}{8} = 250$ mL/hr

b. Step 2: $\frac{\overset{1}{\cancel{15}}}{\underset{4}{\cancel{60}}} \times 250 = \frac{250}{4}$

$= 62.5$ or 63 gtt/min

KNOW   WANT TO KNOW

c. 5 g : 100 mL :: x g : 2000 mL

$x = 5 \times 20 = 100$

$x = 100$ g of dextrose

PROOF

$5 \times 2000 = 10,000$

$100 \times 100 = 10,000$

10. a. $\frac{\overset{3}{\cancel{60}}}{\underset{2}{\cancel{40}}} \times 150 = \frac{450}{2}$

$= 225$ gtt/min is the fastest rate or 225 mL/hr for the infusion device using the microdrip formula

b. $\frac{60}{60} \times 150 = 150$ gtt/min is the slowest rate. Set infusion device for 150 mL/hr using the microdrip formula

6G (PAGE 190)

1. c. KNOW   WANT TO KNOW

2500 mL : 24 hr :: x mL : 1 hr

$24x = 2500$

$x = 104.16$ mL/hr

PROOF

$2500 \times 1 = 2500$

$24 \times 104.16 = 2500 = 104$ mL/hr

KNOW   WANT TO KNOW

15 gtt : 1 mL :: x gtt : 104.16 mL

OR

$\frac{15}{60} \times 104 = \frac{1560}{60} = 26$ gtt/min

$x = 15 \times 104.16 = 1562$

$x = 1562$ divided by 60 min $= 26$ gtt/min

PROOF

$15 \times 104.16 = 1562$

$1 \times 1562 = 1562$

3. d. $\frac{20 \text{ gtt}}{30 \text{ min}} \times 50 = \frac{100}{3} = 33$ gtt/min

2. d. $\frac{15}{15} \times 50 = 50$ gtt/min

4. b. KNOW   WANT TO KNOW

300 mL : 6 hr :: x mL : 1 hr

$6x = 300 \times 1 = 300$

$x = 50$ mL/hr. mL/hr and microdrip gtt/min are the same, so 50 gtt/min is correct

PROOF

$300 \times 1 = 300$

$6 \times 50 = 300$

OR

$\frac{\overset{1}{\cancel{60}} \text{ gtt}}{\underset{6}{\cancel{360}} \text{ min}} \times 300 \text{ mL} = \frac{300}{6} = 50$ gtt/min and 50 mL/hr

5. d. KNOW   WANT TO KNOW
12 mL : 1 hr :: 150 mL : x hr
$12x = 150$
$\quad x = 12.5 = 12$ hr 30 min
PROOF
$1 \times 150 = 150$
$12.5 \times 12 = 150$

6. d. KNOW   WANT TO KNOW
30 gtt : 1 min :: 20 gtt : x min
$30x = 20$
$\quad x = 0.66$ min
PROOF
$1 \times 20 = 20$
$30 \times 0.66 = 20$

KNOW   WANT TO KNOW
1 mL : 0.66 min :: 500 mL : x min
$x = 0.66 \times 500 = 330$
$x = 330$ min $\div\ 60 = 5.5$ hr $= 5$ hr 30 min
PROOF
$1 \times 330 = 330$
$0.66 \times 500 = 330$

7. a. KNOW   WANT TO KNOW
25 gtt : 1 min :: 10 gtt : x min
$25x = 10$
$\quad x = 0.4$ min $= 1$ mL
PROOF
$25 \times 0.4 = 10$
$1 \times 10 = 10$

KNOW   WANT TO KNOW
1 mL : 0.4 min :: 1000 mL : x min
$x = 0.4 \times 1000 = 400$
$x = 400$ min divided by 60
$\quad = 6.66$ hr $= 6$ hr 40 min

8. c. KNOW   WANT TO KNOW
42 gtt : 1 min :: 10 gtt : x min
$42x = 1 \times 10 = 10$
$\quad x = 0.238 = 0.24$ min/mL
PROOF
$1 \times 10 = 10$
$42 \times 0.24 = 10.08 = 10$

KNOW   WANT TO KNOW
1 mL : 0.24 min :: 500 mL : x min
$x = 0.24 \times 500 = 120$
$x = 120$ min divided by $60 = 2$ hr
PROOF
$1 \times 120 = 120$
$0.24 \times 500 = 120$
The transfusion was started at 1100 hours.
The completion time will be 1300 hours.

9. c. KNOW   WANT TO KNOW
30 mL : 1 hr :: 500 mL : x hr
$30x = 500$
$\quad x = 16.66$ hr $= 16$ hr 40 min
PROOF
$30 \times 16.6 = 499.8 = 500$
$1 \times 500 = 500$

10. d. $\dfrac{250}{2} = 125$ mL/hr

CHAPTER 6 FINAL: BASIC INTRAVENOUS CALCULATIONS (PAGE 192)

1. 31 gtt/min

2. 100 mL/hr
17 gtt/min

3. 83 mL/hr
28 gtt/min

4. 150 gtt/min

5. 83 mL/hr
14 gtt/min

6. 125 mL/hr
31 gtt/min

7. 125 mL/hr
125 gtt/min

8. Set infusion device at 267 mL/hr.

9. 83 gtt/min

10. 167 gtt/min or 167 mL/hr if infusion device is used

7 Advanced Intravenous Calculations

7A (PAGE 197)

1. **b.** 9600 mcg/hr or 9.6 mg/hr
   c. 9900 mcg or 9.9 mg/hr (121 lb = 55 kg)
   d. 12,000 mcg/hr or 12 mg/hr
   e. 72,000 mcg/hr or 72 mg/hr

2. **b.** 1 : 1
   c. 1 : 10
   d. 1 : 2
   e. 1 : 2

3. **b.** x = 30 mL/hr (1 : 1 :: 30 : 30)
   c. x = 50 mL/hr (1 : 10 :: 5 : 50)
   d. x = 6 mL/hr (1 : 2 :: 3 : 6)
   e. x = 5 mL/hr (2 : 1 :: 10 : 5)

4. **b.** (2 : 1 :: 12 : 6) 12 mg/hr
   c. (1 : 2 :: 9 : 18) 9 mg/hr
   d. (4 : 10 :: 4 : 10) 4 mg/hr
   e. (2 : 1 :: 36 : 18) 36 mg/hr

5. **b.** (1 : 1 :: 9 : 9) 9 mL/hr
   c. (2 : 1 :: 20 : 10) 10 mL/hr
   d. (1 : 2 :: 1 : 2) 30 mL/hr
   e. (8 : 5 :: 8 : 5) 5 mL/hr

7B (PAGE 199)

1.

	mg/hr	mcg/hr	mg/min	mcg/min
a.	0.050	50	0.050 ÷ 60 = 0.0008	0.8
b.	24	24,000	0.4	400
c.	30	30,000	0.5	500
d.	1.2	1200	0.02	20
e.	7.5	7500	0.125	125

2.

	kg	mg/hr	mg/kg/min	mcg/kg/min
a.	85	25	25 ÷ 85 ÷ 60 = 0.005	5
b.	70	10 × 70 × 60 = 42,000	10	10,000
c.	62	0.37	0.0001	0.1
d.	55	75	0.02	20
e.	48	144	0.05	50

3.

	IV Contents	TD : TV Reduced Ratio	HD (mg/hr)	HV (mL/hr)	mg/mL
a.	500 mg/1000 mL	1 : 2	5	10	0.5
b.	250 mg/500 mL	1 : 2	15	30	0.5
c.	400 mg/250 mL	8 : 5	24	15	1.6
d.	500 mg/500 mL	1 : 1	75	75	1
e.	500 mg/250 mL	2 : 1	16	8	2

7C (PAGE 200)

2. a. $1 : 2 :: x$ mg : 15 mL   ($x = 7.5$ mg/hr)
  PROOF
    $1 \times 15 = 15$
    $2 \times 7.5 = 15$
  b. 7.5 mg $\times$ 1000 = 7500 mcg/hr
  c. 7500 mcg $\div$ 60 = 125 mcg/min
  d. 125 mcg/min $\div$ 50 kg = 2.5 mcg/kg/min

3. a. $2 : 5 :: x$ mg : 5 mL   ($x = 2$ mg/hr)
  PROOF
    $2 \times 5 = 10$
    $5 \times 2 = 10$
  b. 2 mg/hr $\times$ 1000 = 2000 mcg/hr
  c. 2000 mcg/hr $\div$ 60 = 33.3 mcg/min
  d. 33.3 mcg/min $\div$ 55 kg = 0.605 or
    0.6 mcg/kg/min

4. a. $4 : 1 :: x$ mg/hr : 10 mL/hr   ($x = 40$ mg)
  PROOF
    $4 \times 10 = 40$
    $10 \times 4 = 40$
  b. 40 $\times$ 1000 = 40,000 mcg/hr
  c. 40,000 mcg $\div$ 60 = 666.7 mcg/min
  d. 666.7 mcg/min $\div$ 60 kg =
    11.1 mcg/kg/min

5. a. $2 : 1 :: x$ mg : 8 mL/hr   ($x = 16$ mL/hr)
  PROOF
    $2 \times 8 = 16$
    $1 \times 16 = 16$
  b. 16 mg $\times$ 1000 = 16,000 mcg/hr
  c. 16,000 mcg/hr $\div$ 60 = 266.7 mcg/min
  d. 266.7 mcg/min $\div$ 79.5 kg =
    3.4 mcg/kg/min

7D (PAGE 201)

2. a. 60 (132 $\div$ 2.2)
  b. 300 mcg/min $\times$ 60 = 18,000 mcg/hr
  c. 18 mg/hr (decimal moved 3 places
    to left)
  d. $250 : 250 :: 1 : 1$
  e. 18 mL/hr ($1 : 1 :: 18 : x$)
  f. Incorrect flow rate. Should be 18 mL/hr,
    not 36 mL/hr.
  g. Unsafe. Assess patient's vital signs,
    report per hospital policy, and contact
    physician for orders.

3. a. 1000 mg : 500 mL = 2 mg : 1 mL
  b. 4 mg $\times$ 60 = 240 mg/hr
  c. $2 : 1 :: 240 : x$ = 120 mL/hr

4. a. 1 mg : 250 mL
  b. 5 mcg $\times$ 60 = 300 mcg/hr or 0.3 mg/hr
  c. 1 : 250 mL :: 0.3 mg : x mL
  d. 0.3 $\times$ 250 = 75.0 mL/hr

5. a. 1 mg : 250 mL :: x mcg : 50 mL
  b. x = 0.2 mg/hr
  c. 200 mcg/hr
  d. 200 mcg $\div$ 60 = 3.3 mcg/min
  e. 8 to 12 mcg/min
  f. Low; consult with provider

7E (PAGE 203)

2. a. 10,000 milliunits : 1000 mL = 10 : 1
  b. 10 milliunits : 1 mL :: 1200 milliunits
    (hr) : x mL (120) (hr)
  PROOF
    $10 \times 120 = 1200$
    $1 \times 1200 = 1200$
  c. Rate should be 120 mL/hr; obtain order
    to increase.

3. a. 5 : 500 = 1 mg : 100 mL
  b. 10 $\times$ 60 = 600 mcg/hr
  c. 0.6 mg/hr
  d. 1 : 100 :: 0.6 mg : x mL
  PROOF
    $1 \times 60 = 60$
    $100 \times 0.6 = 60$
  e. x = 60 mL/hr (for 30 min) will deliver
    300 mcg total, as ordered.

4. **a.** $2\emptyset : 5\emptyset\emptyset = 1 : 25$
   b. $1 \text{ g} : 25 \text{ mL} :: x \text{ g} : 25 \text{ mL/hr}$
   PROOF
   $1 \times 25 = 25$
   $25 \times 1 = 25$
   c. $x = 1 \text{ g/hr}$
   d. 2 hr

5. **a.** 10 units = 10,000 milliunits
   b. 10 milliunits : 1 mL
   c. 2 milliunits $\times$ 60 = 120 milliunits/hr
   d. $10 : 1 :: 120 : x$
   PROOF
   $10 \times 12 = 120$
   $1 \times 120 = 120$
   e. $x = 12 \text{ mL/hr}$

7F (PAGE 204)

1. **a.** 65 kg
   b. 3250 to 13,000 mcg/min
   c. 195 to 780 mg/hr (mcg/min $\times$ 60 $\div$ 1000)
   d. (5 g = 5000 mg) $10 : 1 :: x \text{ mg} : 39 \text{ mL}$
   e. $x = 390 \text{ mg/hr}$
   f. $390 \div 60 = 6.5 \text{ mg/min}$
   g. 6500 mcg/min
   h. 6500 mcg $\div$ 65 kg = 100 mcg/kg/min
   i. Safe; continue

2. **a.** $5\emptyset \text{ mg} : 5\emptyset\emptyset \text{ mL} = 1 \text{ mg} : 10 \text{ mL} ::$
   $x \text{ mg/hr} : 6 \text{ mL/hr}$
   b. $x = 0.6 \text{ mg/hr}$ (600 mcg/hr)
   PROOF
   $1 \times 6 = 6$
   $10 \times 0.6 = 6$
   c. $1 : 10 :: 0.6 : 6 \text{ mL/hr}$
   d. $0.6 \div 60 = 10 \text{ mcg/min}$
   e. Yes
   f. Safe; continue.

3. **a.** $10\emptyset\emptyset : 5\emptyset\emptyset = 2 : 1 :: x \text{ mg} : 50 \text{ mL}$
   b. $x = 100 \text{ mg/hr}$
   c. 100 mg $\div$ 60 = 1.66 or 1.7 mg
   d. Safe; continue.

4. **a.** $220 \div 2.2 = 100 \text{ kg}$
   b. $0.3 \times 100 \times 60 = 1800 \text{ mcg or } 1.8 \text{ mg/hr}$
   c. $1 : 5 :: 1.8 \text{ mg} : x \text{ mL}$ $x = 9 \text{ mL/hr}$
   d. 15 mL/hr
   e. 3 mg/hr $(1 : 5 :: x \text{ mg} : 15)$ $(x = 3)$
   f. Unsafe; call for order to lower rate to 9 mL/hr.

5. **a.** $125 \text{ mg} : 125 \text{ mL} = 1 : 1 :: 15 : 15 \text{ mL}$
   b. Safe; continue infusion.

7G (PAGE 208)

1. **a.** $5 \times 60 = 300 \text{ sec}$
   $300 \div 50 \text{ lines} = 6 \text{ sec/line}$
   b. $10 \text{ mL} : 5 \text{ min} :: x \text{ mL} : 1 \text{ min}$
   $5x = 10$
   $x = 2 \text{ mL/min}$

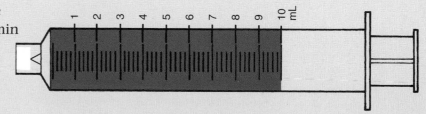

2. **a.** $250 \text{ mcg} : 1 \text{ mL} :: 500 \text{ mcg} : x \text{ mL}$
   $(x = 2 \text{ mL})$
   b. $10 \times 60 = 600 \text{ sec}$
   c. $600 \div 10 \text{ lines} = 60 \text{ sec/line}$
   d. $2 \text{ mL} : 10 \text{ min} :: x \text{ mL} : 1 \text{ min}$
   $x = 0.2 \text{ mL/min}$

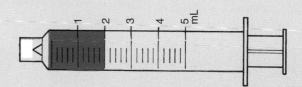

3. a. 100 mg : 1 mL :: 900 mg : x mL
(x = 9 mL)

b. 50 mg : 1 min :: 900 mg : x min
$50x = 900$
$x = 18$ min

c. 9 mL : 18 min :: x mL : 1 min
$18x = 9$
$x = 0.5$ mL/min

4. a. 10 mg : 1 mL :: 20 mg : x mL
(x = 2 mL)

b. $2 \times 60 = 120$ sec

c. $120 \div 10 = 12$ sec/line

d. 2 mL : 2 min :: x mL : 1 min
$2x = 2$
$x = 1$ mL/min

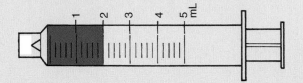

5. a. 5 mL

b. $5 \times 60 = 300$ sec

c. $300 \div 25 = 12$ sec/line

d. 5 mL : 5 min :: x mL : 1 min
$5x = 5$
$x = 1$ mL/min

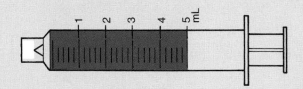

7H (PAGE 210)

1. c
5 mcg : 1 min :: x mcg : 60 min or
$5 \times 60 = 300$ mcg or 0.3 mg/hr

PROOF
$5 \times 60 = 300$
$1 \times 300 = 300$

2. a
250 mg : 1000 mL :: x mg : 1 mL
TD   TV
1 mg : 4 mL :: x mg : 1 mL
$x = 0.25$ mg/mL

PROOF
$1 \times 1 = 1$
$4 \times 0.25 = 1$

3. a
1 g = 1000 mg
TD   TV
1000 mg : 500 mL = 2 : 1

PROOF
1000 mg : 500 mL = 2 : 1 ratio

4. **c**

   8 mcg × 60 min or 480 mcg/hr or
   0.48 mg/hr = minimum drug
   per hour
   TD   TV   HD   HV
   1 mg : 250 mL :: 0.48 mg : x mL
   x = 250 × 0.48 or 120 mL/hr needed
   to infuse 0.48 mg per hour

   PROOF
   1 × 120 = 120
   250 × 0.48 = 120

5. **d**

   Step 1 total volume to be pushed
   10 mg : 1 mL :: 30 mg : x ml
   x = 3 mL
   Step 2 mL/min
   3 mL : 2 min :: x mL : 1 min
   $2x$ = 3 or x = 1.5 mL/min

   PROOF
   10 × 3 = 30
   1 × 30 = 30

   PROOF
   3 × 1 = 3
   2 × 1.5 = 3

6. **b**

   Step 1 Convert milligrams to micrograms
   or micrograms to milligrams by moving
   decimals.
   0.5 mg = 500 mcg OR
   250 mcg = 0.25 mg
   Step 2 Total mL
   On Hand
   250 mcg : 1 mL :: 500 mcg : x mL
   OR
   0.25 mg : 1 mL :: 0.5 mg : x mL
   x = 2 mL total volume to be injected
   over 5 min
   Step 3 mL/min
   2 mL : 5 min :: x mL : 1 min
   $5x$ = 2 or 0.4 mL/1 min

   PROOF
   250 mcg : 1 mL :: 500 mcg : x mL
   $250x$ = 500 or 2 mL
   OR
   $0.25x$ = 0.5 = 2 mL

   PROOF
   2 × 1 = 2
   5 × 0.4 = 2

7. a

Step 1 Calculate SDR for maintenance
for adult

1 mg : 1 min :: x mg : 60 min

x = 60 mg/hr is minimum SDR

6 mg : 1 min :: x mg : 60 min

x = 360 mg/hr is maximum SDR

SDR is 60 − 360 mg/hr.

Step 2 Calculate total drug/total volume
ratio and ordered drug per hour and per
minute.

1 g = 1000 mg

TD   TV   HD   HV

1000 mg : 500 mL :: x mg : 40 mL

2 mg : 1 mL :: x mg : 40 mL

x = 80 mg/hr being infused

80 mg ÷ 60 min = 1.3 mg/min

After reduction of TD : TV ratio,
the answer is apparent.

PROOF

$1 \times 60 = 60$

$1 \times 60 = 60$

PROOF

$6 \times 60 = 360$

$1 \times 360 = 360$

PROOF

$2 \times 40 = 80$

$1 \times 80 = 80$

8. b

Step 1 Change total drug to milligrams to
match hourly drug terms.

TD   TV   HD   HV

1 g : 1000 mL :: 60 mg : x mL

Need to change grams to milligrams
by using memorized conversion

1000 mg = 1 g.

TD   TV

1000 mg :: 1000 mL :: 60 mg : x mL

Step 2 Calculate mL/hr infusing

Simplify: reduce the TD/TV ratio and math
won't be needed to solve this question.

1 : 1 :: 60 : x mL/hr

$1x = 60$ $x = 60$ mL/hr

x = 60 mL/hr

PROOF

$1 \times 60 = 60$

$1 \times 60 = 60$

9. c

TD   HD   HD HV

20 g : 500 mL :: x g : 30 mL

$500x = 600 = 1.2$ g/hr

PROOF

$20 \times 30 = 600$

$600 \times 1 = 600$

1.2 g : 1 hr :: 3 g : x hr

$1.2x = 3$

$x = 2.5$ hr or 2 hr 30 min

10. d

2.5 mcg × 70 kg × 60 min =
10,500 mcg/hr needed
500 mcg : 1 mL :: 10,500 mcg : x mL
500x = 10,500
x = 21 mL/hr flow rate to deliver
10,500 mcg/hr

PROOF

500 × 21 = 10,500
1 × 500 = 500

CHAPTER 7 FINAL: ADVANCED INTRAVENOUS CALCULATIONS (PAGE 212)

1. a. 15,000 mcg (5 mcg × 50 kg × 60 min)
   b. 7.5 mL (2000 mcg : 1 mL :: 15,000 mcg : x mL)

2. a. 20 kg
   b. 60 mEq maximum per 24 hours
   c. 10 mEq
   d. Safe
   e. 5 mL
   f. 105 ÷ 4 = 26.25 or 26 mL/hr (100 mL D5W plus 5 mL KCl)

3. a. 9.6 mg/hr (2 mcg × 80 kg × 60 min = 9600 mcg/hr)
   b. 12 mg/hr (400 mg : 500 mL :: x mg : 15 mL)
      5x = 4 × 15 = 60
      x = 12 mg/hr
   c. 12 mL/hr (4 : 5 :: 9.6 : x mL)
      4x = 48 x = 12 mL/hr
   d. 15 mL/hr infusing
   e. Existing flow rate is too fast. Assess patient for side effects and contact physician for new order.

4. a. 50 kg
   b. 100-500 mcg/min   (2-10 mcg/kg/min)
   c. 200 mcg/min   (4 mcg/kg/min)
   d. Safe
   e. 4 : 5
   f. TD TV   HD HV
      4 : 5 :: x : 15   (x = 12 mg/hr)
   g. TD TV   HD HV
      4 : 5 :: 12 : x (x = 15 mL/hr)
   h. Correct

5. a. 0.4 mL
   b. 5 mL
   c. 3 min
   d. 7.2 = 7 seconds per calibration (approximate)
   e. 1.7 mL/min (1.66 rounded to 1.7)

8 Parenteral Nutrition

8A (PAGE 224)

1. Total grams per bag:
   % × mL = g/L   g/L × TV/L = g/bag
   a. AA 0.055 × 400 = 22 g/L   22 × 1.350 = 29.7 g/bag
   b. Dextrose 0.10 × 350 = 35 g/L   35 × 1.350 = 47.25 g/bag
   c. Lipids 0.10 × 200 = 20 g/L   20 × 1.350 = 27 g/bag

2. Percentages of concentration per bag:
   g/bag ÷ TV = % of concentration
   a. AA 29.7 g ÷ 1350 = 2.2%
   b. Dextrose 47.25 ÷ 1350 = 3.5%
   c. Lipids 27 ÷ 1350 = 2%

3. Percentages for additives per bag:
   mEq/L × TV/L = mEq/bag   mEq/bag ÷ TV = % in bag
   a. Calcium gluconate 5 × 1.35 = 6.75 mEq/bag 6.75 ÷ 1350 = 0.5% Ca gluconate
   b. Magnesium sulfate 10 × 1.35 = 13.5 mEq/bag 13.5 ÷ 1350 = 1% magnesium sulfate
   c. Potassium chloride 20 × 1.35 = 27 mEq/bag 27 ÷ 1350 = 2% K chloride
   d. Sodium chloride 30 × 1.35 = 40.5 mEq/bag   40.5 ÷ 1350 = 3% Na chloride

4. kcal per bag: KNOW
   a. CHO 47.25 × 4 = 189   PRO = 4 kcal/g
   b. PRO 29.7 × 4 = 118.8   CHO = 4 kcal/g
   c. FAT 27 × 9 = 243   FAT = 9 kcal/g
   d. Total kcal 550.8

5. mL/hr to set infusion device

   $\frac{TV}{TT}$ = mL/hr $\frac{1350}{12}$ = 112.5 = 113 mL/hr

8B (PAGE 227)

1. % × mL = g/L   g/L × TV/L = g/bag
   a. 0.085 × 500 = 42.5 g/L AA   42.5 × 1.5 = 63.75 g/bag
   b. 0.50 × 500 = 250 g/L DEX   250 × 1.5 = 375 g/bag
   c. 0.10 × 250 = 25 g/L LIP   25 × 1.5 = 37.5 g/bag

2. Percentage of concentration
   g/bag ÷ TV = % of concentration
   a. 63.75 ÷ 1500 = 4.25% AA
   b. 375 ÷ 1500 = 25% DEX
   c. 37.5 ÷ 1500 = 2.5% LIP

3. Percentage of additives
   mEq/L × TV/L = mEq/bag   MmEq/bag ÷ TV = % in bag
   a. 5 × 1.5 = 7.5 Calcium gluconate   7.5 ÷ 1500 = 0.5% Ca gluconate
   b. 15 × 1.5 = 22.5 magnesium sulfate   22.5 ÷ 1500 = 1.5% magnesium sulfate
   c. 8.3 × 1.5 = 12.45 potassium acetate   12.45 ÷ 1500 = 0.83% K acetate
   d. 35 × 1.5 = 52.5 potassium phosphate   52.5 ÷ 1500 = 3.5% K phosphate
   e. 35 × 1.5 = 52.5 sodium chloride   52.5 ÷ 1500 = 3.5% Na chloride

4. kcal per bag
  a. $63.75 \times 4 = 255$ kcal PRO
  b. $375 \times 4 = 1500$ kcal CHO
  c. $37.5 \times 9 = 337.5$ kcal FAT
  d. Total kcal = 2092.5

g/L $\times$
CHO = 4 kcal/g
PRO = 4 kcal/g
FAT = 9 kcal/g

5. mL/hr to set infusion device

$\frac{TV}{TT} = mL/hr$

$\frac{1500}{12} = 125$ mL/hr

8C (PAGE 229)

Total grams per bag
1. Formula: $5 \times mL = g/L$ **Formula: $g/L \times TV/L = g/bag$**
  Shortcut method: $\% \times mL = g/L \times TV/L = g/bag$
  AA $0.10 \times 900 = 90 \times 1.492 = 134.28$ g/bag
  Dex $0.70 \times 430 = 301 \times 1.492 = 449$ g/bag
  Percentage of concentrate per bag

2. Formula: $\frac{g/bag}{TV} = \%/bag$

  AA $\frac{134.28}{1492.74} = 0.0899 = 9\%$

  Dex $\frac{449}{1492.74} = 0.30 = 30\%$

Percentage of additives
3. Formula $mEq/L \times TV/L = mEq/bag$
  mEq/bag divided by $TV = \%$ in bag
  Shortcut method: $mEq/L \times TV/L$ divided by $TV = \%$ in bag
  a. Sodium chloride $140 \times 1.492 = 209$ divided by $1492 = 0.14 = 14\%$
  b. Potassium phosphate $41 \times 1.492 = 61$ divided by $1492 = 0.040 = 4\%$
  c. Potassium chloride $43 \times 1.492 = 64$ divided by $1492 = 0.042 = 4\%$
  d. Magnesium sulfate $7 \times 1.492 = 10$ divided by $1492 = 0.007 = 0.7\%$
  e. Calcium gluconate $7 \times 1.492 = 10$ divided by $1492 = 0.007 = 0.7\%$

Total kcal per bag
4. a. Protein 134.28 g $\times 4 = 537$ kcal
  b. Carbohydrate 449 g $\times 4 = 1796$ kcal
  c. Total kcal = 2333

5. KNOW   WANT TO KNOW
  55 mL : 1 hr :: 1492 mL : x hr
  $55x = 1 \times 1492 = 1492$
     $x = 27.127 = 27$ hr
  PROOF
  55 mL $\times 27.127 = 1491.9 = 1492$
  $1 \times 1492 = 1492$

8D (PAGE 230)

Total grams per bag
1. **Formulas: % × mL = g/L**
   g/L × TV/L = g/bag
   Shortcut method: % × mL = g/L × TV/L = g/bag
   AA 0.08 × 600 = 48 × 1.246 = 59.8 = 60 g/bag
   Dex 0.20 × 600 = 120 × 1.246 = 149.5 = 150 g/bag
   Percentage of concentrate per bag

2. **Formula: $\frac{g/bag}{TV}$ = %/bag**

   AA $\frac{60}{1246}$ = 0.048 = 4.8%/bag

   Dex $\frac{150}{1246}$ = 0.120 = 12%/bag

   Percentage of additives

3. **Formula: mEq/L × TV/L = mEq/bag**
   mEq/bag divided by TV = %/bag
   Shortcut method: mEq/L × TV/L divided by TV = %/bag
   Sodium chloride 42 × 1.246 = 52.3 divided by 1246 = 0.042 = 4.2%/bag
   Potassium phosphate 26 × 1.246 = 32.3 divided by 1246 = 0.026 = 2.6%/bag
   Potassium acetate 10 × 1.246 = 12.4 divided by 1246 = 0.01 = 1%/bag
   Calcium gluconate 6 × 1.246 = 7.4 divided by 1246 = 0.006 = 0.6%/bag
   Magnesium sulfate 6 × 1.246 = 7.4 divided by 1246 = 0.006 = 0.6%/bag
   kcal per bag

4. **Formula: 1 kcal of protein = 4 g; 1 kcal of dextrose = 4 g; 1 kcal of fat = 9 g**
   a. AA 60 × 4 = 240 kcal
   b. CHO 150 × 4 = 600 kcal
   c. Total kcal = 840

5. KNOW   WANT TO KNOW
   50 mL : 1 hr :: 1246 mL : x hr
   50x = 1 × 1246 = 1246
     x = 24.92   Convert .92 into minutes: 0.92 × 60 = 55 min
     x = 24 hr 55 min
   PROOF
   1 × 1246 = 1246
   50 × 24.92 = 1246

8E (PAGE 230)

1. **d.** $0.085 \times 375 = 31.8 \times 1.500 = 47.8$ g/bag of AA

2. **b.** $\frac{47.8}{1500} = 0.03 = 3\%$ conc. of AA

3. **a.** $0.40 \times 400 = 160 \times 1.450 = 232$ g/bag of dextrose

4. **b.** $\frac{232}{1450} = 0.16 = 16\%$ conc. of dextrose

5. **a.** $0.20 \times 175 = 35 \times 1.200 = 42$ g lipids/bag

6. **b.** $\frac{42}{1200} = 0.035 = 3.5\%$ conc. of lipids

7. **d.** $6 \times 1.350 = 8.1 \div 1350 = 0.006 = 0.6\%$ calcium gluconate

8. **a.** $10 \times 1.258 = 12.5 \div 1258 = 0.01 = 1\%$ magnesium sulfate

9. **c.** $12 \times 1.385 = 16.62 \div 1385 = 0.012 = 1.2\%$ potassium

10. **c.** KNOW   WANT TO KNOW
    110 mL : 1 hr :: 1275 mL : x hr
    $110x = 1275$
          $x = 11.59$ hr $= 11$ hr 35 min
    PROOF
    $1 \times 1275 = 1275$
    $110 \times 11.59 = 1275$
    IV started at 1800 hours plus 11 hr 35 min = 0535 hr

CHAPTER 8 FINAL: PARENTERAL NUTRITION (PAGE 232)

1. **a.** 66.85 g/bag of AA
   b. 267.4 kcal of PRO

2. **a.** 73.62 g/bag of dextrose
   b. 294.52 kcal of CHO

3. **a.** 22.4 g/bag of AA
   b. 89.6 kcal of PRO

4. **a.** 212 g/bag of dextrose
   b. 848 kcal of dextrose

5. 0.4% potassium chloride

6. 2.5% sodium chloride

7. 1559 total kcal

8. **a.** 25 g/bag of lipids
   b. 225 kcal of fat

9. At 0709 hr the infusion will be completed

10. 11 hr to infuse

9 Insulin

9A (PAGE 246)

1. 27 units	**2.** 68 units	**3.** 16 units	**4.** 44 units
5. 32 units	**6.** 78 units	**7.** 42 units	**8.** 39 units
9. 23 units	**10.** 18 units		

9B (PAGE 248)

1. a	**2.** b	**3.** b	**4.** a
5. a			

9C (PAGE 253)

1. Total units: 48
   b is correct

2. Total units: 39
   a is correct

3. Total units: 23
   a is correct

4. Total units: 38
   b is correct

5. Total units: 68
   a is correct
   b insulins are reversed–drawn up incorrectly.

6. 15 units
   Peak: 1 to 3 hr

7. 10 units
   Onset: 15 min

8. 44 units
   Peak: 30 to 90 min and 6 to 10 hr
   Duration: 4 to 5 hr and 10 to 16 hr

9. 50 units
   Duration: up to 24 hr; dose dependent

10. 42 units
   Peak: 2 to 4 hr for R
   Duration: 10 to 16 hr for N

9D (PAGE 258)

1. BGL difference is 20 divided by 10 = 2 units of R
   CHO is 48 g divided by 8 = 6 units R

2. BGL difference is 5 divided by 10 = 0.5 = 1 unit R (rounded to nearest whole number)
   CHO is 71 g divided by 8 = 8.87 = 9 units R

3. BGL difference is 15 divided by 10 = 1.5 = 2 units R
   CHO is 34 g divided by 8 = 4.25 = 4 units R
   Snack: BGL difference is 15 divided by 10 = 1.5 = 2 units R
   CHO is 15 g divided by 8 = 1.87 = 2 units R
   Total insulin for the day = 28 units

4. BGL difference is −5 = 0 units R
   CHO is 43 g divided by 10 = 4.3 = 4 units R

5. BGL difference is 20 divided by 10 = 2 units
   CHO is 93 g divided by 10 = 9.3 = 9 units R

9E (PAGE 260)

1. BGL difference is 30 divided by 20 = 1.5 = 2 units R
   CHO is 98 g divided by 6.5 = 7 units R
   Total = 9 units R

2. BGL difference is 50 divided by 20 = 2.5 = 3 units R
   CHO is 118 g divided by 15 = 7.8 = 8 units R
   Total = 11 units R

3. BGL difference is 20 divided by 20 = 2.5 = 1 unit R
   CHO is 40 g divided by 15 = 2.6 = 3 units R
   Total = 4 units R

4. BGL difference is 90 divided by 3 = 3 units R
   CHO is 58 g divided by 10 = 5.8 = 6 units R
   Total = 9 units R

5. BGL difference is 30 divided by 30 = 1 unit R
   CHO is 120 g divided by 10 = 12 units R
   Total = 13 units R

6. BGL difference is 110 divided by 30 = 3.6 = 4 units R
   CHO is 58 g divided by 10 = 5.8 = 6 units R
   Total = 10 units R

7. BGL difference is 10 divided by 30 = 0.3 = 0 units R
   CHO is 28 g divided by 10 = 2.8 = 3 units R
   Total = 3 units R

8. BGL difference is 10 divided by 20 = 0.5 = 1 unit R
   CHO is 45 g divided by 8 = 5.6 = 6 units R
   Total = 7 units R

9. BGL difference is 30 divided by 20 = 1.5 = 2 units R
   CHO is 80 g divided by 8 = 10 units R
   Total = 12 units R

10. BGL difference is −10 = 0 units R
    CHO is 85 g divided by 8 = 10.6 = 11 units R
    Total = 11 units R

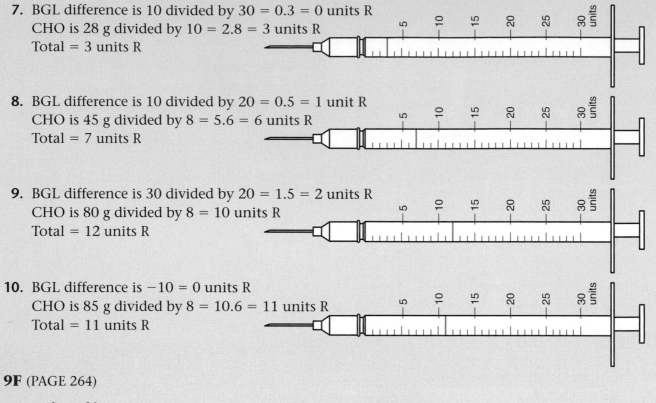

9F (PAGE 264)

1. $\dfrac{\text{total g}}{\text{units}} = \dfrac{26}{13} = 2$ units R

2. $\dfrac{\text{total g}}{\text{units}} = \dfrac{80}{9} = 8.8 = 9$ units R

3. $\dfrac{\text{total g}}{\text{units}} = \dfrac{18}{16} = 1.1 = 1$ unit R

4. $\dfrac{\text{total g}}{\text{units}} = \dfrac{90}{6} = 15$ units R

5. $\dfrac{\text{total g}}{\text{units}} = \dfrac{160}{11} = 14.5$ units = 15 units R for 24 hr

6. $\dfrac{\text{total g}}{\text{units}} = \dfrac{145}{7} = 20.7 = 21$ units R for 24 hr

7. $\dfrac{1}{2}$ of 45 = 22.5 + $\dfrac{3}{4}$ of 75 = 56.25 = 78.75 = 9.8 = 10 units R

8. 50 g divided by 2 = $\dfrac{25\,\text{g}}{10} = 2.5 = 3$ units R

9. Total amount of CHO = 179 g

   $\dfrac{179}{12} = 14.9 = 15$ units for the day

10. $\dfrac{1}{2}$ of 38 = 19 g; $\dfrac{1}{4}$ of 50 = 12.5 g; 13 of 48 = 16 g

    Total CHO grams = 47.5 = 3 units total for the 3 meals

9G (PAGE 266)

1. **a.** 4 mL/hr
   b. 3 units/hr

3. 21 total units

5. **a.** KNOW   WANT TO KNOW
   100 units : 50 mL :: x units : 3 mL
   $50x = 100 \times 3 = 300$
   $x = 6$ units/hr
   PROOF
   $100 \times 3 = 300$
   $50 \times 6 = 300$
   b. 8 hr $\times$ 6 units per hr = 48 units

2. **a.** KNOW   WANT TO KNOW
   100 units : 100 mL :: 2.5 units : x mL
   $100x = 100 \times 2.5 = 250$
   $x = 2.5$ mL/hr
   PROOF
   $100 \times 2.5 = 250$
   $100 \times 2.5 = 250$
   b. Change IV rate to 3 mL/hr
   c. 5.5 units

4. **a.** KNOW   WANT TO KNOW
   50 mL : 100 units :: x mL : 5 units
   $100x = 50 \times 5 = 250$
   $x = 2.5$ mL/hr
   PROOF
   $100 \times 2.5 = 250$
   $50 \times 5 = 250$
   b. 5 units per hour $\times$ 16 hours = 80 units of insulin

6. KNOW   WANT TO KNOW
   100 units : 150 mL :: 10 units : x mL
   $100x = 150 \times 10 = 1500$
   $100x = 1500$
   $x = 15$ mL/hr = 10 units insulin
   PROOF
   $100 \times 15 = 1500$
   $150 \times 10 = 1500$

   KNOW   WANT TO KNOW
   15 mL : 1 hr :: 150 mL : x hr
   $15x = 150$
   $x = 10$ hr to infuse 100 units insulin
   PROOF
   $15 \times 10 = 150$
   $1 \times 150 = 150$

7. KNOW   WANT TO KNOW

50 mL : 50 units :: x mL : 8 units

$50x = 50 \times 8 = 400$

$50x = 400$

   $x = 8$ mL/hr = 8 units of insulin

PROOF

$50 \times 8 = 400$

$50 \times 8 = 400$

KNOW   WANT TO KNOW

8 mL : 1 hr :: 50 mL : x hr

$8x = 50$

   $x = 6.25$ hr to infuse 50 units insulin or

      6 hr 15 min

PROOF

$8 \times 6.25 = 50$

$1 \times 50 = 50$

8. KNOW   WANT TO KNOW

50 mL : 75 units :: x mL : 15 units

$75x = 50 \times 15 = 750$

$75x = 750$

   $x = 10$ mL/hr = 15 units

PROOF

$50 \times 15 = 750$

$75 \times 10 = 750$

KNOW   WANT TO KNOW

67 mL : 1 hr :: 50 mL : x hr

$67x = 50$

   $x = 0.74 = 44$ min to infuse

PROOF

$67 \times 0.74 = 49.58$

$1 \times 50 = 50$

9. KNOW   WANT TO KNOW

100 mL : 120 units :: x mL : 10 units

$120x = 100 \times 10 = 1000$

$120x = 1000$

     $x = 8.33$ mL/hr to deliver 10 units of

       insulin

PROOF

$120 \times 8.33 = 999.6$

$100 \times 10 = 1000$

KNOW   WANT TO KNOW

8 mL : 1 hr :: 100 mL : x hr

$8x = 1 \times 100 = 100$

$8x = 100$

   $x = 12.5$ hr to infuse 120 units of regular

     insulin

PROOF

$8 \times 12.5 = 100$

$1 \times 100 = 100$

10. KNOW   WANT TO KNOW

150 mL : 150 units :: x mL : 12 units

$150x = 150 \times 12$

$150x = 1800$

     $x = 12$ mL/hr to deliver 12 units

       of insulin

PROOF

$150 \times 12 = 1800$

$12 \times 150 = 1800$

KNOW   WANT TO KNOW

12 mL : 1 hr :: 150 mL : x hr

$12x = 150$

   $x = 12.5$ hr to infuse 150 units of regular

     insulin, or 12 hr 30 min

$12 \times 12.5 = 150$

$1 \times 150 = 150$

9H (PAGE 268)

1. 500 mL : 100 units :: x mL : 8 units

  $100x = 500 \times 8 = 4000$

     $x = 40$ mL/hr

PROOF

  $100 \times 40 = 4000$

  $500 \times 8 = 4000$

2. 500 mL : 100 units :: x mL : 10 units

  $100x = 500 \times 10 = 5000$

     $x = 50$ mL/hr

PROOF

  $100 \times 50 = 5000$

  $10 \times 500 = 5000$

3. a. 50 units : 250 mL :: 2 units : x mL
  $50x = 250 \times 2 = 500$
  $x = 10$ mL/hr
  PROOF
  $250 \times 2 = 500$
  $50 \times 10 = 500$

b. 2 units : 1 hr :: 50 units : x hr
  $2x = 50$
  $x = 25$ hr
  PROOF
  $2 \times 25 = 50$
  $1 \times 50 = 50$

4. 500 mL : 15 hr :: x mL : 1 hr
  $15x = 500$
  $x = 33.3 = 33$ mL/hr
  PROOF
  $15 \times 33.3 = 499.9 = 500$
  $500 \times 1 = 500$

5. a. 500 mL : 50 units :: x mL : 3 units
  $50x = 500 \times 3 = 1500$
  $x = 30$ mL/hr
  PROOF
  $50 \times 30 = 1500$
  $500 \times 3 = 1500$

b. 3 units : 1 hr :: 50 units : x hr
  $3x = 50$
  $x = 16.66$ hr
  $0.66 \times 60 = 39.6 = 40$ min
  $x = 16$ hr 40 min
  PROOF
  $3 \times 16.66 = 49.9 = 50$
  $50 \times 1 = 50$
  OR
  30 mL : 1 hr :: 500 mL : x hr
  $3x = 500$
  $x = 16.66$ hr
  $0.66 \times 60 = 39.6 = 40$ min
  $x = 16$ hr 40 min
  PROOF
  $30 \times 16.66 = 499.8 = 500$

c. The IV will be infused at 2340 hours.

6. 20 units : 250 mL :: 1 unit : x mL
  $20x = 250$
  $x = 12.5 = 13$ mL/hr
  PROOF
  $12.5 \times 20 = 250$
  $250 \times 1 = 250$

7. a. 150 mL : 50 units :: x mL : 2 units

$50x = 2 \times 150 = 300$

$x = 6$ mL/hr

PROOF

$50 \times 6 = 300$

$150 \times 2 = 300$

b. 6 mL : 1 hr :: 150 mL : x hr

$6x = 150$

$x = 25$ hr

PROOF

$6 \times 25 = 150$

$1 \times 150 = 150$

8. a. 500 mL : 30 units :: x mL : 4 units

$30x = 500 \times 4 = 2000$

$x = 66.6 = 67$ mL/hr

PROOF

$30 \times 66.6 = 1999.9 = 2000$

$4 \times 500 = 2000$

b. 66.6 mL : 1 hr :: 500 mL : x hr

$66.6x = 500$

$x = 7.5$ hr = 7 hr 30 min

PROOF

$66.6 \times 7.5 = 499.95$

$1 \times 500 = 500$

c. The IV will be infused at 1330 hours.

9. a. 30 units : 250 mL :: x units : 20 mL

$250x = 30 \times 20 = 600$

$x = 2.4$ units/hr

PROOF

$2.4 \times 12.5 = 30$

$1 \times 30 = 30$

b. 2.4 units : 1 hr :: 30 units : x hr

$2.4x = 30$

$x = 12.5$ hr $0.5 \times 60 = 30$ min

$x = 12$ hr and 30 min

PROOF

$2.4 \times 12.5 = 30$

$1 \times 30 = 30$

10. a. 250 mL : 50 units :: x mL : 2 units

$50x = 250 \times 2 = 500$

$x = 10$ mL/hr

PROOF

$50 \times 10 = 500$

$2 \times 250 = 500$

b. 10 mL : 1 hr :: 250 mL : x hr

$10x = 250$

$x = 25$ hr

PROOF

$10 \times 25 = 250$

$1 \times 250 = 250$

9I (PAGE 269)

1. d. 4 units

KNOW   WANT TO KNOW

250 mL : 100 units :: 10 mL : x units

$250x = 100 \times 10 = 1000$

$x = 4$ units/hr

PROOF

$250 \times 4 = 1000$

$100 \times 10 = 1000$

2. b. 25 hr

KNOW   WANT TO KNOW

4 units : 1 hr :: 100 units : x hr

$4x = 100$

$x = 25$ hr

PROOF

$1 \times 100 = 100$

$4 \times 25 = 100$

3. c. 3 mL/hr

KNOW   WANT TO KNOW

100 units : 100 mL :: 3 units : x mL

$100x = 100 \times 3 = 300$

$x = 3$ mL/hr

PROOF

$100 \times 3 = 300$

$100 \times 3 = 300$

4. b. 2.5 units/hr

KNOW   WANT TO KNOW

30 units : 12 hr :: x units : 1 hr

$12x = 30$

$x = 2.5$ units/hr

PROOF

$30 \times 1 = 30$

$12 \times 2.5 = 30$

a. 4 mL/hr

50 mL : 12 hr :: x mL : 1 hr

$12x = 50$

$x = 4.16 = 4$ mL/hr

PROOF

$50 \times 1 = 50$

$12 \times 4.16 = 4.9$

5. a. 50 mL/hr

KNOW   WANT TO KNOW

500 mL : 100 units :: x mL : 10 units

$100x = 500 \times 10 = 5000$

$x = 50$ mL/hr

PROOF

$100 \times 50 = 5000$

$500 \times 10 = 5000$

6. c. Humulin R

7. d. 24 hr

8. b. 4 to 10 hr

9. d. is peakless

10. b. anytime

CHAPTER 9 FINAL: INSULIN (PAGE 272)

1. 15 units

b

2. Sliding scale

Give 8 units.

3. 16 units Humulin R

30 units Humulin N

Total amount is 46 units.

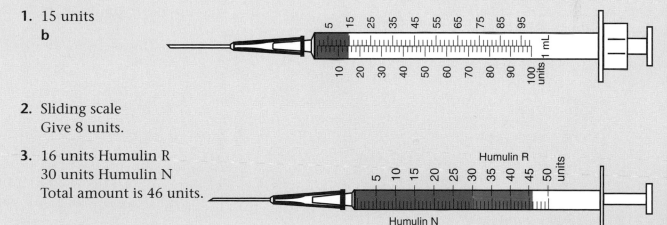

4. 18 units Humalog
   b is easier to read

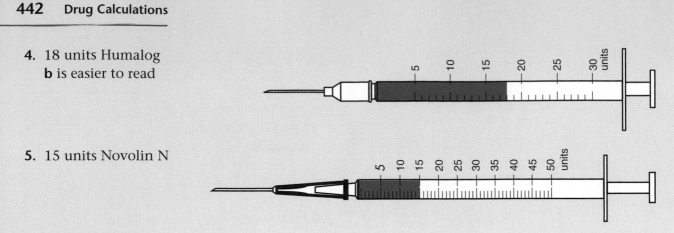

5. 15 units Novolin N

6. 20 mL/hr = 10 units
   25 hr to infuse. An IV solution can hang for only 24 hr (CDC guidelines).

7. 15 mL/hr to infuse 6 units insulin
   16.6 hr to infuse = 16 hr 36 min

8. 20 mL/hr to infuse 8 units insulin
   12.5 hr to infuse = 12 hr 30 min

9. 14 mL/hr to infuse 7 units insulin
   14.28 hr to infuse = 14 hr 17 min

10. 45 mL/hr to infuse 9 units insulin
    11.1 hr to infuse = 11 hr 6 min

10 Anticoagulants

10A (PAGE 280)

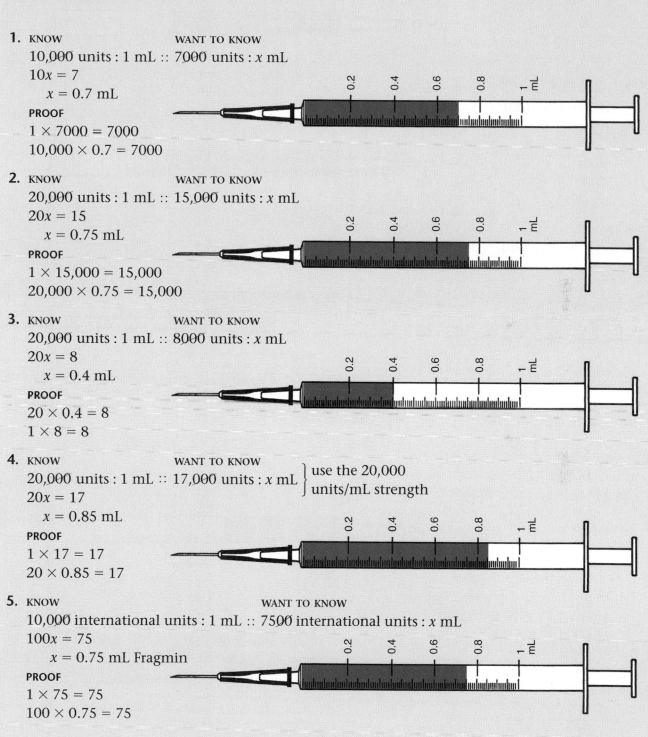

1. KNOW WANT TO KNOW
10,000 units : 1 mL :: 7000 units : x mL
10x = 7
  x = 0.7 mL
PROOF
1 × 7000 = 7000
10,000 × 0.7 = 7000

2. KNOW WANT TO KNOW
20,000 units : 1 mL :: 15,000 units : x mL
20x = 15
  x = 0.75 mL
PROOF
1 × 15,000 = 15,000
20,000 × 0.75 = 15,000

3. KNOW WANT TO KNOW
20,000 units : 1 mL :: 8000 units : x mL
20x = 8
  x = 0.4 mL
PROOF
20 × 0.4 = 8
1 × 8 = 8

4. KNOW WANT TO KNOW
20,000 units : 1 mL :: 17,000 units : x mL } use the 20,000 units/mL strength
20x = 17
  x = 0.85 mL
PROOF
1 × 17 = 17
20 × 0.85 = 17

5. KNOW WANT TO KNOW
10,000 international units : 1 mL :: 7500 international units : x mL
100x = 75
  x = 0.75 mL Fragmin
PROOF
1 × 75 = 75
100 × 0.75 = 75

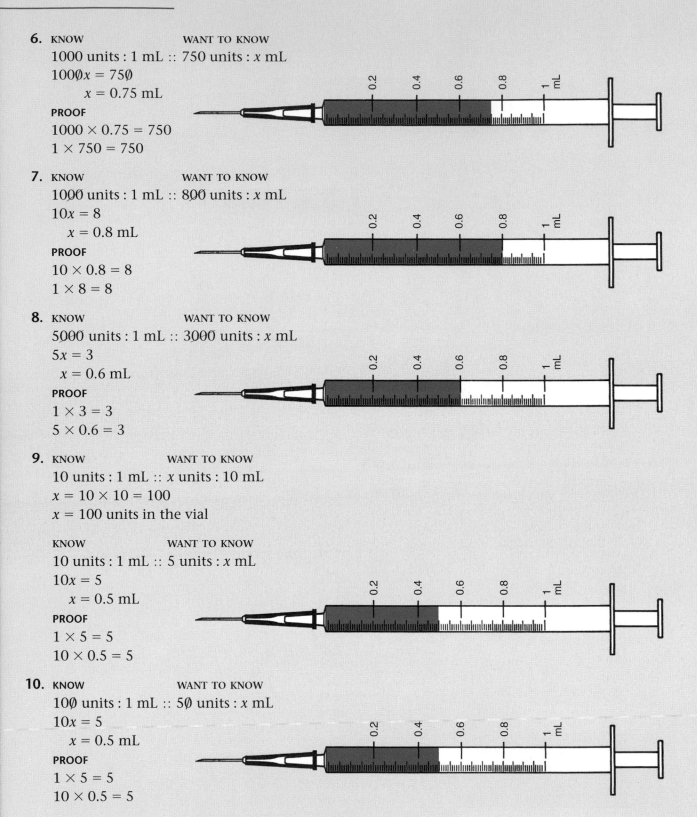

6. KNOW   WANT TO KNOW

1000 units : 1 mL :: 750 units : x mL

1000x = 750

     x = 0.75 mL

PROOF

1000 × 0.75 = 750

1 × 750 = 750

7. KNOW   WANT TO KNOW

1000 units : 1 mL :: 800 units : x mL

10x = 8

     x = 0.8 mL

PROOF

10 × 0.8 = 8

1 × 8 = 8

8. KNOW   WANT TO KNOW

5000 units : 1 mL :: 3000 units : x mL

5x = 3

     x = 0.6 mL

PROOF

1 × 3 = 3

5 × 0.6 = 3

9. KNOW   WANT TO KNOW

10 units : 1 mL :: x units : 10 mL

x = 10 × 10 = 100

x = 100 units in the vial

KNOW   WANT TO KNOW

10 units : 1 mL :: 5 units : x mL

10x = 5

     x = 0.5 mL

PROOF

1 × 5 = 5

10 × 0.5 = 5

10. KNOW   WANT TO KNOW

100 units : 1 mL :: 50 units : x mL

10x = 5

     x = 0.5 mL

PROOF

1 × 5 = 5

10 × 0.5 = 5

10B (PAGE 284)

1. a. KNOW   WANT TO KNOW
20,000 units : 1000 mL ::
1000 units : x mL
$20x = 1000$
$x = 50$ mL/hr = 1000 units heparin
PROOF
$20 \times 50 = 1000$
$1000 \times 1 = 1000$

b. KNOW   WANT TO KNOW
50 mL : 1 hr :: 1000 mL : x hr
$50x = 1000$
$x = 20$ hr
PROOF
$1 \times 1000 = 1000$
$50 \times 20 = 1000$

3. a. KNOW   WANT TO KNOW
20,000 units : 1000 mL ::
1500 units : x mL
$200x = 15,000$
$x = 75$ mL/hr = 1500 units heparin
PROOF
$200 \times 75 = 15,000$
$100 \times 15 = 15,000$

b. KNOW   WANT TO KNOW
75 mL : 1 hr :: 1000 mL : x hr
$75x = 1000$
$x = 13.33$ hr or 13 hr, 20 min
PROOF
$1 \times 1000 = 1000$
$75 \times 13.33 = 999.75$

2. a. $\frac{1000}{12} = 83.3$ or 83 mL/hr
b. KNOW   WANT TO KNOW
20,000 units : 12 hr :: x units : 1 hr
$12x = 20,000$
$x = 1666.6$ units/hr = 1667 units/hr
PROOF
$20,000 \times 1 = 20,000$
$12 \times 1666 = 19,992$

c. KNOW   WANT TO KNOW
83 mL : 1 hr :: 750 mL : x hr
$83x = 750$
$x = 9$ hr remaining
PROOF
$1 \times 750 = 750$
$83 \times 9 = 747$

4. a. KNOW   WANT TO KNOW
10,000 units : 15 hr :: x units : 1 hr
$15x = 10,000$
$x = 666.6$ units/hr = 667 units/hr
PROOF
$15 \times 666.6 = 9999$
$10,000 \times 1 = 10,000$
b. $\frac{1000}{15} = 66.6$ or 67 mL/hr
c. KNOW   WANT TO KNOW
67 mL : 1 hr :: 700 mL : x hr
$67x = 700$
$x = 10.45$ hr or 10 hr 27 min remaining
The IV will be infused at 1727 hours.
PROOF
$1 \times 700 = 700$
$67 \times 10.45 = 700$

5. a. KNOW   WANT TO KNOW

10,000 units : 500 mL ::

      1200 units : x mL

$100x = 6000$

  $x = 60$ mL/hr

PROOF

$500 \times 12 = 6000$

$100 \times 60 = 6000$

b. KNOW   WANT TO KNOW

60 mL : 1 hr :: 500 mL : x hr

$60x = 500$

  $x = 8.33$ hr or 8 hr 20 min

PROOF

$60 \times 8.33 = 499.8$

$1 \times 500 = 500$

6. a. KNOW   WANT TO KNOW

50,000 units : 1000 mL ::

      2500 units : x mL

$500x = 25 \times 1000 = 25,000$

  $5x = 250$

  $x = 50$ mL/hr

PROOF

$500 \times 50 = 25,000$

$1000 \times 25 = 25,000$

b. KNOW   WANT TO KNOW

50 mL : 1 hr :: 1000 mL : x hr

$50x = 1000$

  $x = 20$ hr

PROOF

$50 \times 20 = 1000$

$1 \times 1000 = 1000$

7. a. KNOW   WANT TO KNOW

25,000 units : 500 mL ::

      1500 units : x mL

$250x = 500 \times 15 = 7500$

 $25x = 750$

  $x = 30$ mL/hr

PROOF

$25 \times 750 = 7500$

$500 \times 15 = 7500$

b. KNOW   WANT TO KNOW

30 mL : 1 hr :: 500 mL : x hr

$30x = 500$

 $3x = 50$

 $x = 16.6$ hr = 16 hr 36 min

PROOF

$1 \times 500 = 500$

$30 \times 16.6 = 499.9$

8. a. KNOW   WANT TO KNOW

25,000 units : 500 mL ::

      1300 units : x mL

$250x = 6500$

  $x = 26$ mL/hr

PROOF

$26 \times 250 = 6500$

$500 \times 13 = 6500$

b. KNOW   WANT TO KNOW

26 mL : 1 hr :: 500 mL : x hr

$26x = 500$

  $x = 19.23$ hr or 19 hr 14 min

PROOF

$1 \times 500 = 500$

$26 \times 19.23 = 499.98$

9. a. KNOW   WANT TO KNOW

25,000 units : 250 mL ::

      1800 units : x mL

$250x = 4500$

  $x = 18$ mL/hr

PROOF

$250 \times 18 = 4500$

$250 \times 18 = 4500$

b. KNOW   WANT TO KNOW

18 mL : 1 hr :: 250 mL : x hr

$18x = 250$

  $x = 13.88$ hr or 13 hr 53 min

PROOF

$1 \times 250 = 250$

$18 \times 13.8 = 248.4$

10. a. KNOW   WANT TO KNOW

20,000 units : 250 mL ::

      1000 units : x mL

$20x = 250$

  $x = 12.5$ mL/hr or 13 mL/hr

PROOF

$20 \times 12.5 = 250$

$250 \times 1 = 250$

b. KNOW   WANT TO KNOW

13 mL : 1 hr :: 250 mL : x hr

$13x = 250$

  $x = 19.23$ hr or 19 hr 14 min

PROOF

$1 \times 250 = 250$

$13 \times 19.2 = 249.8$

10C (PAGE 286)

1. lb to kg = 172 ÷ 2.2 = 80 kg

  a. KNOW   WANT TO KNOW

  70 units : 1 kg :: x units : 80 kg

  $x = 70 \times 80 = 5600$ units loading dose

  PROOF

  $1 \times 5600 = 5600$

  $70 \times 80 = 5600$

  b. KNOW   WANT TO KNOW

  20 units : 1 kg/hr :: x units : 80 kg/hr

  $x = 20 \times 80 = 1600$

  $x = 1600$ units/hr

  PROOF

  $1 \times 1600 = 16,000$

  $20 \times 80 = 16,000$

  c. KNOW   WANT TO KNOW

  1000 mL : 25,000 units ::

              x mL : 1600 units

  $250x = 1000 \times 16 = 16,000$

  $250x = 64$ mL/hr

  PROOF

  $64 \times 250 = 16,000$

  $16 \times 1000 = 16,000$

2. lb to kg = 160 lb divided by 2.2 kg =
              $72.7 = 73$ kg

  a. KNOW   WANT TO KNOW

  80 units : 1 kg :: x units : 73 kg

  $x = 80 \times 73 = 5840$

  $x = 5840$ units loading dose

  PROOF

  $1 \times 5840 = 5840$

  $73 \times 80 = 5840$

  b. KNOW   WANT TO KNOW

  1000 mL : 30,000 units ::

              x mL : 1500 units

  $300x = 1000 \times 15 = 15,000$

  $3x = 150$

   $x = 50$ mL/hr

  PROOF

  $50 \times 300 = 15,000$

  $15 \times 1000 = 15,000$

3. lb to kg = 210 lb divided by 2.2 =
              $95.5 = 96$ kg

  a. KNOW   WANT TO KNOW

  90 units : 1 kg :: x units : 96 kg

  $x = 90 \times 96 = 8640$

  $x = 8640$ units loading dose

  PROOF

  $1 \times 8640 = 8640$

  $90 \times 96 = 8640$

  b. KNOW   WANT TO KNOW

  25 units : 1 kg :: x units : 96 kg/hr

  $x = 25 \times 96 = 2400$

  $x = 2400$ units/hr

  PROOF

  $25 \times 96 = 2400$

  c. KNOW   WANT TO KNOW

  1000 mL : 25,000 units ::

              x mL : 2400 units

  $250x = 1000 \times 24 = 24,000$

  $25x = 2400 = 96$

   $x = 96$ mL/hr

  PROOF

  $96 \times 25 = 24,000$

  $24 \times 1000 = 24,000$

4. lb to kg = 300 lb divided by 2.2 =
              $136.3 = 136$ kg

  a. KNOW   WANT TO KNOW

  75 units : 1 kg :: x units : 136 kg

  $x = 75 \times 136 = 10,200$

  $x = 10,200$ units bolus dose

  PROOF

  $1 \times 2720 = 10,200$

  $75 \times 136 = 10,200$

  b. KNOW   WANT TO KNOW

  20 units : 1 kg :: x units : 136 kg

  $x = 20 \times 136 = 2720$

  $x = 2720$ units/hr

  PROOF

  $1 \times 2720 = 2720$

  $20 \times 136 = 2720$

  c. KNOW   WANT TO KNOW

  1000 mL : 50,000 units ::

              x mL : 2720 units

  $5000x = 1000 \times 272 = 272,000$

    $5x = 272$

     $x = 54.4 = 54$ mL/hr

  PROOF

  $1000 \times 272 = 272,000$

  $54.4 \times 5000 = 272,000$

5. lb to kg = 185 divided by 2.2 =
$$84.09 = 84 \text{ kg}$$

  a. KNOW   WANT TO KNOW
    75 units : 1 kg :: x units : 84 kg
    $x = 75 \times 84 = 6300$
    $x = 6300$ units bolus dose
    PROOF
    $1 \times 6300 = 6300$
    $75 \times 84 = 6300$

  b. KNOW   WANT TO KNOW
    17 units : 1 kg/hr :: x units : 84 kg/hr
    $x = 17 \times 84 = 1428$
    $x = 1428$ units/hr
    PROOF
    $1 \times 1428 = 1428$
    $17 \times 84 = 1428$

  c. KNOW   WANT TO KNOW
    1000 mL : 20,000 units ::
                        x mL : 1428 units
    $20,000x = 1000 \times 1428 = 1,428,000$
          $20x = 1428$
             $x = 71.4 = 71 \text{ mL/hr}$
    PROOF
    $1000 \times 1428 = 1,428,000$
    $20,000 \times 71.4 = 1,428,000$

7. **a.** KNOW   WANT TO KNOW
    80 units : 1 kg :: x units : 120 kg
    $x = 80 \times 120 = 9600$
    $x = 9600$ units bolus dose
    PROOF
    $1 \times 9600 = 9600$
    $80 \times 120 = 9600$

  b. KNOW   WANT TO KNOW
    1000 mL : 25,000 units ::
                    x mL : 1000 units
    $25x = 1000$
      $x = 40 \text{ mL/hr}$
    PROOF
    $25 \times 40 = 1000$
    $1 \times 1000 = 1000$

6. lb to kg = 145 divided by 2.2 =
$$65.9 = 66 \text{ kg}$$

  a. KNOW   WANT TO KNOW
    65 units : 1 kg :: x units : 66 kg
    $x = 65 \times 66 = 4290$
    $x = 4290$ units bolus dose
    PROOF
    $1 \times 4290 = 4290$
    $65 \times 66 = 4290$

  b. KNOW   WANT TO KNOW
    15 units : 1 kg/hr :: x units : 66 kg/hr
    $x = 15 \times 66 = 990$ units
    $x = 990$ units/hr
    PROOF
    $1 \times 990 = 990$
    $15 \times 66 = 990$

  c. KNOW   WANT TO KNOW
    500 mL : 30,000 units :: x mL : 990 units
    $30,000x = 500 \times 990 = 495,000$
         $30x = 495$
          $x = 16.5 = 17 \text{ mL/hr}$
    PROOF
    $990 \times 500 = 495,000$
    $30,000 \times 16.5 = 495,000$

8. lb to kg = 194 divided by 2.2 = 88 kg

  a. KNOW   WANT TO KNOW
    70 units : 1 kg :: x units : 88 kg
    $x = 70 \times 88 = 6160$
    $x = 6160$ units bolus dose
    PROOF
    $1 \times 6160 = 6160$
    $70 \times 88 = 6160$

  b. KNOW   WANT TO KNOW
    18 units : 1 kg :: x units : 88 kg
    $x = 18 \times 88 = 1584$
    $x = 1584$ units/hr
    PROOF
    $1 \times 1584 = 1584$
    $18 \times 88 = 1584$

  c. KNOW   WANT TO KNOW
    1000 mL : 30,000 units ::
                    x mL : 1584 units
    $30,000x = 1584 \times 1000 = 1,584,000$
         $30x = 1584$
          $x = 52.8 = 53 \text{ mL/hr}$
    PROOF
    $30 \times 52.8 = 1584$
    $1 \times 1584 = 1584$

9. a. KNOW   WANT TO KNOW

95 units : 1 kg :: x units : 136 kg

$x = 95 \times 136 = 12{,}920$

$x = 12{,}920$ units loading dose

PROOF

$1 \times 12{,}920 = 12{,}920$

$95 \times 136 = 12{,}920$

b. KNOW   WANT TO KNOW

20 units : 1 kg/hr :: x units : 136 kg/hr

$x = 20 \times 136 = 2720$

$x = 2720$ units/hr

PROOF

$1 \times 2720 = 2720$

$20 \times 136 = 22{,}720$

c. KNOW   WANT TO KNOW

1000 mL : 20,000 units ::

$\qquad\qquad x$ mL : 2720 units

$2000x = 1000 \times 272 = 272{,}000$

$\quad 2x = 272 = 136$

$\quad\; x = 136$ mL/hr

PROOF

$2000 \times 136 = 272{,}000$

$1000 \times 272 = 272{,}000$

10. a. KNOW   WANT TO KNOW

1000 units : 1 kg :: x units : 108 kg

$x = 100 \times 108 = 10{,}800$

$x = 10{,}800$ units loading dose

PROOF

$1 \times 10{,}800 = 10{,}800$

$1000 \times 108 = 10{,}800$

b. KNOW   WANT TO KNOW

18 units : 1 kg :: x units : 108 kg

$x = 18 \times 108 = 1944$

$x = 1944$ units/hr

PROOF

$1 \times 1944 = 1944$

$18 \times 108 = 1944$

c. KNOW   WANT TO KNOW

1000 mL : 35,000 units ::

$\qquad\qquad x$ mL : 1944 units

$35x = 1944$

$\quad x = 55.54 = 56$ mL/hr

PROOF

$35 \times 55.54 = 1939$

$1944 \times 1 = 1944$

10D (PAGE 289)

1. c. KNOW   WANT TO KNOW

120 international units : 1 kg ::

$\qquad x$ international units : 84 kg

$x = 120 \times 84 = 10{,}080$

$x = 10{,}080$ international units of

Fragmin

PROOF

$120 \times 84 = 10{,}080$

$1 \times 10{,}080 = 10{,}080$

3. c. KNOW   WANT TO KNOW

1 kg : 2.2 lb :: x kg : 132 lb

$2.2x = 132$

$\quad x = 60$ kg

PROOF

$1 \times 132 = 132$

$2.2 \times 60 = 132$

d. KNOW   WANT TO KNOW

120 international units : 1 kg ::

$\qquad\quad x$ international units : 60 kg

$x = 60 \times 120$

$x = 7200$ international units q12h

PROOF

$1 \times 7200 = 7200$

$60 \times 120 = 7200$

2. b. KNOW   WANT TO KNOW

25,000 international units : 1 mL ::

$\qquad\qquad$ 10,080 : x mL

$25{,}000x = 10{,}080$

$\qquad x = 0.4$ mL

PROOF

$1 \times 10{,}080 = 10{,}080$ (units can be

rounded up or down)

$0.4 \times 25{,}000 = 10{,}000$

4. a. KNOW   WANT TO KNOW

10,000 international units : 1 mL ::

$\qquad$ 7200 international units : L : x mL

$10{,}000x = 7200$

$\qquad x = 0.72 = 0.7$ mL

PROOF

$7200 \times 1 = 7200$

$10{,}000 \times 0.72 = 7200$

5. a. KNOW   WANT TO KNOW

80 units : 1 kg :: x units : 73 kg

$x = 80 \times 73 = 5840$

$x = 5840$ units of heparin

PROOF

$1 \times 5840 = 5840$

$80 \times 73 = 5840$

6. d. KNOW   WANT TO KNOW

18 units : 1 kg :: x units : 80 kg

$x = 18 \times 80 = 1440$

$x = 1440$ units/hr

PROOF

$1 \times 1440 = 1440$

$18 \times 80 = 1440$

d. KNOW   WANT TO KNOW

1000 mL : 20,000 units ::

           x mL : 1440 units

$20,000x = 1000 \times 1440 = 1,440,000$

$x = 72$ mL/hr

PROOF

$1000 \times 1440 = 1,440,000$

$72 \times 20,000 = 1,440,000$

7. b. KNOW   WANT TO KNOW

1000 mL : 25,000 units ::

           x mL : 3000 units

$25,000x = 3,000,000$

$25x = 120$ mL/hr

PROOF

$25 \times 120 = 3000$

$1000 \times 3 = 3000$

8. d. KNOW   WANT TO KNOW

10,000 units : 500 mL :: 500 units : x mL

$10,000x = 250,000$

$x = 25$ mL/hr

PROOF

$25 \times 10,000 = 250,000$

$500 \times 500 = 250,000$

9. a. 220 divided by 2.2 = 100 kg

d. KNOW   WANT TO KNOW

120 international units : 1 kg ::

         x international units : 100 kg

$x = 120 \times 100 = 12,000$

$x = 12,000$ international units Fragmin

PROOF

$1 \times 12,000 = 12,000$

$100 \times 120 = 12,000$

10. c. KNOW   WANT TO KNOW

25,000 international units : 1 mL ::

         12,000 international units : x mL

$25,000x = 12,000$

$x = 0.48$ mL

PROOF

$1 \times 12,000 = 12,000$

$25,000 \times 0.48 = 12,000$

CHAPTER 10 FINAL: ANTICOAGULANTS (PAGE 291)

1. 0.8 mL

2. 0.25 mL

3. 0.2 mL using the 10,000 units/mL strength
or 0.4 mL using the 5000 units/mL strength

4. 0.35 mL using the 20,000 units/mL strength
or 0.7 mL using the 10,000 units/mL strength

5. 0.8 mL

6. 17.5 mL/hr or 18 mL/hr
28 hr, 34 min

7. 30 mL/hr
16 hr, 40 min

8. 42 mL/hr
1041.6 units/hr

9. 42 mL/hr
1458 units/hr

10. 100 mL/hr via infusion device
10 hr to infuse

11 Children's Dosages

11A (PAGE 296)

1. a. Estimate: 7 kg
        Actual: 6.4 kg
    b. Estimate: 6 kg
        Actual: 12.1 lb (2 steps)
                5.5 kg
    c. Estimate: 5 kg
        Actual: 4.5 kg
    d. Estimate: 28 lb
        Actual: 30.8 lb
    e. Estimate: 20 lb
        Actual: 22 lb

2. a. 150 mg × 3 = 450 mg
    b. 200 mg × 4 = 800 mg
    c. 400 mcg × 6 = 2400 mcg or 2.4 mg
    d. 50 mg × 3 = 150 mg
    e. 750 mcg × 2 = 1500 mcg or 1.5 mg

3. a. 1 g or 1000 mg/4 = 250 mg
    b. 750 mg/3 = 250 mg
    c. 2 g or 2000 mg/4 = 500 mg
        2 g or 2000 mg/6 = 333.3 mg
    d. 16 g a day/2 = 8 g
        16 g a day/4 = 4 g
    e. 500 mg/4 = 125 mg

4. a. 10 × 5 = 50 mg
    b. 5 × 7.3 = 36.5 mg (low dose)
        8 × 7.3 = 58.4 mg (high dose)
        SDR is 36.5 to 58.4 mg.
    c. 8 lb = approximately 4 kg estimated
        Step 1: 8 lb = 3.6 kg actual
        Step 2: *Low dose:* 6 × 3.6 = 21.6 mg
                High dose: 8 × 3.6 = 28.8 mg
        SDR is 21.6 to 28.8 mg.
    d. 5 lb, 8 oz = approximately 2.5 kg
        Step 1: *oz to lb:* 8 oz/16 = 0.5 lb
        Step 2: *lb to kg:* 5.5 lb/2.2 = 2.5 kg
        Step 3: *Low dose:* 3 × 2.5 = 7.5 mg
                High dose: 6 × 2.5 = 15 mg
        SDR is 7.5 to 15 mg.
    e. 4 lb, 6 oz = approximately 2 kg
        Step 1: *oz to lb:* 6 oz/16 = 0.37 or 0.4 lb
        Step 2: *lb to kg:* 4.4 lb/2.2 = 2 kg
        Step 3: *Low dose:* 200 mcg × 2 = 400 mcg
                    or 0.4 mg
                High dose: 400 mcg × 2 = 800 mcg
                    or 0.8 mg
        SDR is 400 to 800 mcg or 0.4 to 0.8 mg.

5. a. 36 to 54 mg (2 × 18 = 36)
            (3 × 18 = 54)
    b. 12 to 18 mg (36 ÷ 3)
            (54 ÷ 3)
    c. 150 mg/day; 50 mg per dose
            (50 × 3)   (150 ÷ 3)
    d. Unsafe to give. Overdose ordered. Hold
        and clarify promptly with the physician.

11B (PAGE 298)

1. a. Estimated wt in kg: 10 kg
   b. Actual wt in kg: 9.09 or 9.1 kg
   c. SDR for this child: 18.2 to 36.4 mg/day
      $2 \times 9.1 = 18.2$ mg
      $4 \times 9.1 = 36.4$ mg
   d. Dose ordered: 50 mg daily
   e. Evaluation and decision: Hold and clarify promptly (overdose)

2. a. Estimated wt in kg: 16.5 kg
   b. Actual wt in kg: 15 kg
   c. SDR for this child: 1500 to 3000 mcg/day
      or 1.5 to 3 mg/day
      15×100 mcg = 1500 mcg or 1.5 mg
      15×200 mcg = 3000 mcg or 3 mg
   d. Dose ordered: 0.5 mg tid or 1.5 mg/day
   e. Evaluation and decision: Safe to give

3. a. Estimated wt in kg: 12.5 kg
   b. Actual wt in kg: 11.54 or 11.5 kg
      (25.4/2.2)
   c. SDR for this child: 115 to 345 mg/day
      $10 \times 11.5 = 115$ mg
      $30 \times 11.5 = 345$ mg
   d. Dose ordered: 100 mg tid or 300 mg/day
   e. Evaluation and decision: Safe to give

4. a. Estimated wt in kg: 42.5 kg
   b. Actual wt in kg: 38.63 or 38.6 kg
   c. SDR for this child: 386 mg to 579 mg/day
      in divided doses
   d. Dose ordered: 100 mg q6h or
      $100 \times 4 = 400$ mg/day
   e. Evaluation and decision: Safe to give

5. a. Estimated wt in kg: 2.5 kg
   b. Actual wt in kg: 2.27 or 2.3 kg
   c. SDR for this child: 23-46 mcg/day
      $10 \times 2.3 = 23$ mcg
      $20 \times 2.3 = 46$ mcg
   d. Dose ordered: 0.03 mg $\times 4 = 0.12$ mg/day
      or 120 mcg/day
   e. Evaluation and decision: Hold and clarify promptly (overdose)

11C (PAGE 301)

1. 0.15 m^2
   $10 \times 0.15 = 1.5$ mg

2. 0.20 m^2*
   $15 \times 0.2 = 3$ mg

3. 0.27 m^2
   $5 \times 0.27 = 1.35$ mg

4. $4 \times 10 = 40$ mg

5. $15 \times 6 = 90$ mg

6. $5 \times 10 = 50$ mg

7. $10 \times 1.8 = 18$ mg

8. 2.72 kg
   $2 \times 2.7 = 5.4$ mg

9. $\frac{60 \times 100}{3600} = 1.66$
   $\sqrt{1.66} = 1.29$ m^2

10. $\frac{70 \times 12}{3131} = 0.268$
    $\sqrt{0.268} = 0.517 = 0.52$ m^2

---

*Note: Trailing zeros are seen in BSA square meters. Delete them for math calculations.

11D (PAGE 302)

1. **a.** Estimated wt in kg: 13 kg
   b. Actual wt in kg: 11.8 kg
   c. SDR: 1000 to 2000 mg in
      4 divided doses
   d. Dose ordered: 500 mg × 4 or 2000 mg
   e. Evaluation and decision: Safe to give

2. **a.** SDR for this child: 4.0 to 6.4 mg four
      times daily
      $5 \times 0.8 \text{ m}^2 = 4.0$ mg (low safe dose)
      $8 \times 0.8 \text{ m}^2 = 6.4$ mg (high safe dose)
   b. Dose ordered: 4 mg daily
   c. Evaluation and decision: Safe to give

3. **a.** Estimated wt in kg: 9.5 kg
   b. Actual wt in kg: 8.63 or 8.6 kg
   c. SDR for this child: 0.9 to 2.6 mg in
      2 divided doses or 860 to 2600 mcg in
      2 divided doses
      $0.1 \times 8.6 = 0.86$ mg rounded to 0.9 mg
      (low safe dose)
      $0.3 \times 8.6 = 2.58$ rounded to 2.6 mg
      (high safe dose)
   d. Dose ordered: 2500 mcg bid or
      2.5 mg × 2 = 5 mg/day
   e. Evaluation and decision: Hold and
      clarify promptly (overdose)

4. **a.** Estimated wt in kg: 4.5 kg
   b. Actual wt in kg: 4.09 or 4.1 kg
   c. SDR for this child: 4.1 to 20.5 mcg/day
      $1 \times 4.1 = 4.1$ mcg
      $5 \times 4.1 = 20.54$ mcg
   d. Dose ordered: 0.01 mg or 10 mcg daily
   e. Evaluation and decision: Safe to give

5. **a.** Estimated wt in kg: 7 kg
   b. Actual wt in kg: 6.36 or 6.4 kg
   c. SDR for this child: 0.13 to 0.32 mg/day
      $0.02 \times 6.4 = 0.128$ mg (low safe dose)
      $0.05 \times 6.4 = 0.32$ mg (high safe dose)
   d. Dose ordered: 150 mcg × 2 = 300 mcg/day
      or 0.3 mg/day
   e. Evaluation and decision: Safe to give

11E (PAGE 303)

1. a. Estimated wt in lb: 14 × 2 or 28 lb
    b. Actual wt in lb: 30.8 lb
    c. SDR for this child: For 24 to 35 lb, 1 tsp
    d. Dose ordered: 160 mg
    e. Evaluation and decision: Safe to give
    f. Give: 1 tsp or 5 mL (80 mg per $\frac{1}{2}$ tsp)

2. a. Estimated wt in kg: 66 ÷ 2 = 33 kg
    b. Actual wt in kg: 30 kg
    c. SDR for this child: 300 to 900 mg/day in 3 to 4 doses
       10 × 30 = 300 mg (low safe daily dose)
       30 × 30 = 900 mg (maximum safe daily dose)
    d. Dose ordered: 300 × 3 = 900 mg/day.
    e. Evaluation and decision: Safe to give
    f. Give

       HAVE   WANT TO HAVE
       75 mg : 5 mL :: 300 mg : x mL
       $\frac{\cancel{75}}{\cancel{75}} x = \frac{1500}{75}$

       $x = 20$ mL
       PROOF
       75 × 20 = 1500
       1 × 1500 = 1500

3. a. SDR for this child: 400 to 800 mg/day in 3 to 4 doses
    b. Dose ordered in mg:
       0.25 g = 250 mg × 3 = 750 mg/day
       HAVE   WANT TO HAVE
       1 g : 1000 mg :: 0.25 g : x mg
       $x = 1000 \times 0.25$ or 250 mg
       PROOF
       1 × 250 = 250
       1000 × 0.25 = 250
    c. Evaluation and decision: Safe to give
    d. Give 12.5 mL
       HAVE   WANT TO HAVE
       100 mg : 5 mL :: 250 mg : x mL
       $\frac{\cancel{100}}{\cancel{100}} x = \frac{125\cancel{0}\ (5 \times 250)}{10\cancel{0}}$

       $x = 12.5$ mL
       PROOF
       100 × 12.5 = 1250
       5 × 250 = 1250

4. a. SDR for this child:
       10 × 0.5 × 4 = 20 mg/day
    b. Dose ordered: 20 mg/day
    c. Evaluation and decision: Safe to give
    d. Give 1 tab

5. a. Estimated wt in kg: 13.5
    b. Actual wt in kg: 12.3 kg
    c. SDR for this child: 492 mg/day or 164 mg tid
    d. Dose ordered: 180 mg/dose or 540 mg/day
    e. Evaluation and decision: Slight overdose. Hold and clarify promptly.
    f. Not applicable

11F (PAGE 307)

1. **a.** Estimated wt in kg: 16 kg
   b. Actual wt: 14.7 kg (2 steps)

HAVE	WANT TO HAVE

   16 oz : 1 lb :: 5 oz : x lb

   $$\frac{\cancel{16}}{\cancel{16}}x = \frac{5}{16}$$

   $x = 0.312$ or 0.3 lb
   Child weighs 32.3 lb ÷ 2.2 = 14.68
   or 14.7 kg
   c. SDR for this child: 14.7 to 32.3 mg q4h
   $1 \times 14.7 = 14.7$ mg
   $2.2 \times 14.7 = 32.34$ mg = 32.3 mg
   d. Dose ordered: 30 mg
   e. Evaluation and decision: Safe to give
   f. Give 0.4 mL

HAVE	WANT TO HAVE

   75 mg : 1 mL :: 30 mg : x mL

   $$\frac{\cancel{75}}{\cancel{75}}x = \frac{30}{75}$$

   $x = 0.4$ mL
   PROOF
   $75 \times 0.4 = 30$
   $1 \times 30 = 30$

2. **a.** Estimated wt: 27 kg
   b. Actual wt: 25.2 kg (2 steps)

HAVE	WANT TO HAVE

   16 oz : 1 lb :: 8 oz : x lb
   $16x = 8$
   $x = 0.5$ lb   Child weighs 55.5 lb ÷ 2.2
   or 25.2 kg
   c. SDR for this child: 2.52 to 5.04 mg q4h
   $0.1 \times 25.2 = 2.52$ mg
   $0.2 \times 25.2 = 5.04$ mg
   d. Dose ordered: 5 mg IM
   e. Evaluation and decision: Safe to give
   f. Give 0.5 mL

HAVE	WANT TO HAVE

   10 mg : 1 mL :: 5 mg : x mL

   $$\frac{\cancel{10}}{\cancel{10}}x = \frac{5}{10}$$

   $x = 0.5$ mL
   PROOF
   $10 \times 0.5 = 5$
   $1 \times 5 = 5$

3. **a.** Estimated wt: 8.5 kg
   b. Actual wt: 8 kg (2 steps)

HAVE	WANT TO HAVE

   16 oz : 1 lb :: 9 oz : x lb

   $$\frac{\cancel{16}}{\cancel{16}}x = \frac{9}{16}$$

   $x = 0.56$ or 0.6 lb
   Child weighs 17.6 lb ÷ 2.2 or 8 kg
   c. SDR for this child: between 7 and 9 kg, 0.2 mg
   d. Dose ordered: 0.2 mg
   e. Evaluation and decision: Safe to give
   f. Give 0.5 mL

HAVE	WANT TO HAVE

   0.4 mg : 1 mL :: 0.2 mg : x mL

   $$\frac{\cancel{0.4}}{\cancel{0.4}}x = \frac{0.2\,(1 \times 0.2)}{0.4}$$

   $x = 0.5$ mL
   PROOF
   $0.4 \times 0.5 = 0.2$
   $1 \times 0.2 = 0.2$

4. **a.** Estimated wt : 3.5 kg
   b. Actual wt : 3.2 kg (1 step)
   c. SDR for this child: 320 to 640 mg/day (based on 3.2 kg wt)
   d. Dose ordered: 1000 mg/day
   e. Evaluation and decision: Overdose. Hold and clarify promptly. Also ask whether IV route is preferred.
   f. Not applicable.

5. **a.** Estimated wt: 75 ÷ 2 or 37.5 kg
   b. Actual wt: 75 ÷ 2.2 or 34.1 kg (1 step)
   c. SDR for this child: 1705 to 3410 mg day
   in 4 divided doses
   50 × 34.1 = 1705 mg
   100 × 34.1 = 3410 mg
   d. Dose ordered: 1500 × 3 or 4500 mg/day
   e. Evaluation and decision: Ordered 3 × day.
   Recommendation is to give four times
   daily. Total dose exceeds recommendation.
   Hold and clarify promptly (overdose)
   f. Not applicable

11G (PAGE 312)

1. **a.** Estimated wt in kg: 31 kg
   b. Actual wt in kg: 28.18 or 28.2 kg
   c. SDR for this child: 28.2 to 84.6 kg q24h
   d. Dose ordered: 65 mg IV stat
   e. Evaluation and decision: Safe to give
   f. Dose withdrawn from vial: 0.5 mL
   130 mg : 1 mL :: 65 mg : x mL
   130x = 195
   x = 0.5 mL
   PROOF
   130 × 1.5 = 195
   3 × 65 = 195

2. **a.** Estimated wt in kg: 27.5 kg
   b. Actual wt in kg: 25 kg
   c. SDR for this child: 25 to 150 mg
   (1 to 6 mg/kg)
   1 × 25 = 25
   6 × 25 = 150
   d. Dose ordered: 25 mg IV stat
   e. Evaluation and decision: Safe to give
   (The initial dose must not exceed the
   lowest dose in the SDR.)
   f. Give 2.5 mL
   HAVE   **WANT TO HAVE**
   40 mg : 4 mL :: 25 mg : x mL
   $$\frac{4\cancel{0}}{4\cancel{0}}x = \frac{10\cancel{0}}{4\cancel{0}}\,(4 \times 25)$$
   x = 2.5 mL
   PROOF
   40 × 2.5 = 100
   4 × 25 = 100

3. **a.** Estimated wt in kg: 6.5 kg
   b. Actual wt in kg: 6 kg
   c. SDR for this child: 18 mg q8h
   d. Dose ordered: 18 mg q8h
   e. Evaluation and decision: Safe to give
   f. Amount withdrawn from vial: Give 1.8 mL

   HAVE   WANT TO HAVE
   20 mg : 2 mg :: 18 mg : x mL

   $$\frac{\cancel{20}}{\cancel{20}}x = \frac{36}{20}$$

   $x = 1.8$ mL

   g. Further dilute *to* 50 mL and administer at
   50 mL/hr for 60 min.*

5. **a.** Estimated wt in kg: 13 kg
   b. Actual wt in kg: 11.81 or 11.8 kg
   c. SDR for this child: 590 to 5900 mg
   divided into 4 doses = 1475 mg
   maximum unit dose
   $50 \times 11.8 = 590$
   $500 \times 11.8 = 5900$
   d. Dose ordered: 2 g or 2000 mg q6h
   e. Evaluation and decision: Hold and clarify
   promptly (overdose)
   f. Not applicable
   g. Not applicable

4. **a.** Estimated wt in kg: 17 kg
   b. Actual wt in kg: 15.45 or 15.5 kg
   c. SDR for this child: 775 to 1550 mg/day
   divided by 3 and 4, or 516 mg/max individual dose
   d. Dose ordered: 0.3 g or 300 mg q6h =
   1200 mg total dose per day
   e. Evaluation and decision: Safe to give
   f. First dilution: Mix Zinacef *with* 9 mL and
   withdraw 3.6 mL from the 10 mL total†

   HAVE   WANT TO HAVE
   750 mg : 10 mL :: 300 mg : x mL

   $$\frac{\cancel{750}}{\cancel{750}}x = \frac{300\cancel{0}}{75\cancel{0}}$$

   $x = 4$ mL to be further diluted *to*
   20 mL with IV-compatible solution and administered on an
   IV infusion pump with a volume-
   control device.

   PROOF
   $750 \times 4 = 3000$
   $10 \times 300 = 3000$

   g. Infuse at 40 mL/hr for 30 min

   HAVE   WANT TO HAVE
   20 mL : 30 min :: x mL : 60 min
   $30x = 1200$
   $x = 40$ mL/hr

   PROOF
   $20 \times 60 = 1200$
   $30 \times 40 = 1200$

---

*Dilute *"to"* is interpreted as, "Add diluent to the prepared medicine to make 50 mL total volume."
†Dilution *"with"* a substance adds to the volume. Dilution *"to"* an amount does not add to the volume.

11H (PAGE 315)

1. a. Estimated wt in kg: 16.5 kg
    b. Actual wt in kg: $33 \div 2.2 = 15$
    c. SDR for this child: 300 mg $\div$ 3 or
        100 mg tid
    d. Dose ordered: 100 mg $\times$ 3 or 300 mg/day
    e. Evaluation and decision: Safe to give
    f. Give 2 mL

        HAVE   WANT TO HAVE
        250 mg : 5 mL :: 100 mg : x mL
        $250x = 500$
            $x = 2$ mL
        PROOF
        $250 \times 2 = 500$
        $5 \times 100 = 500$

2. a. SDR for this child: $5 \times 30 = 150$ mg per
        day in 2 or 3 divided doses
    b. Dose ordered: 75 mg bid or
        150 mg per day
    c. Evaluation and decision: Safe to give
    d. Give 11.3 mL

        HAVE   WANT TO HAVE
        100 mg : 15 mL :: 75 mg : x mL
        $100x = 1125$
            $x = 11.25$ rounded to 11.3 mL
        PROOF
        $100 \times 11.25 = 1125$
        $15 \times 75 = 1125$

3. a. Estimated wt in kg: 24.5 kg
    b. Actual wt in kg: 22.27 or 22.3 kg
    c. SDR for this child (IV): 44.6 mcg to
        55.8 mcg ($\frac{1}{2}$ of po dose)
        89.2 mcg po dose $\div$ 2 = 44.6 mcg
        (low safe dose)
        111.5 mcg po dose $\div$ 2 = 55.75 rounded
        to 55.8 mcg (high safe dose)
    d. Dose ordered: 0.1 mg (100 mcg) IV q AM

        HAVE   WANT TO HAVE
        1 mg : 1000 mcg :: 0.1 mg : x mcg
        $x = 1000 \times 0.1 = 100$ mcg
    e. Evaluation and decision: Hold and clarify
        promptly (100 mcg is an overdose for
        IV administration at this child's weight)
    f. Not applicable

4. a. Estimated wt in kg: 33 kg
    b. Actual wt in kg: 30 kg
    c. SDR for this child: 30 to 66 mg
        $1 \times 30 = 30$
        $2.2 \times 30 = 66$
    d. Dose ordered: 35 mg
    e. Evaluation and decision: Safe to give
    f. Prepare 0.7 mL

        HAVE   WANT TO HAVE
        50 mg : 1 mL :: 35 mg : x mL
        $\frac{\cancel{50}}{\cancel{50}} x = \frac{35}{50}$

            $x = 0.7$ mL
        PROOF
        $50 \times 0.7 = 35$
        $1 \times 35 = 35$

5. a. Estimated wt in lb: 27 lb
   b. Actual wt in lb: 29.92 or 30 lb
   c. SDR for this child: 40 mg/0.6 m² =
       24 mg/day
   d. Dose ordered: 30 mg/day
   e. Evaluation and decision: Hold and clarify
       (overdose)
   f. Not applicable

6. a. Estimated wt in kg: 11 kg
   b. Actual wt in kg: 10 kg
   c. SDR for this child: 500 to 1000 mg/day
       in 4 divided doses (250 mg each max)
   d. Dose ordered: 250 mg IV q6h
   e. Evaluation and decision: Safe to give
   f. Give 12.5 mL

   HAVE   WANT TO HAVE
   1000 mg : x mL :: 20 mg : 1 mL

   $$\frac{2\not0}{2\not0}x = \frac{100\not0}{2\not0}$$

   x = 50 mL
   1000 mg : 50 mL :: 250 mg : x mL

   $$\frac{100\not0}{100\not0}x = \frac{12.50\not0}{100\not0}$$

   x = 12.5 mL

7. a. Estimated wt in kg: 3 kg
   b. Actual wt in kg: 2.72 or 2.7 kg
   c. SDR for this child: Up to 8.1 mEq q24h
       3 × 2.7 = 8.1
   d. Dose ordered: 0.9 mEq q8h or 2.7 q24h
   e. Evaluation and decision: Safe to give;
       monitor lab potassium values for thera-
       peutic range, and assess patient's heart
       rate, rhythm, and muscle tone. May be
       underdosed.
   f. Add 0.45 mL KCl to compatible IV and
       mix well.
   HAVE   WANT TO HAVE
   2 mEq : 1 mL :: 0.9 mEq : x mL

   $$\frac{\not2}{\not2}x = \frac{0.9}{2} = 0.45 \text{ mL}$$

   PROOF
   2 × 0.45 = 0.9
   1 × 0.9 = 0.9

8. a. Estimated wt in kg: 15.5 kg
   b. Actual wt in kg: 14.09 or 14.1
   c. SDR for this child: Up to 1410 mg in
       2 doses or 705 mg dose
       100 × 14.1 = 1410
   d. Dose ordered: 600 mg IV q12h or
       1200 mg/day
   e. Evaluation and decision: Safe to give
   f. Use 6 mL after reconstituting
   HAVE   WANT TO HAVE
   100 mg : 1 mL :: 600 mg : x mL
   $$\frac{10\not0}{10\not0}x = \frac{60\not0}{10\not0}$$
   x = 6 mL
   PROOF
   100 × 6 = 600
   1 × 600 = 600
   g. Infuse for 30 min at 60 mL/hr
   HAVE   WANT TO HAVE
   30 mL : 30 min :: x mL : 60 min
   $$\frac{3\not0}{3\not0}x = \frac{180\not0}{3\not0}$$

   x = 60 mL/hr
   PROOF
   30 × 60 = 1800
   60 × 30 = 1800

9. **a.** Draw up 0.2 mL in a 1 mL syringe.
   b. Use enclosed dropper to administer along the inside of the cheek.*

   HAVE   WANT TO HAVE
   80 mg : 0.8 mL :: 20 mg : x mL

   $$\frac{\cancel{80}}{\cancel{80}}x = \frac{16}{80}$$

   $x = 0.2$ mL

   PROOF
   $80 \times 0.2 = 16$
   $0.8 \times 20 = 16$

10. **a.** 2 mg/lb of body weight divided into 2 doses first day
    b. Hold and contact prescriber promptly. Overdose (double the recommended dose for first day).
    c. N/A

11I (PAGE 320)

1. **b**

   This is a *two-step* problem.
   Estimated wt in kg: 25 kg
   Step 1:
   2.2 lb : 1 kg :: 50 lb : x kg
   $x = 50/2.2$ or 22.7 kg
   Step 2:
   20 mg : 1 kg :: x mg : 22.7 kg
   $x = 20 \times 22.7$ or 454 mg

   PROOF
   $2.2 \times 22.7 = 49.94$ or 50
   $1 \times 50 = 50$
   PROOF
   $20 \times 22.7 = 45$
   $1 \times 454 = 454$

2. **c**

   30 mg : 1 m² :: x mg : 1.2$\emptyset$ m²
   $x = 30 \times 1.2\emptyset$ or 36 mg

   PROOF
   $30 \times 1.2\emptyset = 36$
   $1 \times 36 = 36$

3. **b**

   5 mL = 1 tsp
   5 mL : 1 tsp :: x mL : 1.5 tsp
   $x = 7.5$ mL
   Measure 7.5 mL

   PROOF
   $5 \times 1.5 = 7.5$
   $1 \times 7.5 = 7.5$

4. **c**

   This is a *three-step* problem.
   Estimated wt in kg: 25/2 or 12.5 kg
   Step 1:
   2.2 lb : 1 kg :: 25 lb : x kg
   $x = 25/2.2$ or 11.4 kg
   Step 2:
   2 mg : 1 kg :: x mg : 11.4 kg
   $x = 2 \times 11.4$ or 22.8 mg *low safe dose*
   Step 3:
   5 mg : 1 kg :: x mg : 11.4 kg
   $x = 57$ mg *maximum safe dose*
   30 mg is within SDR of 22.8 mg to 57 mg.

   PROOF
   $2.2 \times 11.4 = 25$
   $1 \times 25 = 25$
   PROOF
   $2 \times 11.4 = 22.8$
   $1 \times 22.8 = 22.8$
   PROOF
   $5 \times 11.4 = 57$
   $1 \times 57 = 57$

---

*Note: Concentrated drops are not interchangeable with other liquid medicines.

5. **a**

   Estimated wt: 55/2 or 27.5 kg
   Step 1: lb to kg   PROOF
   2.2 lb : 1 kg :: 55 lb : x kg $2.2 \times 25 = 55$
   $2.2x = 5.5$ $1 \times 55 = 55$
   $x = 25$ kg
   Step 2: SDR   PROOF
   2 mg : 1 kg :: x mg : 25 kg $2 \times 25 = 50$
   $x = 2 \times 25$ or 50 mg *low safe dose* $1 \times 50 = 50$
   Compare low SDR with the order. They are equal for the q8h order.
   No need to calculate high safe dose. Give the medication.

6. **d**

   Estimated wt: 5.5/2 or 2.5 kg
   Step 1: lb to kg   PROOF
   2.2 lb : 1 kg :: 5.5 lb : x kg $2.2 \times 2.5 = 5.5$
   $2.2x = 5.5x = 2.2$ kg $= 2.5$ kg $1 \times 5.5 = 5.5$
   Step 2: SDR   PROOF
   40 mg : 1 kg :: x mg : 2.5 kg $40 \times 2.5 = 100$
   $x = 40 \times 2.5$ or   100 mg/day $1 \times 100 = 100$
   Compare the SDR with the order. The 125 mg order exceeds the 100 mg recommended
   dose. Clarify with the physician promptly and document promptly.

7. **b**

   Estimated wt: 6/2 or 3 kg
   This is a *three-step* problem
   Step 1: lb to kg   PROOF
   2.2 lb : 1 kg :: 55 lb : x kg $2.2 \times 25 = 55$
   $2.2x = 55$ $1 \times 55 = 55$
   $x = 25$ kg
   Step 2: SDR   PROOF
   5 mg : 1 kg :: x mg : 6 kg $5 \times 6 = 30$
   $x = 5 \times 6$ or 30 mg $1 \times 30 = 30$
   Compare the SDR with the order. 30 mg/2 = 15 mg bid. The order is 15 mg bid.
   The order is safe.
   Step 3: Calculate the unit dose.   PROOF
   30 mg : 5 mL :: 15 mg : x mL $30 \times 2.5 = 75$
   $30x = 75x = 2.5$ mL $5 \times 15 = 75$
   Give 2.5 mL using a syringe to measure, if necessary.

8. **d**

   1000 mcg = 1 mg   Metric equivalents
   500 mcg = 0.5 mg
   200 mcg = 0.2 mg
   Estimate: You want to give *more than double* the 10 mL dose.

   HAVE   WANT TO HAVE   PROOF
   200 mcg : 10 mL :: 500 mcg : x mL $200 \times 2.5 = 500$
   $\dfrac{\cancel{200}}{\cancel{200}} x = \dfrac{50\cancel{00}}{2\cancel{00}}$ $1 \times 500 = 500$

   $x = 25$ mL

9. **d**

Estimated wt in kg: 29 kg

Step 1: lb to kg   PROOF

2.2 lb : 1 kg :: 58 lb : x kg $2.2 \times 26.36 = 57.92$ or 58

2.2x = 58 $1 \times 58 = 58$

x = 26.36 kg or 26.4 kg (to *nearest tenth*)

Step 2: low SDR

Low safe dose range is 1 mg/kg or 26.4 mg.

No math is needed for low safe dose range.

The order is for 30 mg; therefore, continue and calculate high SDR.

Step 3: High SDR   PROOF

2.2 mg : 1 kg :: x mg : 26.4 kg $2.2 \times 26.4 = 58.08$

x = 2.2 $\times$ 26.4 or 58.08 or 58.2 mg $1 \times 58.08 = 58.08$

The order for 30 mg is within the SDR of 26.4 mg to 58.2 mg unit dose.

(Step 3 Dose Calculation)   PROOF

You want to give more than 25 mg or 1 mL $25 \times 1.2 = 30$

25 mg : 1 mL :: 30 mg : x mL $1 \times 30 = 30$

$$\frac{\cancel{25}}{\cancel{25}} x = \frac{30}{25}$$

   x = 1.2 mL

10. **b**

Estimated wt in kg is 15 kg.

lb to kg   PROOF

2.2 : 1 kg :: 30 : x kg $2.2 \times 13.6 = 29.92$

$$\frac{\cancel{2.2}}{\cancel{2.2}} x = \frac{30}{2.2}$$ $1 \times 30 = 30$

    x = 13.6

SDR   PROOF

25 mg : 1 kg :: x mg : 13.6 kg $25 \times 13.6 = 340$

x = 25 $\times$ 13.6 or 340 mg day in *4 divided* $1 \times 340 = 340$

doses, or 85 mg per dose

50 mg = 2 times the 25 mg dose of 680 mg/day high safe dose per day

Decision: Hold the order. The drug is supposed to be given 4 times a day, not 3 times a day; and the amount ordered, 750 mg per day, exceeds the recommended safe dose of 680 mg per day.

CHAPTER 11 FINAL: CHILDREN'S DOSAGES (PAGE 322)

1. a. Estimated wt in kg: 21 kg
   b. Actual wt in kg: 19.09 or 19.1 kg
   c. SDR for this child: 477.5 to 955 mg/day in 4 divided doses
   d. Dose ordered: 200 mg × 4 or 800 mg/day
   e. Evaluation and decision: Safe to give
   f. Give 8 mL.

2. a. Actual wt in kg: 19.09 or 19.1 kg
   b. SDR for this child: 573 to 955 mg/day in 4 divided doses
   c. Dose ordered: 175 mg × 4 or 700 mg/day
   d. Evaluation and decision: Safe to give
   e. Give 4.4 mL.

3. a. SDR for this child: 150 mg maximum in 24 hr in divided doses
   b. Dose ordered: 25 mg × 4 or 100 mg/day
   c. Evaluation and decision: Safe to give
   d. Dose to be administered: 2 tsp or 25 mg per dose

4. a. SDR for this child: 400 to 800 mg/day
   b. Dose ordered: 2000 mg/day
   c. Evaluation and decision: Overdose. Hold and clarify promptly.
   d. Dose to be administered: Not applicable

5. a. Estimated wt in kg: 17.5 kg
   b. Actual wt in kg: 15.9 kg
   c. SDR for this child: 0.3 mg (for 12 to 26 kg child)
   d. Dose ordered: 0.3 mg
   e. Safe to give.
   f. Give 0.75 mL in anterolateral thigh.

6. a. Actual wt in kg: 15.9 kg
   b. SDR for this child: 318 to 636 mg/day
   c. Dose ordered: 500 mg × 3 or 1500 mg
   d. Evaluation and decision: Overdose. Hold and clarify promptly.
   e. Dose to be administered: Not applicable

7. a. Actual wt in kg: 15.9 kg
   b. SDR for this child: 95.4 to 119.3 mg/day
   c. Dose ordered: 35 × 3 or 105 mg/day
   d. Evaluation and decision: Safe to give
   e. Volume after dilution: 35 mL
   f. IV flow rate on device: 70 mL/hr for $\frac{1}{2}$ hr

8. a. Actual wt in kg: 15.9 kg
   b. SDR for this child: 0.795 or 0.8 to 1.6 mg q4h
   c. Dose ordered: 5 mg q4h
   d. Evaluation and decision: Hold and clarify promptly (overdose).
   e. Not applicable

9. a. BSA in m²: 1.10 m²
   b. SDR for this child: Up to 44 mg/day 1.10 × 10 × 4 = 44
   c. Dose ordered: 40 mg/day
   d. Evaluation and decision: Safe to give
   e. Give 2 tab.

10. a. Estimated wt in lb: 36 lb
   b. Actual wt in lb: 39.6 lb
   c. SDR for this child: $1\frac{1}{2}$ tsp for children weighing 36 to 47 lb
   d. Dose ordered: 240 mg or $1\frac{1}{2}$ tsp
   e. Evaluation and decision: Safe to give
   f. Give $1\frac{1}{2}$ tsp or 7.5 mL
   g. The enclosed measuring cup

12 Dimensional Analysis

12A (PAGE 329)

1. KNOW   WANT TO KNOW

$$x \text{ mL} = \frac{1 \text{ mL}}{500 \text{ mg}} \times \frac{800 \text{ mg}}{1} = \frac{800}{500} = 1.6 \text{ mL}$$

2. KNOW   WANT TO KNOW

$$x \text{ tabs} = \frac{1 \text{ tab}}{400 \text{ mg}} \times \frac{1000 \text{ mg}}{1 \text{ g}} \times \frac{0.8 \text{ g}}{1} = \frac{800}{400} = 2 \text{ tablets}$$

3. KNOW   WANT TO KNOW

$$x \text{ gtt/min} = \frac{20 \text{ gtt}}{1 \text{ mL}} \times \frac{125 \text{ mL}}{60 \text{ min}} = \frac{2500}{60} = 41.6 = 42 \text{ gtt/min}$$

4. KNOW   WANT TO KNOW

$$x \text{ mL} = \frac{1 \text{ mL}}{2 \text{ mg}} \times \frac{1.5 \text{ mg}}{1} = \frac{1.5}{2} = 0.75 \text{ mL}$$

5. KNOW   WANT TO KNOW

$$x \text{ mL} = \frac{5 \text{ mL}}{200 \text{ mg}} \times \frac{250 \text{ mg}}{1} = \frac{1250}{200} = 6.25 \text{ mL}$$

6. KNOW   WANT TO KNOW

$$x \text{ mL} = \frac{5 \text{ mL}}{200 \text{ mg}} \times \frac{750 \text{ mg}}{1} = \frac{3750}{200} = 18.75 \text{ mL}$$

7. KNOW   WANT TO KNOW

$$x \text{ mL} = \frac{1 \text{ mL}}{10 \text{ mg}} \times \frac{8 \text{ mg}}{1} = \frac{8}{10} = 0.8 \text{ mL}$$

8. KNOW   WANT TO KNOW

$$x \text{ mL} = \frac{2 \text{ mL}}{250 \text{ mg}} \times \frac{300 \text{ mg}}{1} = \frac{600}{250} = 2.4 \text{ mL}$$

9. KNOW   WANT TO KNOW

$$x \text{ mL} = \frac{2 \text{ mL}}{250 \text{ mg}} \times \frac{400 \text{ mg}}{1} = \frac{400}{250} = 1.6 \text{ mL}$$

10. KNOW   WANT TO KNOW

$$x \text{ mL} = \frac{1.2 \text{ mL}}{500 \text{ mg}} \times \frac{700 \text{ mg}}{1} = \frac{840}{500} = 1.7 \text{ mL}$$

12B (PAGE 332)

1. KNOW   WANT TO KNOW

$$x \text{ mL} = \frac{1000 \text{ mL}}{20,000 \text{ units}} \times \frac{1000 \text{ units}}{1 \text{ hr}} = \frac{1,000,000}{20,000} = 50 \text{ mL/hr}$$

2. KNOW   WANT TO KNOW

$$x \text{ units/hr} = \frac{20,000 \text{ units}}{1000 \text{ mL}} \times \frac{50 \text{ mL}}{1 \text{ hr}} = \frac{1,000,000}{1000} = 1000 \text{ units/hr}$$

3. KNOW   WANT TO KNOW

$$x \text{ mg/hr} = \frac{400 \text{ mg}}{500 \text{ mL}} \times 60 \text{ mL/hr} = \frac{24,000}{500} = 48 \text{ mg/hr}$$

4. KNOW   WANT TO KNOW

$$x \text{ mL/hr} = \frac{1000 \text{ mL}}{30 \text{ units}} \times \frac{2 \text{ units}}{1 \text{ hr}} = 66.6 = 67 \text{ mL/hr}$$

5. a. KNOW   WANT TO KNOW

$$x \text{ mL/hr} = \frac{1000 \text{ mL}}{24 \text{ hr}} \times \frac{1 \text{ hr}}{1} = \frac{1000}{24} = 41.6 = 42 \text{ mL/hr}$$

b. KNOW   WANT TO KNOW

$$x \text{ units/hr} = \frac{42 \text{ mL}}{1 \text{ hr}} \times \frac{50 \text{ units}}{1000 \text{ mL}} = \frac{2100}{1000} = 2.1 \text{ units/hr}$$

6. a. KNOW   WANT TO KNOW

$$x \text{ mL/hr} = \frac{250 \text{ mL}}{12 \text{ hr}} \times \frac{1 \text{ hr}}{1} = \frac{250}{12} = 20.8 = 21 \text{ mL/hr}$$

b. KNOW   WANT TO KNOW

$$x \text{ units/hr} = \frac{21 \text{ mL}}{1 \text{ hr}} \times \frac{30 \text{ units}}{250 \text{ mL}} = \frac{630}{250} = 2.5 \text{ units/hr}$$

7. a. KNOW   WANT TO KNOW

$$x \text{ mL/hr} = \frac{250 \text{ mL}}{8 \text{ hr}} \times \frac{1 \text{ hr}}{1} = \frac{250}{8} = 31.2 = 31 \text{ mL/hr}$$

b. KNOW   WANT TO KNOW

$$x \text{ mg/hr} = \frac{31 \text{ mL}}{1 \text{ hr}} \times \frac{300 \text{ mg}}{250 \text{ mL}} = \frac{9300}{250} = 37.2 \text{ mg/hr}$$

8. a. KNOW   WANT TO KNOW

$$x \text{ mL/hr} = \frac{1000 \text{ mL}}{12 \text{ hr}} \times \frac{1 \text{ hr}}{1} = \frac{1000}{12} = 83.3 = 83 \text{ mL/hr}$$

b. KNOW   WANT TO KNOW

$$x \text{ mEq/hr} = \frac{83 \text{ mL}}{1 \text{ hr}} \times \frac{20 \text{ mEq}}{1000 \text{ mL}} = \frac{1660}{1000} = 1.66 \text{ mEq/hr}$$

9. KNOW   WANT TO KNOW

$$x \text{ hr} = \frac{1000 \text{ mL}}{1} \times \frac{15 \text{ gtt}}{1 \text{ mL}} \times \frac{1 \text{ min}}{20 \text{ gtt}} \times \frac{1 \text{ hr}}{60 \text{ min}} = \frac{15,000}{1} \times 20 \times 60 = \frac{15,000}{1200} = 12.5 = 12 \text{ hr } 30 \text{ min}$$

10. KNOW   WANT TO KNOW

$$x \text{ hr} = \frac{1000 \text{ mL}}{1} \times \frac{1 \text{ hr}}{120 \text{ mL}} = \frac{1000}{120} = 8.33 = 8 \text{ hr } 20 \text{ min}$$

12C (PAGE 333)

1. KNOW   WANT TO KNOW

$$x \text{ hr} = \frac{1350 \text{ mL}}{1} \times \frac{1 \text{ hr}}{112 \text{ mL}} = \frac{1350}{112} = 12 \text{ hr}$$

2. KNOW   WANT TO KNOW

$$x \text{ gtt/min} = \frac{500 \text{ mL}}{1} \times \frac{10 \text{ gtt}}{1 \text{ mL}} = \frac{5000}{120} = 41.6 = 42 \text{ gtt/min}$$

3. KNOW   WANT TO KNOW

$$x \text{ mL} = \frac{2000 \text{ mL}}{24 \text{ hr}} \times \frac{1 \text{ hr}}{1} = \frac{2000}{24} = 83.3 = 83 \text{ mL/hr}$$

4. KNOW   WANT TO KNOW

$$x \text{ mL/hr} = \frac{1000 \text{ mL}}{6 \text{ hr}} \times \frac{1 \text{ hr}}{1} = \frac{1000}{6} = 166.6 = 167 \text{ mL/hr}$$

5. a. KNOW   WANT TO KNOW

$$x \text{ mcg/min} = \frac{1 \text{ kg}}{2.2 \text{ lb}} \times \frac{190 \text{ lb}}{1} \times \frac{3 \text{ mcg}}{\text{min/1 kg}} = \frac{570}{2.2} = 259 \text{ mcg/min}$$

b. KNOW   WANT TO KNOW

$$x \text{ mL/hr} = \frac{60 \text{ min}}{1 \text{ hr}} \times \frac{259 \text{ mcg}}{1 \text{ min}} \times \frac{1 \text{ mg}}{1000 \text{ mcg}} \times \frac{250 \text{ mL}}{30 \text{ mg}} = \frac{3,885,000}{30,000} = 129.5 = 130 \text{ mL/hr}$$

c. KNOW   WANT TO KNOW

$$x \text{ gtt/min} = \frac{259 \text{ mcg}}{1 \text{ min}} \times \frac{1 \text{ mg}}{1000 \text{ mcg}} \times \frac{250 \text{ mL}}{30 \text{ mg}} \times \frac{60 \text{ gtt/min}}{1 \text{ mL}} = \frac{3,885,000}{30,000} = 129.5 = 130 \text{ gtt/min}$$

6. KNOW   WANT TO KNOW

$$x \text{ gtt/min} = \frac{1000 \text{ mL}}{4 \text{ hr}} \times \frac{20 \text{ gtt}}{1 \text{ mL}} \times \frac{1 \text{ hr}}{60 \text{ min}} = \frac{20,000}{240} = 83 \text{ gtt/min}$$

7. KNOW   WANT TO KNOW

$$x \text{ gtt/min} = \frac{500 \text{ mL}}{1.5 \text{ hr}} \times \frac{12 \text{ gtt}}{1 \text{ mL}} \times \frac{1 \text{ hr}}{60 \text{ min}} = \frac{6000}{90} = 66.6 = 67 \text{ gtt/min}$$

8. a. KNOW   WANT TO KNOW

$$x \text{ mcg/min} = \frac{5 \text{ mcg/min}}{1 \text{ kg}} \times \frac{110 \text{ kg}}{1} = 550 \text{ mcg/min}$$

b. KNOW   WANT TO KNOW

$$x \text{ mL/hr} = \frac{60 \text{ min}}{1 \text{ hr}} \times \frac{550 \text{ mcg}}{1 \text{ min}} \times \frac{1 \text{ mg}}{1000 \text{ mcg}} \times \frac{250 \text{ mL}}{200 \text{ mg}} = \frac{8,250,000}{200,000} = 41.2 = 41 \text{ mL/hr}$$

9. a. KNOW   WANT TO KNOW

$$x \text{ mcg/min} = \frac{1 \text{ kg}}{2.2 \text{ lb}} \times \frac{160 \text{ lb}}{1} \times 6 \text{ mcg/min} = \frac{960}{2.2} = 436 \text{ mcg/min}$$

b. KNOW   WANT TO KNOW

$$x \text{ mL/hr} = \frac{60 \text{ min}}{1 \text{ hr}} \times \frac{436 \text{ mcg}}{1 \text{ min}} \times \frac{1 \text{ mg}}{1000 \text{ mcg}} \times \frac{500 \text{ mL}}{800 \text{ mg}} = \frac{13,080,000}{800,000} = \frac{1308}{80} = 16.35 = 16 \text{ mL/hr}$$

10. a. KNOW   WANT TO KNOW

$$x \text{ mL/hr} = \frac{1000 \text{ mL}}{12 \text{ hr}} \times \frac{1 \text{ hr}}{1} = \frac{1000}{12} = 83.3 = 83 \text{ mL/hr}$$

b. KNOW   WANT TO KNOW

$$x \text{ units/hr} = \frac{10,000 \text{ units}}{12 \text{ hr}} \times \frac{1 \text{ hr}}{1} = \frac{10,000}{12} = 833.3 \text{ units/hr}$$

12D (PAGE 335)

1. KNOW   WANT TO KNOW

$$mL/hr = \frac{500 \text{ mL}}{250 \text{ mg}} \times \frac{30 \text{ mg}}{1 \text{ hr}} = \frac{15,000}{250} = 60 \text{ mL/hr}$$

2. a. KNOW   WANT TO KNOW

$$lb/kg = \frac{1 \text{ kg}}{2.2 \text{ lb}} \times \frac{80 \text{ lb}}{kg} = \frac{2.2}{80} = 36.4 \text{ kg}$$

$$10 \text{ mcg/kg/min} \times 36.4 \text{ kg} = 364 \text{ mcg/min}$$

b. KNOW   WANT TO KNOW

$$mL/hr = \frac{250 \text{ mL}}{250 \text{ mg}} \times \frac{1 \text{ mg}}{1000 \text{ mcg}} \times \frac{364 \text{ mcg}}{min} \times \frac{60 \text{ min}}{1 \text{ hr}} = 21.8 = 22 \text{ mL/hr to infuse } 10 \text{ mcg/min}$$

3. a. KNOW   WANT TO KNOW

Low range: $\frac{4 \text{ mcg}}{kg/min} \times 75.6 \text{ kg} = 302.4 \text{ mcg/min}$

High range: $\frac{6 \text{ mcg}}{kg/min} \times 75.6 \text{ kg} = 453.6 \text{ mcg/min}$

b. KNOW   WANT TO KNOW

$$mL/hr = \frac{500 \text{ mL}}{50 \text{ mg}} \times \frac{1 \text{ mg}}{1000 \text{ mcg}} \times \frac{302.4 \text{ mcg}}{1 \text{ min}} \times \frac{60 \text{ min}}{1 \text{ hr}} = 181 \text{ mL/hr minimum rate}$$

$$mL/hr = \frac{500 \text{ mL}}{50 \text{ mg}} \times \frac{1 \text{ mg}}{1000 \text{ mcg}} \times \frac{453.6 \text{ mcg}}{1 \text{ min}} \times \frac{60 \text{ min}}{1 \text{ hr}} = 272 \text{ mL/hr maximum rate}$$

The IV must be titrated to between 181 and 272 mL/hr.

c. KNOW   WANT TO KNOW

$$mcg/min = \frac{1000 \text{ mcg}}{1 \text{ mg}} \times \frac{50 \text{ mg}}{500 \text{ mL}} \times \frac{200 \text{ mL}}{1 \text{ hr}} \times \frac{1 \text{ hr}}{60 \text{ min}} = 333.3 \text{ mcg/min}$$

4. a. KNOW   WANT TO KNOW

$110 \text{ kg} \times \frac{0.5 \text{ mcg}}{kg/min} = 55 \text{ mcg/min as the minimum rate}$

$110 \text{ kg} \times \frac{5 \text{ mcg}}{kg/min} = 550 \text{ mcg/min as the maximum rate}$

b. KNOW   WANT TO KNOW

$$mL/hr = \frac{250 \text{ mL}}{75 \text{ mg}} \times \frac{1 \text{ mg}}{1000 \text{ mcg}} \times \frac{550 \text{ mcg}}{1 \text{ min}} \times \frac{60 \text{ min}}{1 \text{ hr}} = 110 \text{ mL/hr to deliver the maximum safe dose}$$

5. a. KNOW   WANT TO KNOW

$\frac{0.2 \text{ mcg}}{kg/min} \times 120 \text{ kg} = 24 \text{ mcg/min as the low dose}$

$\frac{1 \text{ mcg}}{kg/min} \times 120 \text{ kg} = 120 \text{ mcg/min as the high dose}$

b. KNOW   WANT TO KNOW

$$mL/hr = \frac{500 \text{ mL}}{50 \text{ mg}} \times \frac{1 \text{ mg}}{1000 \text{ mcg}} \times \frac{24 \text{ mcg}}{1 \text{ min}} \times \frac{60 \text{ min}}{1 \text{ hr}} = 14.4 = 14 \text{ mL/hr as the lowest rate}$$

$$mL/hr = \frac{500 \text{ mL}}{50 \text{ mg}} \times \frac{1 \text{ mg}}{1000 \text{ mcg}} \times \frac{120 \text{ mcg}}{1 \text{ min}} \times \frac{60 \text{ min}}{1 \text{ hr}} = 72 \text{ mL/hr as the highest rate}$$

6. a. KNOW   WANT TO KNOW

$$\frac{275 \text{ lb}}{2.2} = 125 \text{ kg}$$

$$\frac{2 \text{ mcg}}{\text{kg/min}} \times 125 \text{ kg} = 250 \text{ mcg/min}$$

$$\frac{4 \text{ mcg}}{\text{kg/min}} \times 125 \text{ kg} = 500 \text{ mcg/min}$$

b. KNOW   WANT TO KNOW

$$\text{mL/hr} = \frac{250 \text{ mL}}{500 \text{ mg}} \times \frac{1 \text{ mg}}{1000 \text{ mcg}} \times \frac{250 \text{ mcg}}{1 \text{ min}} \times \frac{60 \text{ min}}{1 \text{ hr}} = 7.5 = 7 \text{ mL/hr for the minimum rate}$$

$$\text{mL/hr} = \frac{250 \text{ mL}}{500 \text{ mg}} \times \frac{1 \text{ mg}}{1000 \text{ mcg}} \times \frac{500 \text{ mcg}}{1 \text{ min}} \times \frac{60 \text{ min}}{1 \text{ hr}} = 15 \text{ mL/hr as the maximum rate}$$

7. KNOW   WANT TO KNOW

$$\text{mL/hr} = \frac{500 \text{ mL}}{500 \text{ mg}} \times \frac{1 \text{ mg}}{1000 \text{ mcg}} \times \frac{5 \text{ mcg}}{1 \text{ kg/min}} \times \frac{60 \text{ min}}{1 \text{ hr}} \times \frac{100 \text{ kg}}{1} = 30 \text{ mL/hr}$$

8. KNOW   WANT TO KNOW

$$\text{mL/hr} = \frac{500 \text{ mL}}{3 \text{ g}} \times \frac{1 \text{ g}}{1000 \text{ mg}} \times \frac{1 \text{ mg}}{1000 \text{ mcg}} \times \frac{100 \text{ mcg}}{1 \text{ kg/min}} \times \frac{60 \text{ min}}{1 \text{ hr}} \times 84 \text{ kg} = 84 \text{ mL/hr}$$

9. KNOW   WANT TO KNOW

$$\text{mL/hr} = \frac{250 \text{ mL}}{100 \text{ mg}} \times \frac{1 \text{ mg}}{1000 \text{ mcg}} \times \frac{6 \text{ mcg}}{1 \text{ kg/min}} \times \frac{115 \text{ kg}}{1} \times \frac{60 \text{ min}}{1 \text{ hr}} = \frac{10,350,000}{100,000} = 103.5 = 104 \text{ mL/hr}$$

10. KNOW   WANT TO KNOW

$$\text{mL/hr} = \frac{1000 \text{ mL}}{5 \text{ g}} \times \frac{1 \text{ g}}{1000 \text{ mg}} \times \frac{1 \text{ mg}}{1000 \text{ mcg}} \times \frac{100 \text{ mcg}}{1 \text{ kg/min}} \times \frac{60 \text{ min}}{1 \text{ hr}} \times 88.4 \text{ kg} = 106 \text{ mL/hr}$$

12E (PAGE 336)

1. c. KNOW   WANT TO KNOW

$$x \text{ (SDR)} = \frac{5 \text{ kg}}{1} \times \frac{10 \text{ mg}}{1 \text{ kg}} = \frac{50}{1} = 50 \text{ mg}$$

a. Yes. 50 mg is the maximum dose for a 5 kg child. The dose ordered is one dose of 25 mg.

2. d. KNOW   WANT TO KNOW

$$x \text{ kg} = \frac{1 \text{ kg}}{2.2 \text{ lb}} \times \frac{8 \text{ lb}}{1} = \frac{8}{2.2} = 3.6 \text{ kg}$$

b. KNOW   WANT TO KNOW

$$x \text{ mg (low dose)} = \frac{6 \text{ mg}}{1 \text{ kg}} \times \frac{3.6 \text{ kg}}{1} = 21.6 = 22 \text{ mg}$$

a. KNOW   WANT TO KNOW

$$x \text{ mg (high dose)} = \frac{8 \text{ mg}}{1 \text{ kg}} \times \frac{3.6 \text{ kg}}{1} = 28.8 = 29 \text{ mg}$$

3. d. KNOW   WANT TO KNOW

$$x \text{ mL} = \frac{2.5 \text{ mL}}{80 \text{ mg}} \times \frac{250 \text{ mg}}{1} = 2.5 \times \frac{240}{80} = \frac{600}{80} = 7.5 \text{ mL}$$

4. b. KNOW   WANT TO KNOW

$$x \text{ mL} = \frac{1 \text{ g}}{1000 \text{ mg}} \times \frac{1 \text{ mL}}{0.5 \text{ g}} \times \frac{600 \text{ mg}}{1} = \frac{600}{500} = 1.2 \text{ mL}$$

5. c. KNOW   WANT TO KNOW

$$x \text{ hr} = \frac{1300 \text{ mL}}{1} \times \frac{1 \text{ hr}}{112 \text{ mL}} \times = \frac{1330}{112} = 11.87 = 11 \text{ hr } 52 \text{ min}$$

a. 2000 hr + 12 hr = 0800 hr

6. a. KNOW   WANT TO KNOW

$$x \text{ mL/hr} = \frac{1000 \text{ mL}}{12 \text{ hr}} \times 1 = \frac{1000}{12} = 83.3 = 83 \text{ mL/hr}$$

d. KNOW   WANT TO KNOW

$$x \text{ units/min} = \frac{50{,}000 \text{ units}}{12 \text{ hr}} \times \frac{1 \text{ hr}}{60 \text{ min}} = \frac{50{,}000}{720} = 69.4 = 69 \text{ units/min}$$

7. a. KNOW   WANT TO KNOW

$$x \text{ kg} = \frac{1 \text{ kg}}{2.2 \text{ lb}} \times \frac{40 \text{ lb}}{1} = \frac{40}{2.2} = 18 \text{ kg}$$

c. KNOW   WANT TO KNOW

$$x \text{ mg (low dose)} = \frac{30 \text{ mg}}{1 \text{ kg}} \times \frac{18 \text{ kg}}{1} = 540 \text{ mg}$$

c. KNOW   WANT TO KNOW

$$x \text{ mg (high dose)} = \frac{50 \text{ mg}}{1 \text{ kg}} \times \frac{18 \text{ kg}}{1} = 50 \times \frac{18}{1} = 900 \text{ mg}$$

8. d. KNOW   WANT TO KNOW

$$x \text{ mL/hr} = \frac{500 \text{ mL}}{40 \text{ units}} \times \frac{3 \text{ units}}{1 \text{ hr}} = \frac{1500}{40} = 37.5 = 38 \text{ mL/hr}$$

9. d. KNOW   WANT TO KNOW

$$x \text{ kg} = \frac{1 \text{ kg}}{2.2 \text{ lb}} \times \frac{195 \text{ lb}}{1} = \frac{195}{2.2} = 88.6 = 89 \text{ kg}$$

b. KNOW   WANT TO KNOW

$$x \text{ units/min} = \frac{89 \text{ kg}}{1} \times \frac{0.5 \text{ units/min}}{1 \text{ kg}} = 44.5 = 45 \text{ units/min}$$

c. KNOW   WANT TO KNOW

$$x \text{ mL/hr} = \frac{45 \text{ units}}{1 \text{ min}} \times \frac{60 \text{ min}}{1 \text{ hr}} \times \frac{500 \text{ mL/hr}}{20{,}000 \text{ units}} = \frac{1{,}350{,}000}{200{,}000} = 67.5 = 68 \text{ mL/hr}$$

10. b. KNOW   WANT TO KNOW

$$x \text{ mL/hr} = \frac{1000 \text{ mL}}{60{,}000 \text{ units}} \times \frac{5000 \text{ units}}{1 \text{ hr}} = \frac{5000}{60} = 83.3 = 83 \text{ mL/hr}$$

CHAPTER 12 FINAL: DIMENSIONAL ANALYSIS (PAGE 338)

1. 0.75 mL

2. 1.6 mL

3. 1.3 mL

4. **a.** 4.0 mL
   b. 300 mg/24 hr

5. 20 tablets of 500 mg scored tablets needed for 10 days

6. 5600 units of heparin for an IV bolus dose

7. 108 mL/hr

8. 33 gtt/min

9. 150 gtt/min

10. **a.** 11.36 kg
    b. 1136 mcg is the low SDR.
    c. 2272 mcg is the high SDR.
    d. Yes, 1500 mcg/day is a safe order.

Multiple-Choice Final (PAGE 339)

1. a	2. c	3. a	4. d
5. d	6. c	7. b	8. c
9. d	10. a	11. c	12. b
13. a	14. c; d	15. a	16. a
17. b	18. c	19. c; d	20. c; d
21. a; d	22. a	23. b	24. b; d
25. d; d	26. b	27. d	28. d
29. a	30. c		

Comprehensive Final (PAGE 349)

1. 2 tab

2. 1 tab

3. 2 tab

4. 2 tab

5. 1 tab

6. 1 tab

7. 7.5 mL

8. 0.7 mL

9. *Error:* 0845 Dose given 45 minutes after prior dose. Order stated q4h intervals prn.

   Current Actions: Prescribe complete bed rest for patient, assess mental status and vital signs, notify supervising nurse/charge nurse and physician immediately, and obtain orders for medication to reverse.

   Establish a patent IV line according to hospital policy in case emergency care may be needed.

   Have crash cart close at hand. Document the error and to whom reported, patient evaluations, and all interventions, and continue to make the above assessments and evaluate. Fill out incident report. Continue to assess and evaluate patient every 10 to 15 minutes until patient is stabilized, then gradually extend assessment time.

   Prevention: prn and stat medications must be charted as soon as possible after administration. Nurse A needed to report to Nurse B orally when her patients were due for their next prn medications. Nurse B needed to state she was too busy to care for additional patients beyond her own caseload. Nurse B needed to check record carefully to see when last medication for pain was given. Nurse B needed to ask patient when last medication for pain was received. (This is a recommended double-check but is not always reliable. The accuracy of response depends on the patient's mental status.)

10. 0.8 mL (grain $\frac{1}{2}$ per mL)

11. 1.3 mL

12. a. 250,000 units/mL
    b. Give 1.6 mL.
    c. 500,000 units/mL
    d. Give 0.8 mL.

13. a. Add 2 mL of diluent
    b. 4 vials per 24 hr
    c. Give 2.4 mL/dose.

14. a. 2.5 mL sterile water for injection
   b. Store in refrigerator. Can be at room temperature for only 24 hr.
        Last dose will be given in 32 hours.
   c. Give 0.8 mL.

15. a. 21 gtt/min
   b. 83 mL/hr on infusion device

16. a. 75 mL/hr
   b. 75 gtt/min

17. a. 104 mL/hr
   b. 17 gtt/min

18. 6 units of Lantus

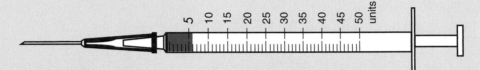

19. 70 mL/hr

20. 25 units of R insulin

21. a. Set infusion rate at 19 mL/hr
   b. IV will be completed at 2339 hours.

22. 0.8 mL Fragmin

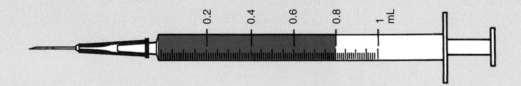

23. a. 50 mL/hr
   b. 20 hr to infuse

24. a. Give 5964 units of heparin for the bolus dose.
   b. 1309 units/hr will infuse
   c. 15 hr 12 min
   d. 33 mL/hr

25. a. 19 g/bag amino acids
   b. 29 g/bag carbohydrates
   c. 14 g/bag lipids

26. a. 76 protein kilocalories
   b. 116 carbohydrate kilocalories
   c. 126 fat kilocalories
   d. Total kilocalories = 318

27. **a.** 2 mEq/mL
    b. 149 mg/mL
    c. 15 mL

28. **a.** 2 mL
    b. 120 seconds
    c. 1 mL/min for 2 min
    d. 12 seconds per calibration

29. 10 mg; 2 tab

30. **a.** 24 mg/hr
    b. 24,000 mcg/hr
    c. 5 mcg/kg/min
    d. Flow rate correct

Index

Page numbers followed by *f*, *t*, and *b* indicate
figures, tables, and boxes, respectively.

Metric Equivalents

Weight
1 mg (milligram) = 1000 mcg (micrograms)
1 g (gram) = 1000 mg (milligrams)
1 kg (kilogram) = 2.2 lb (pounds) = 1000 g (grams)

Volume
1000 mL (milliliters) = 1 L (liter)

Approximate Equivalents of Metric, Household, and Apothecary Measures

Metric	Household	Apothecary
5 mL	1 teaspoon (tsp)	
15 mL	1 tablespoon (tbs)	$\frac{1}{2}$ ounce
30 mL	2 tablespoons (tbs)	1 ounce
240 mL	1 measuring cup	8 ounces
500 mL	1 pint	1 pint or 16 ounces
1000 mL	1 quart	1 quart or 32 ounces

Metric-Apothecary Conversion Clock

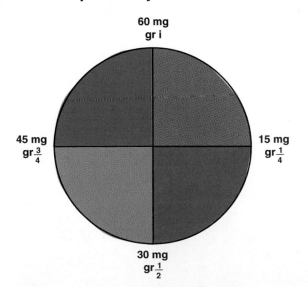

60 mg
gr i

15 mg
gr $\frac{1}{4}$

30 mg
gr $\frac{1}{2}$

45 mg
gr $\frac{3}{4}$